Child Phonology:
Characteristics, Assessment, and Intervention with Special Populations

CURRENT THERAPY OF COMMUNICATION DISORDERS

Series Editor
William H. Perkins, Ph.D.

Child Phonology:
Characteristics, Assessment, and Intervention with Special Populations

John E. Bernthal, Ph.D.

Professor and Chair
Department of Special Education
and Communication Disorders
University of Nebraska
Lincoln, Nebraska

Nicholas W. Bankson, Ph.D.

Professor and Head
Department of Communication
Sciences and Disorders
James Madison University
Harrisonburg, Virginia

1994
THIEME MEDICAL PUBLISHERS, INC.   New York
GEORG THIEME VERLAG   Stuttgart · New York

Thieme Medical Publishers, Inc.
381 Park Avenue South
New York, New York 10016

CHILD PHONOLOGY: CHARACTERISTICS, ASSESSMENT, AND INTERVENTION
  WITH SPECIAL POPULATIONS
John E. Bernthal and Nicholas W. Bankson

Library of Congress Cataloging-in-Publication Data

Child phonology: characteristics, assessment, and intervention with
    special populations / (edited by) John E. Bernthal, Nicholas W. Bankson.
        p.   cm.   (Current therapy of communication disorders.)
        Includes bibliographical references and index.
        ISBN 0-86577-502-8 (Thieme Medical Publishers).—ISBN 3-13-134701-5
    (Georg Thieme Verlag)
        1. Articulation disorders in children.   I. Bernthal, John E.   II. Series.
    [DNLM: 1. Articulation Disorders—in infancy & childhood.   2. Speech
    Intelligibility—in infancy & childhood.   3. Phonetics.   WL 340 C536 1994]
    RJ496.S7C53   1994
    618.92'855—dc20
    DNLM/DLC
    for Library of Congress   94-31616
                                                                         CIP

Printed in the United States of America.

5   4   3   2   1

TMP ISBN 0-86577-502-8
GTV ISBN 3-13-134701-5

Other Volumes in the Series

Contents

Part IV—Cultural Factors

Contributors

John Bernthal, Ph.D.
Department of Special Education and
  Communication Disorders
University of Nebraska—Lincoln
Lincoln, Nebraska

Ken M. Bleile, Ph.D.
Department of Speech Pathology
  and Audiology
School of Medicine
University of Hawaii
Honolulu, Hawaii

Thomas F. Campbell, Ph.D.
Department of Audiology and
  Communication Disorders
Children's Hospital of Pittsburgh
Pittsburgh, Pennsylvania

Li-Rong Lilly Cheng, Ph.D.
Department of Communicative Disorders
San Diego State University
San Diego, California

Susan Clarke-Klein, Ph.D.
Frank Porter Graham Child
  Development Center
University of North Carolina at
  Chapel Hill
Chapel Hill, North Carolina

Christine A. Dollaghan, Ph.D.
Department of Communication
University of Pittsburgh
Pittsburgh, Pennsylvania

Marvin L. Hanson, Ph.D.
Department of Communication Disorders
University of Utah
Salt Lake City, Utah

Margaret M. Kehoe, M.Sc.
Department of Speech and Hearing Sciences
University of Pittsburgh
Pittsburgh, Pennsylvania

Rebecca J. Leonard, Ph.D.
Department of Otolaryngology
Head and Neck Surgery
University of California, Davis
Sacramento, California

Shari A. Miller, M.S.
Children's Seashore House
Philadelphia, Pennsylvania

Karlind T. Moller, Ph.D.
Cleft Palate Maxillofacial
  and Craniofacial Clinics
Division of Pediatric Dentistry
Department of Preventive Sciences
School of Dentistry
University of Minnesota
Minneapolis, Minnesota

Marietta M. Paterson, Ed.D.
Deafness Studies Unit
University of Melbourne
Parkville, Victoria 3052
Australia

Emilio Perez, Ph.D.
Department of Special Education
  and Communicative Disorders
State University
Arkansas State University
Arkansas

Joanne E. Roberts, Ph.D.
Frank Porter Graham Child
  Development Center
Division of Speech and Hearing Sciences
University of North Carolina at
  Chapel Hill
Chapel Hill, North Carolina

Carol Stoel-Gammon, Ph.D.
Department of Speech and
  Hearing Sciences
University of Washington
Seattle, Washington

Kristine Strand, Ed.D.
Department of Neurology
Childrens Hospital
Boston, Massachusetts

Shelley L. Velleman, Ph.D.
Rehabilitation Department
Baystate Medical Center
Springfield, Massachusetts

Walt Wolfram, Ph.D.
College of Humanities and Social Sciences
Department of English
North Carolina State University
Raleigh, North Carolina

Preface

Child Phonology: Characteristics, Assessment, and Intervention with Special Populations grows out of our textbook, *Articulation and Phonological Disorders*, and of our ongoing teaching of courses in phonological disorders. One of the major topics in that book was a chapter entitled "Factors Related to Phonological Disorders," in which we discussed phonological problems associated with four broadly defined factors: (1) structure and function of the speech mechanism, (2) cognitive linguistic factors, (3) psychosocial factors, and (4) hearing and auditory factors. Variables in each of these areas were described as potentially affecting an individual's phonological behavior. The chapter was included because of an abiding interest in the field regarding the identification of variables that may be related to the presence of speech–sound disorders. However, the chapter merely scratched the surface in presenting the nature, impact, and treatment considerations related to certain etiological factors. This new book provides a more extensive coverage of selected variables that merit a more in-depth presentation to students and clinicians. While the chapters in this monograph are primarily focused on children, some discussions focus directly or indirectly on adults.

While our intent in putting together this book was to provide the reader with a state-of-the-art discussion of factors often related to phonological disorders, we had to be judicious about what was selected for inclusion. Two topics one might assume would be covered in a text of this nature are phonological characteristics associated with orofacial anomalies and adult motor speech disorders. We decided not to include discussions of these topics in this book because students typically are exposed to literature in these areas through graduate-level courses or portions of courses focused on these topics.

Child Phonology: Characteristics, Assessment, and Intervention with Special Populations is organized into four sections: (1) Oral Mechanism Factors, (2) Neurological Factors, (3) Sensory Factors, and (4) Cultural Factors. The topics in these sections were selected because we felt there was significant information related to these areas that has not received the depth and/or currency of discussion in the literature that students and clinicians need.

The section on oral mechanism factors includes chapters on three topics: dentition and phonology, myofunctional disorders, and glossectomy. In the first chapter, Karlind Moller, Ph.D., a speech–language pathologist with an academic appointment in a dental college, outlines the relationship between occlusion and speech. He also discusses other dental and oral mechanism factors that may affect phonological productions. In the second chapter, Marvin Hanson, Ph.D., reviews the literature concerning oral myofunctional disorders and their relationship with articulatory productions. Given the shift in posture reflected in the 1974 and 1991 policy statements of the American Speech-Language-Hearing Association regarding the role of the speech–language pathologist with this population (ie, from discouraging to encouraging involvement with oral myofunctional disorders), this topic is especially timely. Dr. Hanson is one of the few speech–language pathologists who has treated, investigated, and written about oral myofunctional disorders and their relationship to articulatory patterns over 30 years. In the third chapter, Rebecca Leonard, Ph.D., discusses speech characteristics and habilitation with individuals evidencing glossectomy and other oral/pharyngeal ablations. Dr. Leonard, a speech–language pathologist, is widely regarded as one of the most experienced and knowledgeable clinicians in our field in this unique area of treatment.

The second topic in this book, neurological factors, includes chapters on toddlers with medical needs, developmental apraxia, and traumatic brain injury (TBI). These areas are grouped under the broad topic of neurological factors because disruptions in the neurological system can result in clients being diagnosed with one of these three conditions. Ken Bleile, Ph.D., and Shari Miller, M.S., have drawn on their experience as speech–language pathologists in a children's medical center to discuss the speech and language concerns and practices with toddlers with medical needs. While phonology cannot be separated from other aspects of communication in this young population, it is nonetheless included as part of the broad mission of professionals in medical environments to prevent speech, language, and other learning problems in those who evidence a medically fragile condition.

A fresh and thought-provoking explanation and treatment approach to developmental apraxia is presented by Shelley Velleman, Ph.D., and Kristine Strand, Ed.D., in this section. These speech–language pathologists have used their clinical experiences and ideas to formulate a "movement-based" approach to what some regard as a "controversial" diagnosis. The third chapter in this section is authored by Thomas Campbell, Ph.D., and Christine Dollaghan, Ph.D., and covers the assessment and treatment of TBI in children. While much is written about TBI in the young adult and adult client, little has appeared in the literature on this disorder in children.

The third section of this book focuses on phonology relating to varying types and levels of hearing impairment. Carol Stoel-Gammon, Ph.D., and Margaret Kehoe, M.Sc., have studied phonological development in hearing-impaired children, and this chapter is a report of their findings and suggestions regarding young children. The abiding interest in the impact that otitis media may have on phonological development and specific implications for the speech–language pathologist are discussed by Joanne Roberts, Ph.D., and Susan Clarke-Klein, Ph.D., in the second chapter of this section. This chapter pulls together data from recent investigations, writings expressing various points of view on this topic, and intervention guidelines for clinicians. Marietta Paterson, Ed.D., discusses phonological behavior of hearing-impaired school-aged children with severe and profound sensorineural hearing losses. Her chapter provides a description of the phonological characteristics of this group and assessment and intervention suggestions for those who work with this population.

The final section of the book is the result of changing U.S. demographics and the need for clinicians to have information about the phonological characteristics of selected linguistic communities that differ from general American English. This section is based on the following understandings: (1) the way children speak is typically a reflection of their linguistic culture; (2) cultural-based linguistic differences are not communication disorders; (3) phonological disorders may, however, exist within cultural differences; and (4) some individuals may wish to learn general American dialect for educational and economic mobility purposes. In light of these understandings, the need for information on dialect variations is critical to speech–language pathologists. The three chapters in this section address phonology in the three dominant subcultures of U.S. society: African-American, Hispanic-American, and Asian-American. Walt Wolfram, Ph.D., a noted scholar in the area of what for some years was identified as Black English Vernacular, presents a scholarly review and discussion of the phonology of African American Vernacular English. In the second chapter in this section Emilio Perez, Ph.D., discusses phonological differences among speakers of Spanish-influenced English. Finally, Li-Rong Lilly Cheng, Ph.D., a widely recognized authority on Asian-American English, discusses the learning of English by Asian/Pacific Islanders. This latter population group probably reflects the greatest heterogeneity of linguistic characteristics of any of the three major linguistic groups discussed in this book. Among other things, Dr. Cheng discusses code-switching, a topic relevant to all clients reflecting culturally based linguistic variation.

We are indebted to the scholars whose writings are included in this book. These are individuals whose phonological expertise is perhaps most easily recognized in specific subpopulations of the larger population of the phonologically impaired. As stated earlier, the kind of extensive discussion they have presented in this narrative is very much needed by those of us who teach and study in the area of phonological impairment in children. We appreciate their willingness to share their expertise.

John E. Bernthal
Nicholas W. Bankson

Part I
Oral Mechanism
Factors

Dental-Occlusal and Other Oral Conditions and Speech

KARLIND T. MOLLER, PH.D.

Introduction

The teeth, upper and lower jaws, lips, and tongue, although used for more primary biologic function, obviously serve as important peripheral structures in the process of speech production. Consideration of certain deviant dental, occlusal, and oral conditions is important to speech–language clinicians for several reasons. First, speech–language clinicians are frequently tempted to attribute a causal relationship between certain sound errors and deviations in dental and oral structures, especially if the response to treatment has been slow or nonexistent. This intuitive clinical thinking persists even though there may be little data for support. Second, the speech–language clinician is frequently called on by our dental and medical colleagues to offer an opinion about the effect of existing structural deviations on speech performance and, perhaps more importantly, to predict the effect of a dental or surgical treatment on speech. Third, parents and caretakers seek knowledgeable explanations about possible dental and speech relationships in their children. Additionally, they may be concerned about the potential effect of certain dental/surgical interventions on speech performance and ask: will treatment make speech better, worse, or have no effect.

It is important to remember there is a wide range of normalcy in dental/occlusal relationships and oral anatomy. "Normals" do not all have perfect alignment of teeth and exacting dental bites (occlusion); their lingual frena are not all attached in the same place; tongue size and range of motion varies; lips come in assorted shapes and thicknesses; and palatal vaults vary in size and configuration. These differences make us individuals. Furthermore, the dental and oral structures change substantially with growth and development from infancy to adulthood. Change is further associated with the aging process and, for some persons, the ultimate attrition and loss of teeth may require prosthetic and/or surgical replacement. It is within that milieu of structural variability and change over time that the speech–language clinician may attempt to assess and modify speech production.

This chapter will focus on certain dental/occlusal and oral conditions in the presence of an intact neuromuscular system and normal cognitive function. Hypo or aglossic conditions are addressed in another chapter and will not be considered here. Oral myofunctional assessment and treatment for swallowing disorders (tongue thrust, reverse swallow, infantile swallow, deviant swallow, etc.), purported by some to influence dental form, are also addressed in Chapter 2. The reader is also referred to the position statements of the American Speech-Language-Hearing Association "The Role of the Speech Pathologist in Assessment and Management of Oral Myofunctional Disorders."[1] and "Orofacial Myofunctional Disorders: Knowledge and Skills."[2] Finally, structural and functional aspects of velopharyngeal closure mechanism are not within the purview of this chapter. However, persons with cleft lip and palate frequently have dental and occlusal deviations in addition to velopharyngeal closure issues that will be considered in this chapter. The following structural conditions will be discussed: (1) dentition—missing, extra, and malpositioned teeth; (2) malocclusion—anterior–posterior, vertical, and transverse discrepancies; (3) tongue—ankyloglossia, size, and shape; (4) palate; and (5) lips. A sensible organization is to initially discuss the nature, pathophysiology, and differentiating or defining features of the conditions as well as special populations in which these characteristics are common. Following this, the research history in this area, the current knowledge base, and some clinical assumptions about speech–dental relationships will be discussed. Next, evaluation and treatment considerations for each condition will be discussed. Finally, the potential effect of dental/surgical treatment such as prosthodontic, orthodontic, and orthognathic surgery on speech performance will be considered.

Nature, Pathophysiology, and Differentiating Features

This section will discuss the nature of each dental and oral condition and the pathophysiologic and defining characteristics.

Dentition

The normal deciduous (primary, baby) dentition and the permanent (secondary, adult) dentition are shown in Figures 1–1 and 1–2. Table 1–1 shows the normal chronological eruption sequence of the deciduous and permanent teeth. Of most importance in relation to speech production are the times when the anterior upper and lower teeth are missing. Edentulous spaces in these areas can create a hazard to acquisition and maintenance of precise articulation. There is a wide variation in the times that deciduous incisor teeth are shed and permanent successors erupt. It is likely there will be some spaces in these areas from age 5 to 9 years. This is what is called the mixed dentition stage. Some children lose deciduous front teeth earlier due to decay or trauma and, therefore, have spaces for longer periods of time. Multiple congenitally missing teeth (incisor area) is a common finding in a variety of craniofacial syndromes (ectodermal dysplasia; ectrodactyly-ectodermal dysplasia-clefting (EEC); oculo-dento-osseous dysplasia,

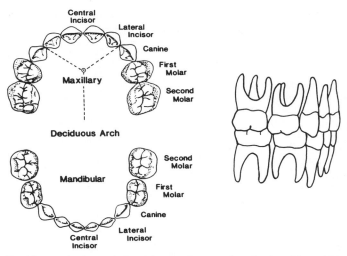

Figure 1–1. Deciduous (primary) dentition and normal occlusion (dental bite).

Hallerman-Streiff, hypoglossia-hypodactylia, Tuomaala-Haapanen, Rieger, Ellis-Van Creveld, Coffin-Lowry, and Rapp-Hodgkin). Lack of eruption of teeth, creating edentulous spaces, is common in cleidocranial dysplasia. Extra or supernumerary teeth may be present and can create a dental crowding situation that can result in malpositioned teeth (ectopic). Single missing teeth (lateral incisors) are common in clefts of the primary palate.

Occlusion (Dental Bite)

The manner in which the teeth in the lower jaw (mandible) contact or occlude with teeth in the upper jaw (maxilla) defines occlusion. The mandible "hinges" to

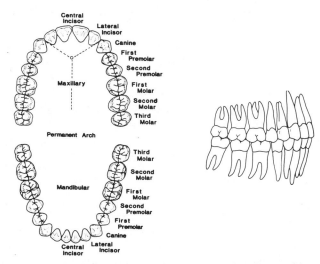

Figure 1–2. Permanent (secondary) dentition and normal occlusion (dental bite).

Table 1–1. Eruption Sequence and Average of Eruption of Deciduous and Permanent Dentition

Tooth	Age of Eruption
Deciduous	
Lower central incisors (2)	6 months
Upper central incisors (2)	7 months
Lower lateral incisors (2)	7 months
Upper lateral incisors (2)	8 months
Lower first molars (2)	12 months
Upper first molars (2)	14 months
Lower canines (2)	16 months
Upper canines (2)	18 months
Lower second molars (2)	20 months
Upper first molars (2)	22 months
Permanent	
Lower first molars (2)	6 years
Upper first molars (2)	6 years
Lower central incisors (2)	6 years
Upper central incisors (2)	7 years
Lower lateral incisors (2)	7 years
Upper lateral incisors (2)	8 years
Lower 1st and 2nd premolars (4)	10–11 years
Upper 1st and 2nd premolars (4)	10–11 years
Lower 2nd molars	12 years
Upper 2nd molars	12 years
Lower and upper 3rd molars	17–25 years

the cranioskeleton via the temporomandibular joint (TMJ) and there are many tissues and muscles interconnecting the two jaws. The TMJ allows the mandible to move up and down (closing and opening the mouth), move from side to side, front to back (protrusion-retrusion), and, to some degree, to rotate. Usually, the teeth fit together so there is reasonable contact of the upper and lower molar and premolar teeth for grinding function and slight anterior positioning (approximately 1 to 2 mm) and overlapping (approximately 1 to 2 mm) of the upper canine and incisor teeth relative to the lowers for incising or cutting function. This is defined as normal occlusion (Class I) and is also illustrated in the deciduous and permanent dentition in Figures 1–1 and 1–2. The upper dentition fits over the lower dentition similar to a lid on a jar.

Malocclusion is defined as excessive deviation from normal and can be caused by individual malignment of teeth (dental malocclusion) or jaw growth discrepancies (skeletal malocclusion). Malocclusion can occur in any plane of space—anterior-posterior, vertical, or side-to-side—and can occur on one side or both.

ANTERIOR–POSTERIOR DEVIATIONS

The upper teeth from the molars forward may be positioned excessively anterior to the lower teeth. This is referred to as Class II malocclusion and results in excessive *overjet*. Or the molar teeth can be in normal occlusion (Class I), but the canines and/or incisors may be positioned excessively anterior to the lowers. In both instances, the upper incisor teeth are excessively forward (overjet) relative to the lower teeth. Again, these deviations may be due to tooth position or jaw growth. Figure 1–3 illustrates this condition.

Conversely, the upper teeth from the molars forward may be positioned posteriorly to the lower teeth. This is referred to as Class III malocclusion and can result in *negative overjet* or *anterior crossbite*. Or, the molar teeth can be in normal occlusion (Class I) but the canines and/or incisors may be excessively posterior to the lowers. In both instances, the incisor teeth are excessively posterior relative to the lower teeth. Again, dental or skeletal factors can contribute to this condition, as is illustrated in Figure 1–4. Maxillary hypoplasia (underdevelopment) or mandibular hyperplasia (overdevelopment or prognathism) may be seen in persons with no other conditions and may be the result of familial growth tendencies. However, maxillary hypoplasia is a common feature in persons with cleft lip and palate; craniosynostoses syndromes (Crouzon, Apert, and Pfeiffer); and other syndromes too numerous to mention. Prognathic (large) mandible occurs in a variety of craniofacial disorders. Micrognathic (small) mandible occurs in numerous disorders. Some of the more frequent include Robin sequence, Stickler syndrome, Velocardiofacial syndrome, Oculo-auriculo-vertebral spectrum, Nager, and Melnick-Needles syndrome.[3]

VERTICAL DEVIATIONS

As discussed previously, normally the upper incisor teeth overlap (lid on a jar) the lower teeth somewhat. Dental factors or skeletal growth can cause a lack of overlap and result in excessive spacing or openness in the front. This defines anterior *openbite* (Fig. 1–5). Conversely, the upper incisors may excessively overlap the lower incisors, and this is defined as excessive overbite or closed bite (Fig. 1–6). Severe openbite is a common finding in craniosynostoses syndromes of Apert, Crouzon, and Pfeiffer; in oculo-auriculo-vertebral spectrum; mandibulofacial dysostosis (Treacher Collins); oro-acral disorders of Nager syndrome and Wildervanck syndrome; and in craniocarpotarsal dysplasia.[3]

TRANSVERSE DEVIATIONS

Transverse or side-to-side malocclusion occurs when the upper posterior teeth (canines and molars) are positioned inside or outside the lower teeth. Usually, it

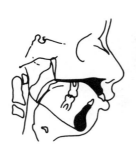 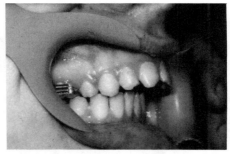

Figure 1–3.   Lateral diagrammatic and clinical view of Class II Division 1 malocclusion. Note the upper molar is excessively anterior to the lower molar and the anterior upper teeth are excessively anterior to the lower teeth (overjet).

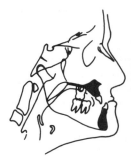
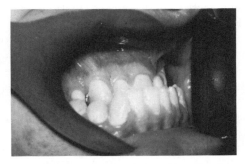

Figure 1–4. Lateral diagrammatic view and clinical view of class III malocclusion. Note the upper molar is excessively posterior to the lower molar and the anterior teeth are posterior to the lower teeth (negative overjet; anterior crossbite).

is the upper teeth that are inside (toward the tongue) of the lowers that present the greater hazard to articulation. This is defined as *posterior crossbite* and results in a transverse constriction of the upper dental arch. This can occur on one side or both. Narrow or constricted dental arches are present in a number of craniofacial anomalies, most notably cleft lip and palate.

Therefore, crossbites, where the upper teeth are inside (toward the tongue) of the lower teeth, can exist in the front from anterior–posterior deviations, and/or in the back from transverse deviations. The resultant structural condition is constriction of the upper dental arch relative to the lower and can be confining to tongue movements involved in speech.

Tongue Conditions

TONGUE-TIE

The medical term ankyloglossia refers to tongue-tie or consolidation of tissues resulting in reduced mobility of the tongue. Commonly, ankyloglossia and tongue-tie refer to a "short" lingual frenum. The frenum or frenulum is an anatomic term to designate a small fold of tissue that checks, curves, or limits the movements of an organ or part. The lingual frenum is a thin vertical fold of

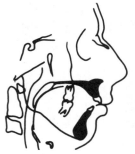
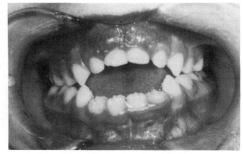

Figure 1–5. Lateral diagrammatic view and clinical view of anterior openbite. Note the upper front teeth do not overlap the lower front teeth.

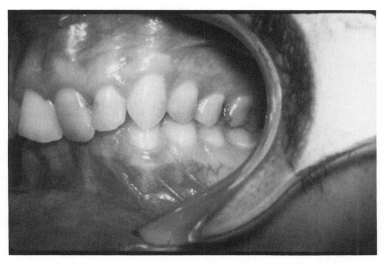

Figure 1–6.   Clinical view of excessive overbite (closed bite). Note the upper front teeth excessively overlap the lower front teeth.

tissue with attachments to the undersurface of the tongue *and* to the floor of the mouth. The term "short" as a pathophysiological condition is unfortunate. It has been intuitively assumed that diagnosis of a short frenum results in restricted tongue movements, most commonly tongue-tip elevation and therefore contributes to faulty production of the tongue-tip sounds (/t/, /d/, /n/, /l/, /s/, /z/). Diagnosis of the condition is frequently made from observation of the speaker's inability to elevate the tongue tip to the maxillary alveolar ridge (just behind the upper incisors) when the mouth is wide open. Clinicians rarely, if ever, "measure" the length of the frenum to make the diagnosis—it is a clinical judgment made during some physiological maneuver. This will be discussed in greater detail later in our discussion of assessment and treatment relative to this condition. For now, consider the lingual frenum as an anatomic tissue connection having two attachments—undersurface of the tongue and the floor of the mouth. Clinical observation of 100 speakers' lingual frena will yield the conclusion that there is impressive variability in the site of the attachments and, indeed, the "length" of the frena.

TONGUE SIZE

Overall bulk or size of the tongue per se is another difficult condition for definitive diagnosis. Perhaps we all too often glibly judge the tongue to be too large. We do not "measure" tongue size. It is a clinical visual judgment made during a physiological maneuver such as rest, speech, swallowing, chewing, etc. Furthermore, it is difficult to divorce the judgment of tongue size from the structural environment in which it functions. Perhaps the anterior and posterior crossbite situations described earlier create a restricted or confining space for a "normal-sized" tongue. Patients with Trisomy 21 (Down's syndrome) are often diagnosed with large tongues, or macroglossia, but this may be the result of habitual forward positioning of the tongue (physiologic) and a restricted oral space, a situation not uncommon in this population. Similarly, macroglossia has been a clinical finding in Angelman syndrome but, again, this observation may be related to the protrusive tongue positioning as well as midfacial retrusion noted in these patients. This is also true in mucopolysaccharidoses syndromes such as Maroteaux-Lamy type VI and Hurler's type I-H. Probably the best recognized syndrome involving a true macroglossia is Beckwith-Wiedemann syndrome. These patients have also been observed to have a remarkable ability to protrude the tongue (Fig. 1–7). Also, severely enlarged tonsils can contribute to a forward tongue carriage.

TONGUE SHAPE

The shape or configuration of the tongue varies in normals. Certain deformities are characteristic of certain disorders involving the orofacial structures. Deformities in shape can result from atrophy of one side of the tongue seen in hemifacial atrophy (atrophy process usually plateaus in adolescence); neoplastic growths seen in Cowden's syndrome, epidermal nevus syndrome, Maffucci syndrome, multiple endocrine neoplasias, and neurofibromatosis; or tongue clefts seen in some of the oral-facial-digital syndromes.[3]

As noted previously, it is not within the scope of this chapter to discuss orofacial myofunctional swallowing disorders referred to variously as tongue thrust, reverse, visceral, infantile, or deviant swallow. However, the importance of this issue for speech–language clinicians is that dental and medical colleagues frequently seek diagnosis, evaluation, and treatment of deviant swallow patterns. The rationale for our services is to modify the swallowing pattern to allow for more favorable dental/skeletal growth and successful orthodontic/oral surgical treatment. The reader is referred to position statements of the American Speech-

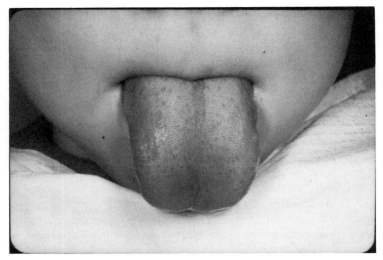

Figure 1–7.   Macroglossia in a patient with Beckwith-Wiedemann syndrome.

Language-Hearing Association[1-2] and Chapter 2 on myofunctional disorders in this volume.

Palate Conditions

Deviant palate conditions usually refer to the vault or configuration of the hard palate. The high and narrow or wide and shallow palatal vault is not an uncommon observation in medical, dental, and speech reports. Although technically measurable, the diagnosis is usually based on visual observation and clinical judgment. Palatal height is difficult to judge independent of width. That is, a narrow palatal width due to a number of factors (transverse jaw discrepancies due to constricted maxilla, posterior crossbite, or excessive thickening of gum tissues) often yields concomitant judgments of high palatal vault (Fig. 1–8). For our purposes, palatal configuration and potential effect on speech will relate to the extent to which space for tongue function might be restrictive. There are certain craniofacial disorders having a very characteristic palatal vault, for example a very narrow, byzantine vault in Apert, Crouzon, and Pfeiffer syndromes and very high and narrow vaults in myotonic dystrophy.

Lips

Obviously, there are a number of neuromuscular conditions affecting lip approximation and coordination (notably Moebius syndrome) that have implications for speech. However, we will consider only those structural conditions affecting lip approximation during speech. Problems with approximation could occur with excessive lip shortness or other structural conditions, making it difficult for approximation to occur. In some disorders, the lips are excessively large and bulky (Coffin-Lowry syndrome, Hughes syndrome, Ackerman syndrome, and in several of the mucopolysaccharidoses syndromes) and can contribute to imprecise bilabial approximation.

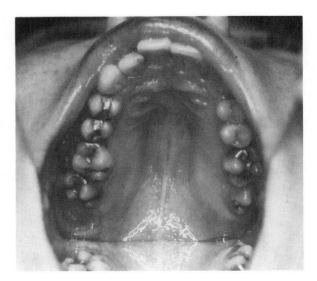

Figure 1–8. Clinical view of a high, narrow palatal vault.

Lip incompetence is a term utilized by dental practitioners to describe a habitual lip-apart posture at rest and perhaps during function. However, this may be the result of a dental-occlusal condition rather than a muscular problem, as the term seems to suggest. The dental-occlusal situations most frequently associated with a lip-apart posture are excessive anterior openbite and/or overjet.

Historic Aspects, Assumptions, and Issues

The effect of dental-occlusal and oral conditions on speech performance has been the subject of several reports in the speech and dental literature for over 60 years.[4-29] In most instances, the independent variable has been the subjects' dental-occlusal status, and the dependent variable has been speech performance. For example, articulatory characteristics (dependent variable) of subjects with missing maxillary central incisors (independent variable) have been investigated. However, some studies have identified and classified subjects on the basis of speech performance (independent variable) and assessed their dental-occlusal status (dependent variable).

Methods used to evaluate speech performance have ranged from clinical observation and judgment by one listener, to multiple listener ratings of speech, to instrumental speech assessment. Additionally, the rigor applied to the subjects' dental-occlusal and oral status has likewise varied. For the most part, adult speakers have been studied, although there have been studies of younger speakers.[15,23,27] Several of the reports are based more on clinical experience and opinion than on data generated. Some authors' conclusions conflict with others and sample size varied considerably between the studies. It must be recognized that experimentation in this area is problematic due to the large number of variables that are difficult, if not impossible, to control (variability in speaker/subject cognitive functioning, neuromuscular control, severity of the dental-occlusal deviation, and concomitant existence of other conditions). In general, the research suggests that although some relationships between dental-occlusal conditions and speech performance do exist, the nature and extent of the relationship is far from clear.

Several authors have reviewed research pertaining to the relationship between dental-occlusal conditions and their effect on speech as well as the effect of surgical/prosthetic treatment on speech.[30-33] Based on the results of previous investigations and prevailing clinical opinion, the following statements are offered as a framework for the speech–language clinician in approaching speech function in the presence of dental-occlusal and oral deviations.

1. Although there appears to be some relationship (coexistence) between dental-occlusal and oral conditions and speech performance, this does not imply cause and effect.
2. Single dental deviations for the most part do not prevent the acquisition of acceptable articulation; however, these deviations can present hazards to acceptable speech.
3. Severe dental-occlusal and oral conditions, or in combination with other structural conditions, may limit acquisition of acceptable speech.

4. Some speakers do very well in the presence of rather significant dental-occlusal deviations.

With these statements in mind, the treatment implication is that defective speech articulation can be modified in the presence of structural deviations. A fruitful area of investigation is to study how some speakers with existing dental-occlusal deviations or who have oral or dental appliances are able to produce acceptable speech. What strategies do they utilize to produce perceptually accurate articulation? And based on this information, is application of a particular strategy appropriate for the client we might be treating? Several studies[23,24,28,34-38] have generated data that are helpful in this regard and will be discussed later.

It is important to understand that dental-occlusal, as well as other oral deviations, may have a different, perhaps greater effect on a speaker *acquiring* articulation than a speaker *maintaining* acceptable articulation. That is, a dental-occlusal condition constituting a hazard to precise articulation for a child acquiring articulation may not be similar to an adult whose normal articulation has been acquired and a dental hazard (loss of teeth, prosthetic appliance) has been introduced.

Speech Assessment and Treatment for Existing Dental-Occlusal and Oral Conditions

The following discussion will focus primarily on articulation effects of dental-occlusal and oral conditions. There is no strong evidence at this time to suggest that vowel variations are significantly affected by the kinds of structural deviations considered here. However, in some patients with craniofacial syndromes resulting in severe maxillary/mandibular disproportion and severely constricted palatal vaults in combination with nasal deformities and velopharyngeal problems, vowel articulation may be distorted, and there may be concomitant resonance and voice disorders. The dental-occlusal and oral conditions have been described, the following sections will discuss assessment and treatment considerations.

Dentition

MISSING TEETH

The general wisdom concerning the effect of missing teeth is that edentulous or excessive spaces make it more difficult to achieve the sharpness or sibilancy associated with the /s/ and /z/ sounds.[30,31] In general, it is the absence of the anterior dentition (upper and lower) that accounts for the hazards. Fymbo[5] studied three groups of college students who were rated as superior, average, or defective speakers. He classified the subjects in each group according to their dental-occlusal status (missing teeth, occlusion, palatal vault). He found that edentulous spaces in the upper and lower incisor areas occurred more frequently in the defective speaker group, but there were other concomitant occlusal discrepancies in those speakers. Snow[15] found that first grade children with one or more missing upper incisors made more errors on the /s/ and /z/ sounds than a control group with central incisors. However, some children produced these sounds correctly. Other sounds assessed (/f/, /v/, and the /th/ sounds) revealed no differences between the groups. Bankson and Byrne[21] assessed the articulation of a large group (304 subjects) of kindergarten and first-grade children who had all deciduous anterior incisors and cuspid teeth and then reassessed them 4 months later. Children who produced normal /s/ sounds on the first assessment and had missing teeth on the second assessment made more errors on the /s/ sounds. Other sounds tested (/f/, /sh/, and /z/) were not affected. Again, not all children were affected by the loss of teeth. Riekman and El Badrawy[27] reported on the degree of "speech impairment" in 14 children (ages 5 to 11 years) who had premature loss of the maxillary four incisor teeth. The age at which the incisors were removed ranged from 15 to 54 months. They found that 4 of the 14 children, or 40%, had some degree of speech impairment, but the type was unspecified. In three of the four who had speech impairment, the incisors were removed before age 2. Speech was not assessed at the time of extraction of the teeth.

Weinberg[23] investigated mandibular and tongue tip positioning during /s/ sound production in the following three groups of speakers ages 5 to 9: (1) normal /s/ production and missing central incisors; (2) defective /s/ production and missing central incisors; and (3) normal /s/ production and normal dentition. All subjects had normal occlusion (molar relationships). Speakers who produced the /s/ normally positioned the tongue tip below and behind the cutting or incisal edge of the lower incisor teeth. The speakers with defective /s/ production protruded the tongue tip beyond the incisors.

Replacement of missing teeth with fixed bridgework, implants and crowns, removable partial dentures, and complete dentures restores patients occlusion and facial and dental esthetics and can provide a more optimal mechanism for speech production. There is little argument that speech is adversely affected in edentulous patients. Prosthodontic and speech reports[25,39–43] are in agreement that replacement of missing teeth facilitates speech. Although it may require some time to adapt to the change in structure, speech performance typically returns to pretreatment status. However, specific tooth positioning, anterior-posterior and vertical relationships, in complete denture patients may be significant for speech, and this will be discussed later in this chapter.

It can be concluded that: (1) Missing anterior upper and lower teeth create hazards for normal speech; (2) the sounds most frequently affected are the sibilants /s/ and /z/; (3) adequate /s/ production can be achieved in the presence of missing teeth; and (4) replacement of teeth for edentulous patients facilitates articulation improvement.

The speech–language clinician may choose not to treat a sibilant distortion if tooth loss is temporary and there will be replacement either naturally (permanent incisor eruption) or prosthodontically. However, tongue tip positioning for the /s/ and /z/ sounds should not protrude beyond the cutting edge of the incisors to achieve the most accurate /s/ production. The clinician needs to recognize and appreciate the range of tongue tip positioning (tongue tip up or down) in producing normal sibilants with or without missing teeth. With missing upper anterior teeth, it may be easier to achieve the sharpness for the sibilants with a tongue tip down, behind the lower incisors. It makes good sense with other occlusal conditions to encourage adaptive strategies consistent with what is planned structurally for the patient. Anticipation of tooth replacement would suggest encouraging a postdental tongue tip position. Some tongue tip protrusion may be evident with frontal distortion of /s/ (lisping) in certain patients. However, this protrusion may diminish following normal eruption of the incisors or following prosthodontic replacement. The adaptive process needs to be monitored by the speech–language clinician.

SUPERNUMERARY/MALPOSITIONED TEETH

The extent to which extra teeth or malpositioned individual teeth contribute to speech has not been systematically investigated. The eruption of single teeth out of position probably presents minimal, if any, risk to articulation. However, in severe cases (teeth erupted midpalatally) or when multiple teeth are malpositioned, distortions of sibilants might be anticipated. This would depend on the extent to which the tongue is restricted in movement to achieve precise production of sibilants and palatal fricatives and affricates such as /ʃ/,/+ʃ/, and /ʤ/ and /ʒ/). Treatment may involve extraction of selected teeth and/or orthodontic treatment that may facilitate speech improvement if errors are noted.

Occlusion

ANTERIOR-POSTERIOR DEVIATIONS

Upper teeth excessively anterior or posterior to the lower teeth, either due to dental variations or skeletal jaw growth discrepancies, can create a hazard to precise articulation. There is no evidence to suggest that molar or posterior teeth deviations alone present significant hazards, but the molar malrelationships or jaw discrepancies can contribute to excessive overjet or underjet (negative overjet, anterior crossbite) in the cuspid/incisor areas, and these can affect articulation.

We noted that in Class II, division 1 malocclusions the upper incisors are excessively anterior to the lower incisors. The sounds most frequently affected perceptually are the sibilants sounds. However, not all speakers with this situation are similarly affected, and some have normal articulation. Subtelny, Mestre, and Subtelny[24] studied the three following groups of adolescents: (1) normal /s/ production and Class II, division 1 malocclusion; (2) normal /s/ production and normal occlusion; (3) defective /s/ production and Class II, division 1 malocclusion. Cephalometric radiographs were taken during sustained /s/ production and during occlusion. The authors measured the tongue position relative to the upper and lower incisor teeth. Results indicated the group with normal /s/ production, but Class II, division 1 malocclusion positioned the tongue more posterior to the upper incisors than the group with normal occlusion. Also, the speakers with malocclusion who produced /s/ correctly positioned the tongue tip more posterior to the lower incisors and raised the lower jaw more than speakers with defective /s/ production.

Starr[31] pointed out the importance of tongue tip positioning relative to the upper and lower incisors during /s/ production. Distortion of the /s/ sounds in speakers with Class II, division 1 malocclusion have also been reported by other authors.[13,30] Turet[34] compared tongue and mandibular positioning in speakers with normal occlusion and Class II, division 1 malocclusion during normal /s/

production. He found that "successful adaptation" was the result of mandibular protrusion and tongue positioning more anterior and superior relative to the maxilla. Interpretation of his report does not suggest that the tongue tip protruded beyond the lower incisors, but that the lower incisors approximated the upper incisors anteriorly-posteriorly with mandibular protrusion. No indication of severity of the malocclusion was reported.

We can conclude that there is no cause-and-effect relationship between Class II, division 1 malocclusion or overjet and speech performance, but that sibilant sounds are distorted by some speakers. Based on the data, successful adaptation to the situation might involve mandibular protrusion to more closely approximate the upper and lower incisors anteriorly–posteriorly. It may be helpful for some speakers to produce the /s/ sound with a more passive tongue tip down position and create the constriction with the blade of the tongue in the maxillary anterior area. This may be especially appropriate if orthognathic surgery (jaw surgery) is planned because speakers who utilize a tongue tip up position to create the constriction may have more difficulty compensating when the maxillary anterior–posterior dimension is structurally modified. This also applies to placement of dental prostheses and appliances that will be discussed later in this chapter. Depending on the severity of the malocclusion, the patient may not seek orthodontic or surgical correction, and speech treatment may be helpful.

In severe situations, protrusion of the upper incisors relative to the lower incisors may make bilabial approximation difficult for /p/, /b/, and /m/ production, and speech treatment may be indicated.[30,44] Although bilabial approximation is encouraged generally, the discrepancy may be of sufficient severity that bilabial approximation is not feasible. Perceptually, adequate /p/, /b/, and /m/ production can be accomplished with labiodental approximation (lower lip to upper teeth). However, the visual effect of this pattern is not as favorable.

Class III malocclusion or situations described previously that result in the upper anterior teeth being posterior to the lower teeth probably constitute the most significant hazards to precise articulation. The reason is that it is more difficult for the tongue to accommodate to a restricted or confining space and to retrude the mandible to achieve more normal anterior–posterior incisor relationships. Guay, Maxwell, and Beecher[28] studied speakers with Class III malocclusions (full anterior crossbite) radiographically to determine tongue posture at rest and during /s/ production. They reported that only 1 of their 12 subjects was judged to produce normal /s/ during a spontaneous speech sample, although 4 speakers produced normal /s/ in single words. Cephalometric analyses (group data) revealed a more inferior and posterior resting tongue posture when compared with normals. Also, during sustained /s/ production the tongue was retruded, there was greater mandibular depression, and increased distance was noted between the tongue tip and lower incisors. It would have been interesting to compare the one subject who produced normal speech with the overall group measurements. Other authors have commented about the posterior positioning of the maxillary anterior teeth relative to the lower anterior and the effect on sibilants.[30–32]

Witzel, Ross, and Munro[44] found that patients with severe Class III anterior relationships reversed labiodental approximation for the /f/ and /v/ sounds. I have observed this reversal in patients with cleft lip and palate and similar occlusion and also noted bilabial approximation for /f/ and /v/. Generally, these sounds are judged to be perceptually correct, but appear deviant visually.

Although it can be concluded that Class III malocclusions more frequently are related to sibilant distortions, some speakers do reasonably well. In severe situations, however, compensation becomes more difficult and some distortion of the sibilants is expected. Generally, I have found that a tongue tip down posture with tongue blade constriction yields more optimal sibilant production rather than attempting to achieve tongue tip constriction behind the maxillary incisors. The tongue tip sounds /t/, /d/, /n/, and /l/ may be produced off the upper incisal edges with the tongue tip or tongue blade. This adaptation is reasonable if orthodontic and/or orthognathic surgery to improve the dental-occlusal situation is planned. Speech assessment for patients with dental-occlusal situations that appear to be presenting significant hazards to articulation might result in the following statement: "the speaker may be capable of improved articulation with the present structure; however, a more favorable dental-occlusal situation should facilitate improved production." Structural treatment may be a surgical one to advance the maxilla or middle third of the face or to set the mandible back. Obviously, the primary reason for doing the surgery is not speech; however, the benefits of the surgery for more favorable articulation should not be discounted.

VERTICAL DEVIATIONS

As noted previously, vertical deviations include excessive overlap of the upper anterior teeth to the lower teeth (overbite or closed bite) or no overlap at all (openbite). Generally, isolated overbite situations do not result in significant speech hazards; however, openbite can create significant hazards. In the openbite situation, it is more difficult to use the cutting edges of the upper incisors to achieve the sharpness or sibilancy for the /s/ and /z/ sounds. Fairbanks and Lintner[11] studied the relationship between articulation proficiency and dental-occlusal measurements and judgments. Subjects were college students selected on the basis of their performance on an articulation test. A "superior" and an "inferior" articulation group were compared on the basis of maxillary arch width and palatal height as well as judgments of molar occlusion, anterior teeth occlusion, alignment of incisors and cuspids, and spacing of anterior teeth. None of the measurements or judgments were significant; however, the additional judgment of "one or more marked dental-occlusal deviations" was significantly more frequent in the inferior speech group. Openbite was only found in the inferior articulation group. Bernstein[12] studied 137 elementary school children with speech defects and then assessed their occlusion according to Classes I, II, and III and openbite. He also utilized a control group of 446 children. He concluded that only the openbite was related to lisping. He also reported that the severity of lisping was not related to the severity of the openbite.

As with the other single occlusal deviations discussed, it can be concluded that although the openbite condition may place precise sibilant production at risk, this situation does not prevent acceptable production. There are many speakers with anterior openbite who have normal speech. I am not aware of studies that have focused on tongue or mandibular positioning of speakers with openbite who have compensated successfully. In patients I have observed, it appears easier to produce acceptable sibilants with a tongue tip down position and tongue blade constriction in the maxillary alveolar area. Furthermore, following orthodontic manipulation and/or a surgical procedure to close the openbite (maxillary impaction and/or anterior mandibular repositioning), adaptation appears to be easier. In severe anterior openbite situations, lip approximation also may be difficult, if not impossible. A reasonable compensation to produce acceptable /p/, /b/, and /m/ is a labiodental approximation for these sounds.

Speech–language clinicians need to be aware of the natural change in openbite situations that occurs with growth and development. There is a marked decrease in anterior openbite from ages 7 to 9 and from 10 to 12.[45] This knowledge is important for at least two reasons. First, the clinician might defer speech services for certain patients with mild sibilant distortions in the presence of openbite until further growth and development has occurred. Second, if the treatment goal is to modify a forward tongue positioning (tongue-thrust) during speech and perhaps swallowing and to contribute to closure of the anterior openbite, we might not be the one to take credit. According to Worms, Meskin, and Isaacson, "openbites represent, at least in part, a dynamic condition subject to change" (p. 592).[45]

TRANSVERSE DEVIATIONS

Occlusal discrepancies from side to side can occur in isolation and they can occur on one or both sides. The transverse deviation of most concern to us is when the maxillary arch is constricted so as to restrict or confine tongue movement. Fairbanks and Lintner[11] found that reduced maxillary width in the canine and molar areas was related to defective articulation of sibilants. Similar to Class III malocclusions, tongue restriction in the maxillary arch can present hazards to precise sibilant production. The modifiability of the distortion is likely dependent on the severity of the discrepancy as well as other coexisting conditions.

In summary, single dental and occlusal deviations, while presenting hazards to articulation, rarely prevent the acquisition of acceptable articulation. Many speakers produce normal speech in the presence of single and sometimes multiple dental-occlusal deviations. Some compensatory strategies have been described. More information is needed about successful adaptation to better determine appropriate treatment. However, in severe situations, and/or when there are other concomitant physical deviations, any compensatory strategy may not be totally successful, and speech deviations may be anticipated. Clinicians need to know what can be accomplished by the speaker and what limitations there may be. Clinicians must appreciate the speaker's current stage of physical growth and development to understand how this can, and perhaps will, change, aid, or hinder treatment efforts. We need to keep in close interdisciplinary contact with surgical and dental colleagues to know what is being planned and what can be done to help the patient develop appropriate skills to prepare for that change and to facilitate successful adaptation.

Tongue Conditions

TONGUE-TIE

As noted previously, the lingual frenum has two attachments: undersurface of the tongue and the floor of the mouth.

Figure 1–9 shows a patient in whom the lingual frenum is attached at the tongue tip (above) and at the gum tissue behind the lower central incisors (below). This patient could not protrude the tongue tip beyond the lower incisal edges nor elevate the tongue tip to the maxillary alveolar ridge for the sounds /t/, /d/, and /l/, yet these sounds were judged to be normal in all speech contexts. The patient effectively utilized the blade of the tongue for lingua-alveolar approximations. All other sounds were judged to be normal. In spite of the appearance of a "short" lingual frenum, or tongue-tie, there were no speech indications for a surgical procedure (frenectomy). However, there was a dental or periodontal (gum tissue) indication for surgery. The anterior attachment of the frenum caused the gum tissue to be separated or stripped away from the teeth. Therefore, a frenectomy was done and Figure 1–10 shows the two attachments following surgery.

This example points out several things. First, although the frenum may appear to be "short" or attached close to the tongue tip, a frenectomy may not be indicated on the basis of speech. Many patients in whom the frenum is attached close to the tongue tip on the undersurface of the tongue do not exhibit articulation deviations. Just because a speaker cannot elevate the tongue tip to the maxillary alveolar ridge with the mouth wide open, or even in close approximation with the maxilla such as biting on a tongue blade, does not mean that a frenectomy is necessary. Second, the attachment in the floor of the mouth should also be assessed to determine if there is a dental-periodontal indication for surgery. Third, if there are no speech or dental indications, a frenectomy is definitely contraindicated. Frenectomy surgery has the potential for possible complications and there are

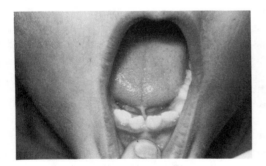
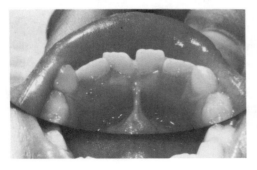

Figure 1–9. Photographs showing lingual frenum attached to the tongue tip (above) and to the gum (gingival) tissue behind the lower central incisors (below).

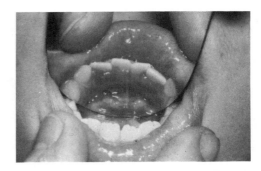

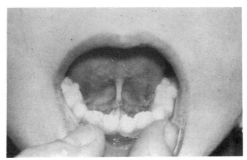

Figure 1–10. Photographs showing lingual frenum attachments following a frenectomy. Above, lower attachment; below, under surface of tongue.

other costs and patient discomfort. The procedure involved is not a "simple clipping" of the frenum, but more involved tissue resection and a "Z-plasty" for optimal results. I have occasionally recommended a frenectomy to release the lower attachment to the gum ridge for speech purposes. In some instances, this attachment can restrict the retroflexive motion of the tongue required for the approximant /r/ sound. However, this recommendation would be made only after a sufficient period of speech treatment without a favorable response.

As speech–language clinicians, we are requested by our medical and dental colleagues to assess speech and recommend appropriate treatment. Our task is to determine what the patient is doing with the present structures and what the patient *potentially* can do. Recommendations for surgery need to be based on identification of a significant limitation for speech, lack of success at modifying the problem with treatment, and clear expectations that the surgery will provide a more favorable mechanism to bring about desired speech change.

TONGUE SIZE

The judgment of excessive tongue size must always be considered in the context of space available and makes the assessment of the contribution of tongue size to articulation problems difficult. As we have noted, anterior–posterior and transverse discrepancies can result in restrictive oral environments for tongue function and present hazards to speech, but the tongue is a very malleable and adaptive structure. Frequently, judgments of large tongue are made when it is visible during rest and function. This can be due to more forward tongue carriage that may be viewed as a behavioral pattern and/or due to poor neuromuscular control. Excessively large tonsils and adenoids may result in more forward tongue positioning. To assess tongue size and its potential influence on speech articulation, it is suggested that the speaker be asked to position the tongue within the confines of the oral space (postdentally), occlude the teeth, and to breathe nasally for approximately 10 seconds. This will aid in identifying the presence of possible airway obstruction problems. Observation of the manner in which the lingua-alveolar sounds /t/, /d/, /n/, and /l/ and sibilants are produced should reveal whether the tongue tip or blade is utilized for these productions. Tongue blade productions can result in acceptable articulation. If the tongue tip is used for the sounds /t/, /d/, and /n/, they may be produced off the incisal edges of the upper teeth. This place of articulation can also result in acceptable production perceptually, but more posterior (postdental-alveolar) placement with the tongue tip or blade should be tried. In general, an attempt should be made to determine the patient's capability with the postdental placement. The determination of whether this is realistic must be balanced with the potential distraction of tongue visibility during speech.

Macroglossia is a constant feature of Beckwith-Wiedeman syndrome (Fig. 1–7). For most of these patients, the tongue cannot be positioned within the oral space during rest or function. In addition to articulation problems and constant visualization of the tongue, dental changes such as labioverted anterior teeth and openbite can occur. Surgical tongue reduction is frequently beneficial for these patients. The speech–language pathologist can provide the surgeon with important information that may suggest the most appropriate type of surgical procedure and extent of reduction. For example, noting the site on the dorsal surface of the tongue that approximates the maxillary alveolar area during production of /t/, /d/, /n/, and /l/ may suggest the extent of tongue tissue desirable to remove.

TONGUE SHAPE

Tongue asymmetry due to atrophy, neoplastic changes, postsurgical effects, or tongue clefts can interfere with precise articulation. As mentioned previously, the tongue is extremely adaptive and depending on severity of the anomaly, speech can be quite intelligible. However, speech treatment can be helpful to optimize articulation.

Palate Conditions

Frequently, medical, dental, and speech–language professionals speculate about the relationship between a high, narrow palatal vault and speech. There has been little evidence of a relationship except that severe deviations result in restricted oral space for tongue function during speech. The concern for speech articulation is more with transverse discrepancies (narrowness) rather than "highness." Unusual palatal vault configurations, such as those seen in Apert, Crouzon, and Pfeiffer syndromes, may result in unusual resonance; however, this has not been systematically assessed.

The clinician needs to be an astute observer of the hard tissue structures such as the palate and alveolar ridge and function of the tongue within that environment. Again, adaptation is the rule and the clinician may experiment with ways to optimize articulation with the patient's present oral mechanism. Articulation focus in most instances is on sibilant production.

Lips

Neuromuscular concerns and lip function, such as occurs in a number of congenital and acquired disorders, will not be considered here. Rather, structural characteristics of lip size and concomitant conditions affecting lip approximation will be discussed. Very few existing lip conditions result in either the upper or lower lip being too short for bilabial approximation. Some patients with cleft lip, especially repairs carried out many years ago, exhibit short, tight upper lips. Additionally, they might have muscle diastasis or a separation of the circular orbicularis oris muscle. If there is insufficient tissue for easy approximation for the bilabial consonants /p/, /b/, and /m/, the sounds can be satisfactorily produced with labiodental approximation.

Severe anterior openbite or overjet are concomitant conditions that can make bilabial production difficult, if not impossible, for some speakers. The term lip incompetence has been applied to these situations. Again, labiodental approximation (lower lip to upper teeth) is a very reasonable adaptation until the dental-occlusal condition has been corrected. At that time, speech intervention with a focus on bilabial production may be indicated.

Effect of Dental and Orthognathic Surgical Treatment on Speech

It is important for speech–language clinicians to be aware of the potential effects of dental-surgical procedures on speech. Although specific effects may vary from patient to patient, this section will discuss previous research findings and clinical experience.

Throughout this chapter, I have alluded to physical treatment required to correct a given structural deviation, which might be beneficial for speech as well. However, certain procedures may adversely affect speech, at least temporarily. Speech–language clinicians may be requested to offer input and opinions regarding potential beneficial or deleterious effects of dental-surgical procedures on speech.

Prosthodontic/Orthodontic

Prosthodontics, or prosthetic dentistry, is the branch of dentistry that restores or replaces missing or lost structures and function. Most speech–language pathologists are familiar with speech prostheses to obturate oronasal fistulae and palatal lifts, and speech bulbs used to improve velopharyngeal function. These are made specifically to improve speech. Removable partial dentures, fixed bridgework, and complete dentures are made to replace missing teeth and restore dental function and facial harmony. Although speech is an important consideration, it is not the primary reason this treatment is done. However, these patients (most frequently older adults) are often concerned about the effect of these prostheses on speech. Usually, their expectations are for speech to be status quo. That is, they are not expecting better speech but certainly do not want speech to worsen. The prosthodontist follows principles of restorative procedures designed to achieve optimal form and function, including speech. However, sometimes, patients are dissatisfied with speech. Prosthodontists and patients may seek a speech–language pathologist's assessment and treatment.

For the most part, single or even multiple tooth bridges seldom present significant speech concerns; however, removable partial dentures and complete dentures can result in a speech concern for the patient. The speech–language clinician is unlikely to encounter large numbers of prosthodontic patients for assessment and treatment before or after reconstruction. The clinical dental literature suggests most patients adapt readily to dentures and do not experience significant speech problems.[25,39,42,43,46]

The most frequent complaint following placement of removable partial dentures or complete dentures is with the sibilant sounds /s/ and /z/. Patients who have learned to produce the sibilants with the tongue tip actively constricting the air stream centrally in the maxillary alveolar area can experience difficulty adapting to prostheses that have reduced the anterior–posterior dimension in the upper incisor area. Conversely, patients who have learned to produce the sibilants with the tongue tip more passive (positioned behind the lower incisors), with the blade of the tongue actively constricting the air stream centrally in the maxillary alveolar area, can experience difficulty adapting to a prosthesis that has reduced the anterior–posterior dimension in the lower incisor area. It is not always well recognized that the consistent feature of sibilant production is *where* the constriction occurs (maxillary alveolar ridge area just behind the central incisors). The inconsistent feature for speakers is *what* portion of the tongue actively participates in the constriction. For many, it is the tip of the tongue; for many others, it is the blade of the tongue. How readily speakers adapt, and perhaps if they ever satisfactorily do, to anterior teeth replacement may be dependent on these individual patterns. Recognition of these patterns preceding prosthodontic reconstruction might alleviate some speech difficulty encountered after placement. Hamlet and Stone[47] studied physiologic and acoustic compensation that occurred in four normal speakers after an experimental maxillary alveolar-palatal prosthesis was inserted. The speakers wore the prosthesis for 1 week. Mandibular movements, resonance characteristics, and articulation were assessed. They noted that compensatory patterns occurred within the first 15 minutes after placement, and that after 1 week, increased jaw opening and mild sibilant distortions were observed. Some speakers adapted more readily than others. However, there was no information about individual speakers' tongue tip positioning prior to or following the duration of the study. They concluded that speech compensation is an adaptory ability that permits new patterns to be learned following surgery or placement of dental prosthesis. Hamlet and her colleagues have investigated speech adaptation to prostheses in other studies.[35–38,48,49]

Garber et al[50] noted wide individual variability in articulation proficiency following placement of maxillary palatal prosthesis (1.5- and 3.5-mm thicknesses) in normal adult speakers with normal occlusion. Some speakers' articulation was essentially unchanged, and others demonstrated marked increase in articulation errors. They speculated and presented some data for support that speakers develop different strategies when adapting to appliances. An alternate explanation could be that the specific tongue positioning for sibilant production allowed for smoother adaptation for some speakers. I examined two speakers in the Garber et al study and found that one speaker clearly employed a tongue tip up position for sibilants and one employed a tongue tip down position. The speaker utilizing the tongue tip up position demonstrated marked changes (deterioration) in articulation with the maxillary prosthesis, whereas the speaker with the tongue tip down position demonstrated essentially no change. Garber et al[51] conducted a similar study using 5-year-old children to determine the effect of an anterior palatal appliance (1-mm thickness) on a high and low articulation skill group. Findings were similar to the adult group study; both group's articulation errors increased with the prosthesis, but there was marked individual variation. As previously mentioned, further investigation of how speakers compensate for changes in oral morphology is fertile area for further investigation. To be most informative, however, variations in individual articulation patterns need to be specified carefully before dental-surgical changes are made.

Speech–language clinicians may see children who are wearing temporary, very bulky intraoral appliances that can interfere with precise articulation and may impede efforts to bring about positive speech change. They include transpalatal arch expansion devices and biometric devices. It may be appropriate to defer articulation treatment during the time these appliances are being worn. The clinician needs to judge whether progress can be made or maintained in the presence of such appliances.

Orthodontic retainers, obturators, and other temporary removable appliances that are constructed for children and adolescents should not present unmanageable problems. As a general principle, if an anterior palatal prosthesis needs to be in place for dental treatment, it should minimize negative effects on speech. There are two areas of concern that speech–language clinicians should be aware of. First, the prosthesis should fit well with the dental-oral structures, in contact with the palatal tissues and be well retained. Prostheses/appliances that fit poorly and/or are loose can hinder speech treatment efforts. Because the speech–language clinician sees patients on a frequent and regular basis, monitoring of fit and retention is helpful. When problems are identified, the appropriate dental specialist should see the patient and make the necessary adjustments. A second concern is with thickness or bulk of the prosthesis. Some prostheses are unnecessarily thick in areas that may be creating hazards to articulation. Direct communication with the dental specialist is strongly encouraged. It is not wise for speech–language clinicians to assume that once a prosthesis is made it cannot be modified. I and others[25,52] have found that dental specialists are interested and most willing to cooperate to achieve optimal dental as well as speech function.

Orthognathic Surgery

Orthognathic surgery combines orthodontic treatment and surgical repositioning of all or a portion of the upper and/or lower jaws. As we have discussed, surgery is sometimes required to correct a skeletal jaw or facial discrepancy because orthodontic treatment alone cannot achieve the desired result. Procedures to correct skeletal Class II, Class III, openbite, and transverse discrepancies are now common procedures performed by oral and maxillofacial surgeons. The specific surgical plan for a patient is designed to achieve more optimal dental and facial form and function. In general, these efforts can provide the speaker with more favorable oral structures to produce speech. Speech intervention for patients for whom jaw procedures are planned needs to take into account the anticipated occlusion. Our previous discussion of compensatory adaptive strategies used by speakers with malocclusions is pertinent here. Speech–language clinicians should be familiar with the effect of surgical procedures on speech to have realistic expectations.

MAXILLARY ADVANCEMENT PROCEDURES

Studies investigating speech performance following advancement of the maxilla focus primarily on changes in velopharyngeal capabilities.[53] The reported results have been ubiquitous. Witzel and Munro[54] described a patient with cleft palate who developed velopharyngeal inadequacy following this procedure. McCarthy, Coccaro, and Schwartz[55] reported on a series of 40 patients who underwent maxillary advancement; none developed velopharyngeal inadequacy. Steinhauser and Moller[56] found no perceptual changes in resonance characteristics following maxillary advancement in six patients, although velopharyngeal structure and function were modified. Other reports[57–59] also found no effect on velopharyngeal function. I have seen some patients having mild velopharyngeal inadequacy and mild hypernasality before maxillary advancement surgery who demonstrated improved velopharyngeal function and resonance following surgery. This appeared to be the result of more extensive medial movement of the lateral pharyngeal walls. The variability of findings could be due to several factors: extent of advancement, presurgical velopharyngeal status, and specific surgical procedure. Surgeons and speech–language clinicians need to be aware of the range of changes in velopharyngeal function and speech characteristics that can occur, and patients and families need to be informed about these possibilities before surgery.

The effect of maxillary advancement on articulation performance has also been investigated. Again, results have been somewhat variable and are difficult to interpret for the same reasons cited above. Favorable effect for labiodental production[57] and improved sibilant production[54] have been reported. For some patients with reduced velopharyngeal space due to severe midfacial hypoplasia (such as occurs in the craniosynostosis syndromes of Apert and Crouzon) maxillary advancement can have a favorable effect on resonance as well as articulation of the nasal consonants.

MANDIBULAR PROCEDURES

Surgical repositioning of the mandible and its effect on speech has also been studied and results have ranged from no change in speech[60] to improved sibilant production[61,62] following mandibular setback. Ewan[62] also observed improvement in sibilant production following mandibular advancement.

OPENBITE

Turvey, Journet, and Epker[63] found improvement in sibilant production following surgical closure of anterior openbite. Ruscello et al[6] reviewed and summarized the literature from 1973 to 1984 on the effect of a variety of orthognathic surgical procedures on speech. They found that in general, articulation returns to normal with time, and almost 90% of patients having articulation errors presurgically showed improvement in articulation following surgery. That orthognathic procedures do not have a lasting negative effect on articulation is supported by other investigations.[65–67] It seems reasonable to conclude that: (1) For normal speakers, orthognathic surgical procedures do not have a lasting deleterious effect on articulation; and (2) speakers who have articulation deviations may demonstrate improved speech performance following surgery.

In anticipation of orthognathic surgery, speech–language clinicians need to evaluate current speech production patterns, anticipate the structural outcome of the correction, and plan speech treatment that will be most helpful in adapting to the correction. For example, it makes little sense to teach tongue tip positioning posterior to the upper incisors if plans are being made for a surgical maxillary advancement. Tongue tip to upper incisor approximation or tongue blade productions may be more reasonable for the lingua-alveolar sounds prior to surgery. If acceptable articulation has been achieved before surgery, it may be appropriate to dismiss the patient from active speech services and periodically monitor speech until the surgery has been completed. Following the surgery and an approximately 3- to 6-month adaptation period, the speech–language clinician should re-evaluate articulation status. Reinitiation of active treatment to optimize articulation may be beneficial at that time, if successful adaptation has not occurred.

Summary

Dental, occlusal, and other oral conditions can present hazards to precise articulation but generally do not prevent the acquisition of acceptable articulation. The extent of the hazard is dependent on the severity of structural conditions and perhaps other conditions that are present. Compensatory or adaptive strategies are available to help the patient optimize articulation in the presence of most dental, occlusal, and oral conditions.

Dental prosthetic treatment can create difficulties in articulation, but generally basic, common sense construction/fabrication principles will minimize negative effects and maximize successful adaptation. Orthognathic surgical procedures may result in a temporary negative effect on articulation in normal speakers. For speakers who exhibit articulation errors presurgically, a more favorable dental-oral environment postsurgically should facilitate articulation. The speech–language clinician needs to be aware of what procedures are planned for individual patients to teach appropriate strategies in the presence of structural deviations and in anticipation of structural outcome.

References

1. American Speech-Language-Hearing Association: The role of the speech–language pathologist in management of oral myofunctional disorders. *ASHA* 1991; 33(suppl 5):7.
2. American Speech-Language-Hearing Association: Oral myofunctional disorders: Knowledge and skills. *ASHA* 1993; 35(suppl 10):21–23.

3. Gorlin RJ, Cohen MM, Levin LS (eds): *Syndromes of the Head and Neck,* 3rd ed. New York, Oxford University Press, 1990.
4. Tench R: The influence of speech habits on the design of full artificial dentures. *J Am Dent Assoc* 1927; 14:644–647.
5. Fymbo L: The relation of malocclusion of the teeth to defects of speech. *Arch Speech* 1936; 1:204–217.
6. Greene J: Speech defects and related oral anomalies. *J Am Dent Assoc* 1937; 224:1969–1974.
7. Wolf IJ: Relation of malocclusion to sigmatism. *Am J Dis Child* 1937; 54:521–528.
8. Frowine V, Moser H: Relationship of dentition to speech. *J Am Dent Assoc* 1944; 31:1081–1090.
9. Palmer M: Orthodontics and the disorders of speech. *Am J Orthodont* 1948; 34:579–588.
10. Gardner A: Dental, oral and general causes of speech pathology. *Oral Surg* 1949; 2:742–751.
11. Fairbanks G, Lintner MA: A study of minor organic deviations in functional disorders of articulation. *JSHD* 1951; 16:253.
12. Bernstein M: The relation of speech defects and malocclusion. *Am J Orthod* 1954; 40:149–150.
13. Blythe P: The relationship between speech, tongue behavior, and occlusal abnormalities. *Dent Pract* 1959; 10:11–22.
14. Rathbone JS, Snidecor JC: Appraisal of speech defects in dental anomalies with reference to speech improvement. *Angle Orthodont* 1959; 29:54.
15. Snow K: Articulation proficiency in relation to certain dental abnormalities. *JSHR* 1961; 4:361–372.
16. Benediktsson E: Variation is tongue and jaw position in "s" sound production in relation to front teeth occlusion. *Acta Odont Scand* 1957; 15:275–303.
17. Hopkin GB, McEvan JD: Speech and the orthodontist. *Dent Pract* 1957; 7:313–326.
18. Jaffe P: Speech problem and its effect on the developing situation. *NY State Dent J* 1962; 28:198–200.
19. Jaffe P: Lisping and malocclusion. *NY State Dent J* 1964; 30:279–281.
20. Kessler HE: The relationship of dentistry to speech. *J Am Dent Assoc* 1954; 48:44–49.
21. Bankson N, Byrne M: The relationship between missing teeth and selected consonant sounds. *JSHD* 1962; 27:341–348.
22. Harrington R, Brienholt V: Relation of oral-mechanism malfunction to dental and speech development. *Am J Orthodont* 1963; 49:84–93.
23. Weinberg B: A cephalometric study of normal and defective/s/ articulation and variations in incisor dentition. *JSHR* 1968; 11:288–300.
24. Subtelny J, Mestre J, Subtelny J: Comparative study of normal and defective articulation of /s/ as related to malocclusion and deglutition. *JSHD* 1964; 29:264–285.
25. Chierici G, Lawson L: Clinical speech considerations in prosthodontics: Perspectives of the prosthodontist and speech pathologist. *J Prosthet Dent* 1973; 29:29–39.
26. Kent R: The effects of dental abnormalities on speech production. *Quintessence Int* 1982; 12:1353–1362.
27. Riekman GA, Elbadrawy HE: Effect of premature loss of primary maxillary incisors on speech. *Pediatr Dent* 1985; 7:119–122.
28. Guay A, Maxwell D, Beecher R: A radiographic study of tongue posture at rest and during the phonation of /s/ in class III malocclusion. *Angle Orthod* 1978; 48:10–22.
29. Vallino LD, Tompson B: Perceptual characteristics of consonant errors associated with malocclusion. *J Oral Maxillofac Surg* 1993; 51:850–856.
30. Bloomer H: Speech defects associated with dental malocclusions and related abnormalities, in Travis L (ed): *Handbook of Speech Pathology and Audiology.* New York, Appleton-Century-Crofts, 1971, p 715.
31. Starr C: Dental and occlusal hazards to normal speech production, in Bzoch K (ed): *Communicative Disorders Related to Cleft Palate.* Boston, Little, Brown, 1979, pp 90–99.
32. Peterson-Falzone SJ: Speech disorders related to craniofacial structural defects: Part 1, in Lass NJ, McReynolds LV, Northern JL, Yoder DE (eds): *Handbook of Speech–Language Pathology and Audiology.* Philadelphia, BC Decker, 1988, pp 442–476.
33. Witzel MA, Vallino LD: Speech problems in patients with dentofacial or craniofacial deformities, in Bell WH (ed): *Modern Practice in Orthognathic and Reconstructive Surgery.* Philadelphia, W.B. Saunders Co., 1992, pp 1686–1735.
34. Turet SE: A preliminary cephalometric investigation of adaptive physiologic adjustment in class II, div. I, malocclusion during "s" sound production. *Am J Orthodont* 1962; 181:64.
35. Hamlet SL: Speech adaptation to dental appliances: Theoretical consideration. *J Balt Coll Dent Surg* 1973; 28:52–63.
36. Hamlet SL, Stone M: Compensatory vowel characteristics resulting from the presence of different types of experimental dental prostheses. *J Phonet* 1976; 4:199–218.
37. Hamlet SL, Stone M: Compensatory alveolar consonant production induced by wearing a dental prosthesis. *J Phonet* 1978; 6:227–248.

38. Hamlet SL, Stone M, McCarty T: Conditioning prostheses viewed from the standpoint of speech adaptation. *J Prosth Dent* 1978, 40:60–66.
39. Ylippo A, Sovijarvi A: Sonographic and palatographic studies of full denture, half denture, and edentulous cases. *Acta Odontol Scan* 1962; 20:257–299.
40. Pound E: The mandibular movements of speech and their seven related values. *J Prosth Dent* 1966; 16:845–843.
41. Sherman H: Phonetic capability as a function of vertical dimension in complete denture wearers. *J Prosth Dent* 1970; 23:621–632.
42. Tanaka H: Speech patterns of edentulous patients and morphology of the palate in relation to phonetics. *J Prosth Dent* 1973; 29:16.
43. Chierici G, Parker M, Hemphill C: Influence of immediate dentures on oral motor skill and speech. *J Prosth Dent* 1978; 39:21–28.
44. Witzel MA, Ross RB, Munro I: Articulation before and after osteotomy. *J Maxillofac Surg* 1980; 8:195–202.
45. Worms FW, Meskin LH, Isaacson RJ: Open-bite. *Am J Orth* 1971; 59:589–595.
46. Cheney SA, Moller KT, Goodkind RJ: Effects of immediate dentures on certain structural and perceptual parameters of speech. *J Prosth Dent* 1978; 40:8–12.
47. Hamlet SL, Stone M: Reorganization of speech motor patterns following prosthodontic changes in oral morphology, in Fant G (ed): *Speech Communication Seminar*. New York, John Wiley & Sons, 1974, pp 79–86.
48. Hamlet SL, Geoffrey VC, Bartlett DM: Effect of a dental prosthesis in speaker specific characteristics of voice. *JSHR* 1976; 19:639–650.
49. Hamlet SL, Stone M: Compensatory vowel characteristics resulting from the presence of different types of experimental dental prostheses. *J Phonet* 1976; 4:1199.
50. Garber SR, Speidel TM, Siegel GM, Miller E, Glass L: The effects of presentation of noise and dental appliances on speech. *JSHR* 1980; 23:838–852.
51. Garber SR, Speidel TM, Siegel GM: The effects of noise and palatal appliances on the speech of five-year-old children. *JSHR* 1980; 23:853–863.
52. Leeper HA, Sills PS, Charles DH: Prosthodontic management of maxillofacial and palatal defects, in Moller KT, Starr CD (eds): *Cleft Palate: Interdisciplinary Issues and Treatment*. Austin, TX, Pro-Ed, 1993, pp 145–188.
53. Mason R, Turvey T, Warren D: Speech considerations after maxillary advancement procedures. *J Oral Surg* 1980; 38:752–758.
54. Witzel MA, Munro I: Velopharyngeal insufficiency after maxillary advancement. *Cleft Palate J* 1977; 14:176–180.
55. McCarthy JG, Coccaro PJ, Schwartz MD: Velopharyngeal function following maxillary advancement. *Plast Reconstruct Surg* 1979; 64:180–189.
56. Steinhauser E, Moller KT: The effect of maxillary advancement on certain structural and perceptual parameters of speech. *Deutsche Zahnartzliche Zeitschrift* 1972; 27:203–207.
57. Schwarz C, Gruner E: Logopedic findings following advancement of the maxilla. *J Maxillofac Surg* 1976; 4:40–55.
58. Bralley RC, Schoeny ZG: Effects of maxillary advancement on the speech of a submucosal cleft palate patient. *Cleft Palate J* 1977; 14:98–101.
59. Schendel SA, Oeschlager M, Wolford LM, Epker BN: Velopharyngeal anatomy and maxillary advancement. *J Maxillofac Surg* 1979; 7:116–124.
60. Goodstein D, Cooper D, Wallace L: The effect on speech of surgery for correction of mandibular prognathism. *Oral Surg Oral Bio Oral Pathol* 1974; 37:846–849.
61. Glass L, Knapp J, Bloomer H: Speech and lingual behavior before and after mandibular osteotomy. *J Oral Surg* 1977; 35:104–109.
62. Ewan A: Aspects of speech and orthognathic survey, in Lass N (ed): *Speech and Language: Advances in Basic Research and Practice*, 4th vol. New York, Academic Press, 1980, pp 239–289.
63. Turvey T, Journot V, Epker B: Correction of anterior open bite deformity: A study of tongue function, speech changes, and stability. *J Maxillofac Surg* 1976; 4:93–101.
64. Ruscello D, Tekieli M, Van Sickels J: Speech production before and after orthognathic surgery: A review. *J Oral Surg Med Oral Pathol* 1985; 59:10–14.
65. Garber S, Speidel T, Marse G: The effects on speech of surgical premaxillary osteotomy. *Am J Orthod* 1981; 79:54–62.
66. Dalston R, Vig P: Effects of orthognathic surgery on speech: A prospective study. *Am J Orthod* 1984; 86:291–298.
67. Bowers J, Tobey E, Shaye R: An acoustic-speech study of patients who received orthognathic surgery. *Am J Orthod* 1985; 88:373–379.

2

Oral Myofunctional Disorders and Articulatory Patterns

MARVIN L. HANSON, PH.D.

The evaluation and treatment of defective speech articulation have evolved from focusing on individual speech sounds to searching for patterns of errors. Identifying existing patterns and exploring interrelationships among articulatory errors and between phonemic and phonological deviations have resulted in more efficient treatment plans. Children whose articulatory errors form patterns may have accompanying nonspeech oral motor patterns, attention to which may contribute to the efficiency of the remediation of articulation.

Mitigating factors in the development of normal articulatory movements might also be abnormal resting postures of the orofacial musculature, atypical chewing and swallowing patterns, dental malocclusions, inefficient nasal airways, maladaptive self-images, and inaccurate perceptions by other people.

For example, in newborns the jaw, lips, and tongue function as a single unit to move milk into the esophagus. There is no independent movement of any of the three parts. If all the parts are essentially normal in size, in sensory and motor innervation, and in shape, and are afforded normal stimulation and nourishment, they eventually gain independence of function. Each structure grows at a different rate and for a different period of time, but the structures function together smoothly and together contribute to the development of discrete vegetative and communicative skills. Any or all such functions might be affected adversely by the following conditions: (1) the presence of an intrusive object, such as tissue swollen chronically from allergies, enlarged tonsils and adenoids, or a sucked thumb; (2) abnormal growth patterns, such as a severe lingual crossbite, a skeletal openbite, a narrow palatal arch, or a deep overbite; or (3) a deprivation of listening, talking, or chewing opportunities.

Developmental irregularities in structures and functions may contribute to the emergence of faulty oral motor patterns. Travis wrote in 1931,[1] "An entirely new total reaction pattern must be acquired in overcoming an articulatory difficulty. The correction does not amount to altering the activity of a single group of muscles, such as those of the lips or tongue, but equals an entirely new move-ment on the part of the entire speech apparatus" (p 256). The more holistically the speech–language pathologist views the client with defective articulation, the more effective will be the treatment administered.

This chapter focuses on the interrelationship of structures, functions, facial appearance, oral motor behaviors, and self-concept. Factors to be discussed include the fronting of lingua-alveolar consonants, abnormal lip and tongue rest-ing postures, occluded or partially occluded nasal airways, dental malocclusions, tongue thrusting during chewing and swallowing, and digit-sucking habits. Not all children with faulty articulation demonstrate faulty oral structures or abnor-mal nonspeech oral motor patterns, but some do. Little time is required to inves-tigate their possible co-occurrence.

The Patterns

A number of orofacial muscle activities may accompany improper production of articulated sounds. Foremost among these is the behavioral pattern traditionally referred to as "tongue thrust," which consists of resting and pushing the tongue against or between the anterior teeth. Other accompanying oral-motor activities include thumb or finger sucking, lip licking, lip or cheek biting, leaning the hand against the chin or cheek, tongue sucking, and excessive breathing through the mouth. Of these, the most detrimental to speech is probably resting the tongue abnormally low and forward in the mouth. In many children, the tongue remains in that position during speech, possibly resulting in the anteriorization of lingua-alveolar consonants. The bilabials may be produced labiodentally when anterior malocclusions accompanying the myofunctional disorders make lip approximations difficult. General imprecision in the production of any conso-nants, with the exception of the /h/, may be a part of a disorder involving improper tongue and lip resting postures and forward tongue movements for vegetative functions.

Definitions of Terms

The following terms relevant to oral functioning will be defined because some are not routinely encountered by speech–language pathologists.

TONGUE THRUST

Habitual or frequent resting or pushing of the tongue against the lingual surface area of the incisors or cuspids, or protrusion between the upper and lower anteri-or teeth.

OROFACIAL MYOLOGY

The study of relationships among dentition, speech, and nonspeech tongue and facial muscle activities.

DIASTEMA

A space between two teeth within the upper or lower arch.

GINGIVA

The gum; fibrous tissue covered by mucous membrane that covers the alveolar processes of the jaws and surrounds the necks of the teeth.

OVERJET

Distance on the *horizontal* plane between the lingual surfaces of the upper incisors and labial surfaces of the lower incisors.

OPENBITE

Vertical distance between incisal or occlusal surfaces of upper and lower teeth during habitual occlusion.

OVERBITE

When upper incisors extend *vertically* to cover more than one third of the labial surfaces of the lower incisors.

CROSSBITE

When one or more teeth are positioned toward the tongue, (lingual crossbite) or toward the lips or cheeks (buccal crossbite).

Prevalences

TONGUE THRUST

Due to the undifferentiated muscle activity of lips, tongue, and jaws during sucking and swallowing, tongue thrust during infancy approaches 100% prevalence. Longitudinal research done by the author found the following prevalences by age (Hanson and Barrett)[2]:

Years of Age	Prevalence (%)
4	58
5	43
6	52
7	35
8	35
12	38
18	43

At age 4, 225 subjects participated. By age 18, 61 subjects remained in the study. The presence or absence of tongue thrust within individuals was not constant over the years. Commonly, at ages 5 and 6 years, and again at 11 and 12 years, when the loss of primary incisors and cuspids creates open spaces for the tongue to explore, a temporary tongue thrust was observed.

RELATED ARTICULATORY ABNORMALITIES

Hale and associates[3] examined 137 kindergarten students for articulatory and myofunctional disorders. Dentalized articulation of one or more phonemes was found in 74% of the subjects. Dentalized resting postures of the tongue occurred in 65% of the subjects. Twenty-seven percent manifested both dentalized resting postures and tongue thrusting. In a subsequent study (Hale and associates),[4]

84.3% of 133 second-grade students were found to dentalize lingua-alveolar sounds. Except for sibilant sounds, this dentalization rarely results in speech that *sounds* different. In this writer's private practice, 30% of 320 children referred for therapy for tongue thrust were found to have a frontal lisp.

In a study by Fletcher, Casteel, and Bradley,[5] a significant relationship was found between the presence of lisping and tongue thrust swallowing among 1615 school-age children. The lisping occurred relatively frequently at all age intervals: 76 children (28%) in the 6- to 7-year-old group and 27 (30%) in the 12- to 18-year-old group were lisping. Studies by Shelton, Haskins, and Bosma,[6] Ronson,[7] Jann, Ward, and Jann,[8] Bell and Hale,[9] and Subtelny, Mestre, and Subtelny[10] found that children with abnormal swallowing patterns are much more likely to have lisps than those without a tongue thrust.

History

The Beginnings

In 1918, Rogers,[11] an orthodontist, began advocating corrective exercises for developing tonicity in facial muscles to aid in proper eruption of the teeth. He devised a program of myofunctional therapy for correcting malocclusions that incorporated devices such as bite plates, rubber exercise straps, and a metal orbicularis oris exerciser. He was not particularly interested, however, in swallowing.

In 1937, the Truesdells[12] applied Rogers' theories on the effects of muscle behaviors on teeth to the process of swallowing. They contended that the voluntary (oral) stage of swallowing contributed to teeth positioning and could be altered with training. They then formulated a treatment program, which included training the patient to bite down while swallowing.

In 1946, Rix, a British orthodontist, published a series of articles describing a condition characterized by protruded upper incisors and a high, narrow palatal arch, resulting from a "teeth-apart swallow."[13] He attributed the manner of swallowing to a delay in muscular maturation.

Training Programs

Concern over the return of anterior teeth to preorthodontic treatment positions stirred the interest of Walter Straub, considered to be the father of modern oral myofunctional therapy. In 1960, Straub[14] published the first of a series of three articles on malfunction of the tongue and began teaching myofunctional therapists to retrain orofacial muscles. The exercises he devised and promulgated formed the basis for most of the current treatments. His theory that bottle feeding was responsible for most tongue thrusting was later challenged and repudiated by Hanson and Cohen,[15] who found no significant relationship between manner of feeding and presence or absence of tongue thrusting in a group of 225 4 year olds.

Two speech–language pathologists trained by Straub as oral myofunctional therapists in the late 1950s were Richard Barrett and William Zickefoose. They trained many other therapists, and by the 1970s referrals by orthodontists and other dental specialists to individuals referred to as "oral myofunctional therapists" were quite common.

The Joint Committee Statement

This new specialty, oral myofunctional therapy, required no special degree for clinicians to treat patients. Many people began treating clients after only a few days' exposure to the field of "tongue thrust." Their therapy was often unsuccessful, and a great deal of antipathy and distrust were engendered among referring dentists. In 1974, an official statement of the Joint Committee on Dentistry and Speech Pathology was issued, which included the following statement: "Consequently, the Committee urges increased research efforts, but cannot recommend that speech pathologists engage in clinical management procedures with the intent of altering functional patterns of deglutition"[16] (p 331).

The shadow cast on the treatment of tongue thrust by this "statement" resulted in a near-arrest of new training programs. In addition, there was a marked diminution of research on the topic, as research funding in this area became less available. Interestingly, more funded research was carried out during the decade prior to the official statement calling for more research in the area than in the decade following the statement.

The International Association of Orofacial Myology

A small group of oral myofunctional therapists and dentists, seeing a need for additional research and improved diagnostic and therapeutic procedures, formed a professional organization in 1972. The organization eventually assumed the name "International Association of Orofacial Myology" (IAOM). Soon after its inception, the IAOM began publishing the *International Journal of Orofacial Myology*.

ASHA's Revised (1990) Position Paper

The American Speech–Language Hearing Association (ASHA) re-examines its position papers at least every 20 years. In accordance with this policy, a committee was formed in 1989 that developed a revised position paper on orofacial myology. The paper, published in 1990, provided suggestions to clinicians interested in preparing themselves to provide treatment in this area. It includes the following statement: "Oral myofunctional phenomena, including abnormal fronting of the tongue at rest and during swallowing, lip incompetency, and sucking habits can be identified reliably. These conditions co-occur with speech misarticulations in some patients." And, later, "There is published research that demonstrates that oral myofunctional therapy is effective in modifying disorders of tongue and lip postures and movement"[17] (p 7).

Particularly pertinent to the present chapter is the sentence in the 1990 ASHA position paper: "The speech–language pathologist performing oral myofunctional therapy should collaborate with an orthodontist, other dentists, or with medical specialists, such as otolaryngologists, pediatricians, or allergists, as needed." The paper urges further investigation into the nature, evaluation, and treatment of oral myofunctions and disorders. Approved by ASHA's Executive Board and

Legislative Council following extensive peer review, the position statement "The Role of The Speech–Language Pathologist in Assessment and Management of Oral Myofunctional Disorders" was made official in 1991, superseding the 1974 paper.

To assist professionals in assessing their competence and needed supplementary training to provide oral myofunctional therapy, an "Ad Hoc Joint Committee" consisting of representatives of ASHA and IAOM prepared a "Knowledge and Skills" statement, which was published in *ASHA* in March 1993.[18] ASHA has begun to sponsor training courses in this area of study in the United States.

Pathophysiology

Research on Oral Form and Function

Do children and adults have dental malocclusions partly because of lingual pressures against the teeth, or is the tongue thrusting the result of dental occlusal abnormalities? The answer as provided by research with humans and monkeys, as well as by clinical experience, is that, in all likelihood, form (occlusion, maxillary, and mandibular arch configurations; tongue size; and patency of nasal airway) and function (resting postures and functions of lips and tongue) affect one another reciprocally. Research with human subjects has consistently demonstrated a strong relationship between form and function, and research with monkeys provides good evidence that tongue thrust can create anterior malocclusions.

RESEARCH WITH HUMAN SUBJECTS

A number of studies done prior to 1985 found significant relationships between oral myofunctional disorders and structural deviations. The disorders studied were tongue thrust, digit-sucking and pacifier-sucking habits, and chronic mouth breathing. Structural deviations include anterior malocclusions, narrow palatal arches, lateral lingual crossbite, and restricted nasal passages. Information on these studies may be found in Hanson and Barrett[2] and will not be presented here. They include research by Rix,[13] Rogers,[19] Hanson and Cohen,[15] Lowe and Johnston,[20] Lowe,[21] Lamberton,[22] Larsson and Konnerman,[23] Modeer,[24] and Bresolin.[25]

Research done with human subjects during the past decade substantiated results obtained from the earlier studies.

Dental Occlusion and Pacifier Use.   Three studies have examined relationships between pacifier, or "dummy" sucking, and dental occlusion. Larsson[26] found the prevalence of crossbite to be five times as high in a group of 4 year olds with a history of dummy-sucking as in a group with no history of sucking habits. Twelve years later, an examination of the same groups of children, now age 16, found no significant correlation between the early sucking habits and the presence of crossbite in the permanent dentition. Hannuksela and Vaananen[27] found more posterior crossbites in 217 7 year olds among children who sucked a pacifier beyond the age of 4 years than in those who did not. (Children with frequent upper respiratory infections also were found to have more posterior crossbites than those with no history of those infections.) Lindner and Modeer[28] studied 76

4 year olds with crossbites to determine any relationships between those malocclusions and dummy-sucking and finger-sucking. They found high positive correlations between the degree of narrowing of the palatal arch and the intensity and duration of sucking habits, with dummy-sucking more strongly correlated to the narrow arches than finger-sucking. More research is needed to determine whether the co-occurrence of pacifier-sucking and lingual crossbite persists into adolescence and adulthood.

Tongue Thrust and Malocclusion in Adults. Little research has been done with adults. Hanson and Andrianopoulos[29] reported a pilot study on 24 subjects, ages 35 to 52, selected at random from a university telephone directory. The presence of tongue thrust was studied with respect to Angle classification dental occlusion, wherein class I represents normal molar relationships; class II, upper first molars positioned anteriorly to their normal locations; and class III, upper first molars positioned posteriorly to normal. Of the 15 with normal tongue resting postures and functional movements, 13 had normal molar occlusion. Of the nine with tongue thrust, only one demonstrated normal molar occlusion. A significantly greater number of subjects with class II exhibited tongue thrusting, and, collectively, a significantly greater number of persons with malocclusions displayed tongue thrusting.

Mouth Breathing and Malocclusions. Behlfelt and associates[30] compared the dentition of children with enlarged tonsils and mouth breathing to that of control children. They found that children with enlarged tonsils had more retroclined lower incisors, more anteriorly positioned upper incisors, more openbite, larger overjets, shorter lower dental arches, narrower upper dental arches, and an increased frequency of lateral crossbite. They postulated that the open posture of the mouth and lowered tongue resting posture resulting from the obstruction of the oropharynx by the enlarged tonsils might be an important factor in the malocclusions and altered palatal configurations. Melsen and associates[31] studied 824 children, ages 13 and 14, in Italy. Among the 5.5% who breathed orally, significantly more subjects had overjets, openbites, crossbites, and anterior crowding of teeth.

A review of research finds significant relationships between malocclusion and tongue thrust, pacifier use, and mouth breathing. None of the research with human subjects has been designed to determine whether these relationships demonstrate that the oral motor patterns *caused* the malocclusions. Only research done with animals has provided evidence of causation.

RESEARCH WITH ANIMALS

Effects of lingual pressures on dentition have been demonstrated in a number of investigations involving animals. In 1965, Negri and Croce[32] performed total glossectomies on 10 rats. Three months after surgery, the diameters of both jaws in the rats were smaller than those of a group of control rats. The tongues had apparently maintained the integrity of the dental arches. In 1973, Harvold et al[33] inserted acrylic bite blocks over the posterior palates of five rhesus monkeys, resulting in a more anterior resting and functioning position of the tongue. The experimental animals developed anterior openbites during the 9 months of the study, along with changes in the width of the dental arch.

In 1981, Harvold et al[34] induced nasal passage obstruction in 21 rhesus monkeys. The monkeys adapted variably, exhibiting an open-mouth posture, a protruding tongue, and, gradually, some type of malocclusion. Increased orofacial muscle activity was observed. In most cases, the mandibular arch narrowed and the length of the maxillary arch decreased. An anterior crossbite developed. In 1982, Miller et al[35] induced oral respiration in rhesus monkeys. There was an observed increase in activity of the mandibular depressor muscles, in the muscles that protrude or alter the shape of the tongue, and the muscles that raise the upper lip.

In 1987, Bernard and Simard-Sovoie[36] reported on a monkey that had spontaneously developed an anterior openbite coincident with a pattern of eating that involved an almost continuous tongue thrust. Instead of chewing food, he licked it. In an attempt to close the openbite, a partial glossectomy was performed after 28 months of observation. After the surgery, the bite gradually returned to its original normalcy. These studies involving monkeys, whose dentition and dental supportive structures are similar to those of humans, demonstrate oral form changes do occur as a result of forced changes in resting postures and functional movements of the tongue.

Psychosocial Considerations

Both malocclusions and speech problems may bring psychosocial consequences. Mowrer and associates[37] found that listeners rated adult male speakers with frontal lisps lower than nonlispers in five categories: speaking ability, intelligence, education, masculinity, and friendship. A similar result, related to dentition rather than to speech, was reported by Shaw.[38] Forty-two children and 42 adults viewed photographs of an attractive boy and girl and an unattractive boy and girl. Each photo was modified so that, for each face, five different dentofacial arrangements were presented. Children with normal dental appearances were judged to be better looking, more desirable as friends, more intelligent, and less likely to behave aggressively.

Most people who seek orthodontic treatment do so to improve their appearances. Helm and associates[39] re-examined subjects who had been examined 15 years earlier for occlusal status. None of these 977 Danish adolescents had received orthodontic care at the time of the initial examination. A questionnaire was mailed to the subjects, and 841 responded. The 10% who had since received orthodontic treatment were excluded from the report. The questions dealt with the subjects' perceptions of their dental appearance and of reactions of people to their appearance. In both adolescence and adulthood, unfavorable perceptions by others of the subjects' teeth were expressed significantly more often by subjects with extreme overjet, deep overbite, and anterior crowding. The authors concluded that conspicuous malocclusions may adversely affect body image and self-concept in adolescence and in adulthood.

Sperry[40] found that people with class II and class III malocclusions typically alter the rest posture of the mandible to assume a more normal appearance. By displacing the mandible anteriorly or posteriorly at rest, they produce a more normal profile. Sperry postulated potential strain on the temporomandibular joint and possible subsequent dysfunction and pain.

Etiologic Factors

Bottle Feeding

Straub[14] reported that of 478 tongue thrusters he had treated orthodontically, only two had been breast-fed, and the mothers reported they had provided these two infants with an overabundant flow of milk. The Hanson and Cohen study[15] failed to find any evidence linking breast feeding or bottle feeding of infants to the perpetuation of tongue thrusting beyond the age of 5 years. No subsequent research has reported any etiologic significance for bottle feeding.

Pacifier Use

Pizarro and Honorato[41] found a significant relationship between pacifier use beyond the age of 2 years and the persistence of "bad oral habits" in 5-year-old children. Vaidergorn[42] studied feeding patterns and pacifier use in a group of 160 7 to 10 year olds in Sao Paulo, Brazil. Of these children, 77.2% had used a pacifier. In a matched control group, significantly fewer (23.0%) children with no tongue thrust had a history of pacifier sucking.

Genetic Influences

Certain factors would seem to predispose a child to persist in forward tongue positioning:

1. A tendency toward allergies and upper respiratory congestion.
2. An extremely high or narrow palatal arch.
3. An unusually large tongue.
4. A restricted nasal passageway, such as from small nares or a deviated septum.
5. An imbalance between the number or size of teeth and the size of the oral cavity.

The relative size and shape of the mandible and maxilla, the sizes of the teeth, and growth patterns of oral structures are all determined by genetic constitution. The forces that establish and maintain occlusion act within physiologic limits established by heredity. These factors may predispose a child to persist in lingual resting and motoric patterns present at birth throughout life. The presence of specific genetic factors in the persistence of these patterns is speculative and unsubstantiated by carefully controlled research.

Open Spaces During Mixed Dentition

Hanson and Cohen[15] measured the total diastema and edentulous spaces in each child in a longitudinal study. No significant difference in total space was found between children who retained a tongue thrust pattern through the age of 8 years and those who demonstrated normal patterns at that age.

Tonsils and Adenoids

Theoretically, the presence of enlarged tonsils and adenoids might promote a forward posturing of the tongue. Large adenoids make oral breathing preferable, and large tonsils block the isthmus from the oral pharynx to the oral cavity, fostering a dropped jaw and lowered tongue. Hanson and Cohen[15] found a significant relationship between enlarged tonsils and the retention or development of tongue thrust in children.

Allergies

Research has not found significant correlations between allergies and tongue thrust, but when the effects of allergies in a given child preclude efficient nasal breathing, closed-lips resting postures and corrected swallowing patterns are difficult to achieve.

Mouth Breathing

Holik[43] found 85% of a group of children who breathed habitually through the mouth to have underdeveloped oral musculature. Watson and associates[44] found that children with long, narrow faces or high, narrow palates have a mean greater nasal resistance to breathing than those with short, wide faces or low, broad palates. Hanson and Cohen[15] found a significant relationship between the presence of mouth breathing and the occurrence of tongue thrust.

Tongue Size

No controlled research has been done relating tongue size to presence of tongue thrust. Tongues that appear to be excessively large due to their visibility in resting positions appear much smaller following training to rest more posteriorly; they have not shrunk but have become less obvious.

Orthodontic Treatment

When there is a severe class II malocclusion with resulting anteriorized positioning of the incisors or a class III with posteriorized positioning of the incisors, while orthodontics are moving molars posteriorly or anteriorly over cusps of molars in the opposing jaw, there is a period of time when cusps meet cusps, creating open spaces between upper and lower teeth. Cusp-to-cusp contacts make firm occlusion uncomfortable and encourage the tongue to become a pad between opposing sets of teeth. A tongue thrust pattern might be induced during such a time.

Oral Sensory Deficiencies

Some investigators have postulated that the more complex lingual movements involved in "adult" chewing and swallowing patterns might not be developed in a child whose oral sensory skills are inadequate. Similarly, deficiencies in oral sensory discrimination might impede the development of normal articulation. Ringel[45] reviewed four investigations that found that children and adults with defective articulation have poorer form recognition ability than normal speakers. Silcox[46] found no significant differences between performances of tongue thrusters and normal swallowers on oral stereognostic tasks. These studies and other similar ones use small geometric forms placed on the tongue and require that the subject identify their shapes. The serious limitation of these tests is that they do not test functions pertinent to sensory abilities of people with tongue thrust. What needs to be determined is whether such people can tell what part of the tongue is contacting what part of the oral cavity, both at rest and during chewing and swallowing. Research designed to make this determination has employed pseudopalates, which cover the anterior palate and alter the perceptions being studied. Clinically, many patients with tongue thrust are unable to tell precisely where tongue contacts are being made and whether the tongue is being narrowed or widened. After repeated attempts some still are unable to place the tongue tip on the same spot on the palate twice. While attempting to achieve elevation of the posterior tongue, as for the /k/, many patients are unable to discern where or whether the contact is being made. There may well be sensory deficiencies in the tongue or palate in people with tongue thrust, but more research is needed.

A Developmental Theory

A theory explaining the persistence of tongue thrust as representing alterations in developmental changes in the oral cavity was proposed by Hanson and Barrett[2] and will be briefly summarized here. Eating patterns in infants are totally reflexive and become more complex, eventually under voluntary control. Gradually a relatively greater portion of the time spent on eating is devoted to preparatory phases, rather than to swallowing. Solids, unlike milk, must be bitten, chewed, formed into a bolus, moved posteriorly, and propelled into the esophagus. Some important developmental changes take place in the oral cavity and pharynx during infancy and early childhood:

1. The oral cavity enlarges. At rest, most of the dorsum of the tongue ceases to contact the palate.
2. Movements of the tongue, lips, and mandible, once undifferentiated, gain independence.
3. Movements of the posterior wall of the pharynx that assist swallowing diminish.
4. Mandibular and maxillary growth provides more anterior space for the tongue, allowing it to rest more posteriorly away from the lips and later away from the teeth.
5. Vertical mandibular growth, along with eruption of the teeth, provide more vertical space for the tongue.
6. The oral-pharyngeal airway is opened by enlargement and growth of the oral cavity.
7. The preparatory phases of swallowing are cortically controlled, and eating becomes partly voluntary and partly reflexive.

Any factors that interrupt these developmental processes may encourage persistence of infantile handling of saliva, liquids, and food. Some of these are:

1. Tongue size increases disproportionately to the size of the oral cavity.

2. Bottle feeding persists beyond the time when solids should be introduced into the diet of the child. Motor patterns developed through activities of biting, chewing, and food moving do not emerge when they normally would. The disruption of developmental timing may result in permanent retention of infantile patterns.

3. Mandibular or maxillary growth, or both, are retarded or inhibited, limiting the amount of space available for the tongue.

4. Insufficient or delayed eruption of the teeth restricts vertical expansion of the oral cavity. The crowded tongue persists in moving anteriorly.

5. Enlarged adenoids, swollen membranes, or deviated septa restrict the diameter of the nasal passages, fostering mouth breathing and forward-resting tongue postures.

6. Neurophysiological abnormalities preclude the development of skills required for the development of normal, adult oral skills.

Hanson and Cohen[15] found considerable variability in maturational changes in children in their longitudinal research. When first examined at age 4, for example, 75 of the 225 children were swallowing normally. At age 8 years, 25 of these 75 were manifesting tongue thrust patterns. Some may have reverted to earlier patterns due to missing teeth over a prolonged period of time.

Anything that fosters a low, forward resting posture of the tongue can contribute to the retention or development of tongue thrusting patterns. Mouth breathing is particularly influential. Generally, any factor that restricts the oral space available to the tongue in any of the three planes may contribute to a tongue thrust.

Summary of Etiologic Factors

Some of the terminology and procedures used in the investigations reviewed reflect difficulties in quantification. Terms such as "mouth breathing," "narrow maxillary arch," and "abnormal swallow" often involve subjective determinations. Certainly more longitudinal research is needed. There is a common thread in results reported, however, and a correlation between form and function seems to emerge. The following patterns seem to emerge: (1) There are co-occurrences of malocclusion and mouth breathing and of malocclusion and tongue thrust; (2) there appears to be a relationship between orofacial morphology and tongue strength; (3) there is a relationship between sucking habits and openbite and crossbite.

Clinical Evaluation

Information from parents or family members and from medical, dental, and other relevant specialists should be received prior to the consultation appointment, consistent with standard evaluative procedures for clients with any type of speech or language disorders. At the initial session, the clinician should observe the client's oral resting patterns before calling any attention to them. Structures should be examined prior to direct evaluation of functions.

Structures

The general appearance of the face from the front and in profile provides clues about the presence of anterior malocclusions and deviations in relative heights of the lower and upper face. Some habitual mouth breathers have a narrow nose and keep the corners of the mouth drawn downward. The smiles of some children may reveal a great deal of "gum" tissue, or gingiva, possibly related to a steep mandibular plane and anterior openbite.

THE NOSE

The speech–language pathologist or orofacial mycologist does not usually examine the nostrils or choanae. Explorations of the nasal chambers are generally the realm of the physician. A few speech–language pathologists, however, do become proficient with the use of nasendoscopy. If the nostrils are unusually small, obviously filled with mucous, or asymmetric, excessive mouth breathing may be present.

THE LIPS

The lips may give evidence of injury or surgery. The lower lip may appear to be full due to eversion or protrusion. This is often indicative of lips-apart resting postures.

THE ORAL VESTIBULE

The upper medial labial frenum may be restricting movement of the upper lip. At times a tough membrane extends between the maxillary central incisors, creating a wide diastema (space) that may encourage forward positioning of the tongue. The jaw may be dropped at rest, and the tongue visibly resting against the lower front teeth or between the upper and lower front teeth. In children with a moderate-to-severe overjet, there may be strain on the circumoral musculature at rest, affecting appearance negatively.

THE TEETH

Within a dental arch, any unusual crowding of teeth, the presence of large or numerous diastemas, or teeth that have erupted lingual to their normal locations may help foster a tongue-thrusting pattern. Anterior or lateral openbites, lateral lingual crossbites, and anterior overjets and overbites are all associated with a greater tendency for a tongue thrust. When cusps on molars are worn down, there may be a bruxing habit occurring. Openbites may also be indicative of a digit-sucking habit.

THE TONGUE

A forward-resting tongue often appears to be excessively large. True macroglossia is extremely rare; the tongue is more likely lacking in muscle tone and resting low and forward. Any discoloration or fissures on the tongue are usually harmless and unrelated to orofacial muscle disorders.

THE HARD PALATE

The palate that is unusually narrow, high, or, in its posterior aspect, flat, may contribute to lingual crowding. As is the case in some persons with repaired palatal clefts, it may be difficult to produce the fine positions and movements required for the sibilant sounds, and a frontal or lateral lisp may result, with or without a tongue thrust.

THE SOFT PALATE

Mason and Grandstaff[47] suggested that the velar "dimple" should be found at a point about four fifths of the distance from the anterior border of the velum to its posterior border. If the dimple is located near the halfway point of the front-to-back distance, the effective length of the soft palate may be so limited that therapy to increase its motility may prove futile. If the voice is hypernasal, velar motility may be inadequate to close off the velopharyngeal port for vegetative purposes as well. The person may depend on an exaggeratedly strong lingua-dental and lingua-palatal seal to propel the food into the esophagus.

An examination of the structures gives direction for the evaluation of oral functions. For example, it is common to break the labial seal as swallowing is initiated to observe tongue position. The location for the parting of the lips should be determined by the location of the accompanying malocclusion. A lateral openbite would prompt a lateral parting of the lips.

Functions

Four functions are assessed: resting postures of tongue and lips, predominant breathing pattern, vegetation (including the handling of saliva), and speech.

LABIAL AND LINGUAL RESTING POSTURES

Most people, including those who breathe predominantly through the nose, rest with the lips slightly parted some of the time. The tongue may rest low in the mouth and lightly touch the lower margins of the mandibular teeth, or it may rest against the upper gums. Only when the tongue contacts a large portion of the lingual surface of a number of front teeth or protrudes between upper and lower teeth during most of the time at rest should there be concern. Observation of the client, plus, in the case of a child, asking the child or parent whether the lips are usually closed at rest, helps in the determination of the nature of lip and tongue resting postures. A postural evaluation of the head, neck, and trunk is advocated by Saboya.[48] Extremes in bodily postures affect general health, respiratory patterns, and swallowing.

BREATHING PATTERNS

Only when mouth breathing is the usual pattern, rather than the exception, does it become diagnostic. Habitual manner of breathing is not always easy to determine, particularly in children, who often have never pondered the issue. Observe the child during the consultation. If a determination is difficult to make, assign parent and child to be aware at certain times and in certain situations during the week and keep a record of their findings. Listen to the patient breathe. Noises in the throat or nasal passage may suggest a constriction of the passage and signal a need for a referral to an otolaryngologist.

EATING

During eating, the patient may demonstrate any of the following: The tongue reaches out of the mouth to meet the approaching food; the lips are parted during chewing or may protrude, pucker, or generally show greater than normal activity. Unusual chewing patterns may be characterized by very brief or unusually prolonged chewing. During swallowing the circumoral muscles may contract vigorously. As the lips part following the swallow, the tongue may be seen to leave the front teeth. By placing a finger on the thyroid notch to detect the upward movement as the swallow begins and placing another finger and thumb at the margins of the upper and lower lips, the lips may be separated, and the tongue observed in a forward position.

DRINKING

During drinking, the tongue may reach out as the glass nears the mouth. The subject's head may be exaggeratedly tipped forward, and the lips may be active. While checking sip-at-a-time drinking, the clinician can part the lips as the swallow begins to check for tongue fronting.

HANDLING SALIVA

The saliva swallow examination requires that the lips be parted as for food and liquid swallows. If the lips resist spreading as the clinician attempts to break the labial seal, a tongue thrust pattern is probably present. Experience is required to achieve skill in the timing of breaking the labial seal. If the seal is broken too early, water is emitted; if it is broken too late, the tongue may have returned to its preswallow position.

ARTICULATION

The examination of structures, resting postures, and swallowing helps prepare the clinician to look for sound errors and for patterns in those errors. Lingual crossbites and narrow palatal arches may result in difficulties with the production of sibilants and affricates, which may be reflected as lateral or frontal lisps. The fronting of the tongue at rest often contributes to excessive protrusion of the tongue during the production of the /θ/ and /ð/, or to the dentalization of the lingua-alveolars /t, d, n, l, s, and z/. The first four of these six lingua-alveolars may be within normal perceptual limits, but their anteriorized productions may make habituation of corrected /s/ and /z/ sounds more difficult.

Severe anterior malocclusions also signal possible articulatory errors. The /θ/ and /ð/ may be produced with the tongue contacting the upper teeth and lower lip, instead of contacting the lower teeth, in the case of a severe overjet. The /f/ and /v/ may be produced bilabially, or, in the case of a severe class III occlusion, with upper teeth on lower lip. A frequent report of parents is the visually and auditorily apparent presence of excessive saliva in the child's mouth during speech due to impaired awareness of its presence or difficulty in handling it quickly and efficiently. The search for articulatory patterns is aided by deep-testing consonants that are produced incorrectly.

Any abnormal articulatory patterns found among persons with normal dentition and swallowing may, of course, also be found in people with oral myofunctional disorders. The same procedures followed in identifying those patterns in children in general should be applied with this special population.

Prognostic Considerations

Two prognostic questions may be asked following the initial evaluation session: (1) What is the likelihood of spontaneous correction of aberrant swallowing or resting patterns without intervention? (2) What is the prognosis for treatment of the disorder? Prognostic factors contributing to answers to these questions are similar. In younger children, particularly those with a full set of primary teeth, any conditions that crowd the tongue in any direction, any obstructions to the oral-pharyngeal or nasal passages, any moderate-to-severe anterior malocclusions, and sucking or biting habits in addition to the tongue thrust mitigate against spontaneous correction of tongue thrust. These same factors can impede the progress of treatment in patients of all ages.

Most people referred for an oral myofunctional evaluation have crooked teeth. Either the patient, parent, or friend wants to have the teeth straightened, primarily to improve appearance. Persons whose malocclusions affect their profile or the handsomeness of their smile are usually more highly motivated to comply with treatment regimens and hence have a better prognosis. Children who care little about their teeth and whose speech is essentially normal are more difficult to treat successfully. The success rate for therapy in most practices, however, is high: between 80 and 95%, based on the author's experience.

Treatment

When an oral myofunctional disorder is present in a patient, and some kind of treatment is indicated, five choices are available: oral surgery, oral reminder appliances, palatal arch expansion, orthodontic treatment alone, and oral myofunctional therapy.

Choices

SURGICAL REDUCTION OF TONGUE SIZE

True macroglossia is rare, but there are several reports, all on very limited numbers of subjects, on the effects of surgical reduction of the tongue. These have included alterations in sensitivity, nonspeech oral motor skills, and speech.

Effects of Sensitivity.   Impaired ability to discern shapes of small objects placed on the tongue following partial glossectomy was reported by the six investigators reviewed by Ingervall and Schmoker.[49] One other study failed to find such effects. Ingervall and Schmoker's own research on 27 subjects found no statistically significant difference in the number of form misidentifications following surgery.

Nonspeech Oral Motor Skills.   Ingervall and Schmoker's literature review found that impaired rapidity of tongue movements following partial glossectomy was reported in seven studies. Their own research found no significant change in this function. They did not study presurgical or postsurgical speech of their subjects.

Effects on Speech.   Lynch[50] (p 60) reviewed speech effects of surgery on tongues of children with Down syndrome. Lynch concluded that parents tend to perceive improvements in speech following tongue-reduction surgery in their children, but research does not support those perceptions. Studies reviewed include those of Parsons and associates[51] and Margar-Bacal.[52] Both investigations failed to find any reduction in number of consonant errors following surgery.

Speech–language pathologists may be consulted regarding advisability of surgery for tongue reduction for the purpose of improving speech. Lynch's warning, although directed primarily to considerations for persons with Down syndrome, is appropriate for all children. Lynch advises that consideration of alternate procedures to surgery, such as trial speech intervention, procedures to secure a clear airway, and increased acceptance by parents and others of imperfections in handicapped children, should be a part of the decision-making process. "More information is needed regarding criteria to distinguish true macroglossia from pseudomacroglossia, and tongue size is most difficult to measure objectively."

MAXILLARY ARCH EXPANSION

Hanson and Cohen[15] found that factors that tended to decrease oral space available to the tongue appeared to contribute to the retention of infantile swallowing patterns. Laterally, a narrow palatal arch and a lingual crossbite were found to foster forward tongue resting and pushing behaviors. Expansion of the maxillary arch is not an infrequent part of orthodontic treatment. Ohkiba and Hanada[53] reported on seven subjects with repaired unilateral clefts and two subjects with complete lingual crossbite (both class III patients). All nine subjects wore expansion devices in the maxillary arch. Following expansion, all nine subjects were found to be contacting the posterior palate with the tongue over a greater area and for a longer time during swallowing. At rest, the tongue maintained a more posterior position.

REMINDER APPLIANCES

Some orthodontists attempt to eliminate forward tongue posturing and movement by attaching prongs to the anterior teeth. The prongs protrude into the oral cavity and discourage the tongue from pushing forward. Huang and associates[54] reported on 33 openbite patients whom they had treated for tongue thrust with these "cribs." The sample was divided into two groups, one composed of 26 "growing" patients (children), and the other of 7 "nongrowing patients." Prior to treatment, the mean openbite in the growing group was 2.88 mm and in the adult group 2.71 mm. Following treatment, both groups had essentially normal anterior occlusion, with overbites of 1.8 and 1.5 mm, respectively. Mean vertical closure in both groups exceeded 4 mm. Altered occlusion essentially remained stable in both groups throughout a maintenance period. The investigators concluded that crib therapy was successful, with or without complete orthodontic treatment, in closing and maintaining anterior openbites in children and in adults. However, only one of four studies cited by Huang et al[54] found cribs to be effective in closing openbites (Justus[55]). Haryett[56] found cribs to be effective in reducing or eliminating thumbsucking in children under 6 years of age, but did not report effects on anterior occlusion. He also found that several side effects accompanied cessation of the sucking habit, including nightmares, bedwetting, and speech problems.

ORTHODONTIC TREATMENT

Movement of teeth toward their preorthodontic treatment positions was the reason Straub and other orthodontists began to seek methods of eliminating unwanted tongue pressures against teeth and normalizing lip resting postures. In 1981, Uhde[57] reported unacceptable occlusion in 49.2% of 72 orthodontically treated patients examined 12 years after the completion of treatment. Lopez-Gavito and associates[58] found that more than 35% of a group of 41 subjects seen an average of 9 years and 6 months after orthodontic retention demonstrated an openbite of 3 mm or more. Andrianopoulos and Hanson[59] found significantly less orthodontic relapse in 17 patients seen an average of 7.4 years postretention who had received therapy for tongue thrust than in 17 patients a like number of years following treatment who had not received therapy for tongue thrust. All patients had class II, division 1 malocclusions prior to orthodontic treatment. Those with therapy for tongue thrust had a mean relapse in overjet of 0.59 mm; those with no therapy relapsed a mean of 1.94 mm.

Pancherz[60] reported on 45 patients who had successfully completed treatment at least 5 years earlier with an orthodontic appliance called the Herbst appliance. All had class II, division 1 malocclusions prior to treatment. Pancherz observed two relapse-promoting factors: (1) A lip-tongue dysfunction pattern (eg, an atypical swallowing pattern) at the end of the total observation period was noted in nine (64%) of the relapse cases but in none of the stable cases; and (2) an unstable class I cuspal interdigitation existed in eight (57%) of the relapse cases but in only two (13%) of the stable cases.

ORAL MYOFUNCTIONAL THERAPY

Of 15 studies reported in the literature regarding the effectiveness of therapy for tongue thrust, 14 reported that swallowing and resting patterns were altered successfully. Most of the studies reviewed patients at least 1 year following the completion of treatment. Representative findings, including the one study that failed to find significant results of therapy, are as follows:

1. Subtelny[61] studied five subjects with "abnormal swallows," three of whom exhibited tongue thrust. He found therapy to be ineffective in correcting the disorder.

2. Robson[62] reported on 666 subjects who received tongue thrust therapy; 520 retained a corrected swallowing pattern when seen from 6 months to 31 months following therapy.

3. Stansell's[63] 54 subjects with malocclusion were divided into three groups of 18 each. One group received speech therapy, another received swallowing therapy, and the third group received neither treatment. Speech training alone was accompanied by decreased overjets. Tongue thrust therapy was reported to prevent an increase in overjet, whereas the overjets of untreated patients increased in several cases.

4. Overstake,[64] using surface electromyography (EMG), studied the strap muscles on the neck in 12 normal swallowers, 12 tongue thrusters, and six corrected tongue thrusters. The EMG patterns of the corrected thrusters resembled closely those of normal swallowers. He summarized that there was a

significant difference between EMG patterns of these two groups and those of tongue thrusters.

5. Cooper[65] found both oral myofunctional therapy and cribs to be effective in correcting tongue thrust. In two experimental groups anterior dental overjet decreased. In the control group (no therapy or cribs) the overjet increased.

6. Christensen and Hanson[66] studied 10 6-year-old children, all with frontal lisps and tongue thrust. Five received speech therapy plus tongue thrust therapy, and five received articulation therapy alone. Children in both groups made equal progress on /s/ remediation. Those who received tongue thrust therapy also corrected the tongue thrust. Tongue thrust persisted in children who did not receive oral myofunctional therapy. Equal amounts of total therapy time were given both groups.

7. Bigenzahn and associates[67] examined 45 patients before and after therapy for tongue thrust. All had either openbite or crossbite, or both. Prior to therapy, 84% demonstrated misarticulations of lingua-alveolar sounds. Sixty-nine percent had both lisps and dentalization of the other lingua-alveolars. Articulation therapy was included in the regimen. Tongue resting postures improved in 91% of the patients. "Hyperactivity of the tongue, diagnosed in 57% of the patients, was reduced to normal tonicity in three out of four cases." Sixty-six percent of the patients attained normal articulation.

Fourteen of the 15 studies on the effectiveness of tongue thrust therapy found it to be effective. Several of the studies employed an "ex post facto" analysis. This is a weak design, but it is often used because of the difficulties of withholding treatment from members of a control group. Seven of the studies employed appropriate control procedures. Although more closely controlled research is needed, the preponderance of clinical research that finds therapy to be effective, coupled with the single study using only three tongue thrusting subjects, which finds it to be ineffective, provide convincing evidence that it is possible to effect permanent changes in oral myofunctional patterns through therapy.

Principles of Therapy

The incorporation of certain treatment principles into the myofunctional training regimen assures the clinician that therapy will be optimally efficacious. A factor that impedes success is the application of a cut-and-dried program of treatment to every patient, regardless of individual needs. Some of the more important principles are:

1. The approach should be individualized, taking into account the specific needs of the client. For example, a typical exercise involves strengthening the masseter muscle. The exercise should be withheld from the treatment of the patient whose masseter is already competent.

2. Changes in behavior achieved through treatment must reach the automatic level and be incorporated into daily behaviors consistently.

3. The cooperation of family members and specialists who treat the patient in observing and providing feedback to the clinician is essential to successful treatment.

4. Treatment should be modified in response to new findings from clinical experience and research.

5. The elimination or reduction of factors that promote retention of infantile patterns can begin in children as young as 3 years old.

6. Sucking and biting habits should be eliminated early in therapy.

7. Timing of treatment procedures must be coordinated with planned treatment by other specialists, such as orthodontists, oral surgeons, and otolaryngologists.

8. Home practice must be organized, with appropriate feedback secured, throughout all stages of treatment.

9. In most cases, several weeks of attention to resting postures during the early part of treatment prepares the client optimally for work on correcting articulatory problems involving the lingua-alveolar sounds. This provides solid kinesthetic awareness and tongue-elevating practice that serve as precursors for correct positioning of the tongue tip for the production of these sounds.

Procedures

Most clinicians work with children with one or both parents in the treatment room or in an observation room. Exceptions occur, but having a parent watch closely as exercises are taught helps ensure their correct execution at home. Typically, clinicians ask clients to practice assignments two or three times each day, in practice sessions of 10 minutes or less. Treatment can be divided into four phases: (1) developing new muscle movements through exercises; (2) integrating these movements into functional patterns; (3) making corrected patterns automatic; and (4) retaining learned patterns.

EXERCISES

Most clients overuse genioglossus and circumoral muscles and underuse muscles that raise the tongue to the roof of the mouth. This is true for speech as well as for chewing and swallowing. Exercises are employed to correct these dysfunctions. Attention is first given to learning and maintaining correct tongue and lip resting postures, with the tongue resting lightly against the upper alveolar ridge anteriorly and maintaining a small space between itself and the palate posteriorly, with the lips lightly closed. Although a tongue tip down posture is also acceptable, training the tongue to rest superiorly is more conducive to subsequent training of the tongue for functions, including proper production of the lingua-alveolar sounds. Only infrequently are stretching exercises for the lips or tongue tip elevation exercises for the tongue required for rest posture purposes.

Also infrequent is the need for muscle-strengthening exercises. The need for such is identified by having the child imitate basic tongue and lip movements necessary for retraining purposes. Movements must be retrained and awareness of these new patterns maximized. Most clinicians begin by teaching elevation of tongue tip and progress with exercises for elevating middle and back portions of the tongue. Exercises are used that permit easy observation of the elevation of the posterior tongue. Awareness of molar occlusion during swallowing is included in the training. The lips and cheeks are trained to suck against the teeth to assist in food collecting and saliva gathering prior to swallowing. For preparing the musculature for swallowing, exercises combining these elements in proper sequences are used. In most programs this portion of training takes from 3 to 6 weeks to accomplish. (For examples of specific exercises, see Hanson and Barrett[2], chapter 11.)

Within 2 or 3 weeks of beginning muscle retraining, attention to articulatory errors can begin. Any need for muscle retraining aside from the procedures inherent in teaching new patterns of sound production is usually taken care of by the exercises for the oral myofunctional disorder. Approaches that are useful for treatment are the Multiple Phoneme, McDonald Sensory-Motor, Paired Stimuli, Distinctive Feature, and Ingram Phonological approaches, all described in Hanson[68] and in Bernthal and Bankson.[69] When a child receiving oral myofunctional therapy has only a frontal lisp affecting the /s/ and /z/ only, this writer provides by the second or third session of treatment conventional instruction procedures, relating the positioning of the tongue for the production of these sounds to the "spot" on the alveolar ridge that is very familiar to the patient. Instructions are given for either occluding the posterior teeth until the sound is learned in syllables and words or for keeping the teeth minimally apart at the outset. Practice with speech becomes a part of each practice session during the week.

When a patient contacts the anterior teeth during the production of the /t/, /d/, /n/, or /l/ sounds as well as on the /s/ and /z/, a distinctive features approach is often followed. If the patient can read, an assignment is given for 1 week to read with the tongue retroflexed in such a manner as to make the lingua-alveolar sounds sound abnormal. This step, using the "opposite extreme" approach, has been very effective. The child reads very slowly and focuses attention on exaggeratedly posterior position of the tongue. During the second week, the reading assignment continues to stress keeping the tongue up and back, but now the retroflexing is eliminated and the words must sound normal. During subsequent weeks, rate is increased and the corrected tongue placement and movements are systematically incorporated into conversational speech. Additional training is sometimes needed on the /s/ and /z/ and is provided after 3 weeks or so of work on the feature of lingua-alveolar placement. The retraining of articulatory patterns can proceed concurrently with the next two stages of oral myofunctional therapy.

TRAINING FUNCTIONS

The client is taught to keep the tongue away from the anterior teeth during biting, chewing, moving, and swallowing food. Attention to each of these phases of eating helps assure efficiency of swallowing and precludes the necessity for "clean-up" swallows that might follow. Instruction in continuous drinking precedes attention to "sip-at-a time" drinking and use of a straw. For continuous drinking, the child is taught to keep the tongue away from the front teeth, to keep the head straight, and to gradually tip the glass or cup as the liquid flows into the mouth. The lips are trained to be passive during drinking. Sip-at-a-time drinking is much like eating without biting or chewing. The tongue remains on the alveolar ridge as a small sip is taken. The molars occlude, the lips suck back against the teeth, moving the liquid posteriorly. The tongue tip remains on its "spot" while the posterior portions of the tongue raise to propel the liquid posteriorly. Instruction in moving saliva posteriorly in the mouth by occluding the molars and sucking in with cheeks and lips precedes saliva-swallow training.

"The only time your tongue need touch your front teeth, day or night, is when you say the `th' sound." This is frequent instruction, and albeit a requirement beyond the limits of normal function, it serves to emphasize the need for attention to all oral functions, including speech. By the end of this second stage of treatment, usually 4 to 6 weeks, most clients can perform the necessary movements with lingual and facial musculature to begin the next phase of treatment without difficulty.

GENERALIZING PATTERNS

This phase, although formally begun after phase 2, has beginnings throughout the first two phases of treatment. Resting postures begin to become automated during the first intervention session. As eating, drinking, and saliva skills are taught, assignments help to begin their automatization. In phase 3 all practice and awareness time is devoted to increasing the frequency of their utilization. Charts are kept; reminders used; peers, family members and teachers assist; rewards are given; and the patterns are incorporated into daily use in a very organized manner. It is not unusual for patients to report after 3 months or so of training that former patterns now feel awkward. The patterns they have acquired are similar to those learned without training by two thirds or more of the population; thus, they become very natural, particularly if they have become more efficient than previous tongue thrust patterns.

MAINTENANCE

The patient, along with other concerned people in his or her life, uses reminders and signals to continue awareness of postures and movements. Follow-up visits to the clinician at gradually increasing intervals of time are scheduled, until all phases of orthodontic treatment are complete or for a period of at least 1 year if no orthodontic treatment is undertaken.

Chapter Summary

A holistic approach to the evaluation and treatment of oral myofunctional disorders and accompanying phonological disturbances is advocated. Proper tongue and lip resting postures, permitted by a competent nasal airway and the absence of detrimental sucking, biting, or grinding habits, form a sound foundation for retraining of tongue and facial muscles for proper vegetative and communicative functioning. Retraining of eating and drinking patterns can occur simultaneously with the correction of articulatory errors. The cooperative efforts of patient, clinician, family members, friends, teachers, and medical and dental professionals maximize progress toward automatization of corrected patterns. Improvements in cosmesis, self-esteem, communication skills, and oral vegetative functioning can accrue from this concerted program of remediation of patterns.

References

1. Travis LE: *Speech Pathology*. New York, D. Appleton and Company, 1931.
2. Hanson ML, Barrett RH: *Fundamentals of Orofacial Myology*. Springfield, IL, Charles C. Thomas, 1988.
3. Hale ST, Kellum GD, Nason MS, Johnson MS: Analysis of orofacial myofunctional factors in kindergarten subjects. *Int J Orofac Myol* 1988; 14:12–15.
4. Hale ST, Kellum GD, Richardson JF, Messer SC, Gross AM, Sisakun S: Oral motor control, posturing, and myofunctional variables in 8-year-olds. *JSHR* 1992; 35:1203–1208.
5. Fletcher SG, Casteel RL, Bradley DP: Tongue thrust swallow, speech articulation, and age. *JSHD* 1961; 26:219.
6. Shelton RL, Haskins RC, Bosma JF: Tongue thrusting one of monozygotic twins. *JSHD* 1959; 24:105–117.
7. Ronson I: Incidence of visceral swallow among lispers. *JSHD* 1965; 30:318–324.
8. Jann GR, Ward MM, Jann HW: A longitudinal study of articulation, deglutition, and malocclusion. *JSHD* 1964; 29:424–435.
9. Bell D, Hale A: Observations of tongue-thrust swallow in preschool children. *JSHD* 1963; 28:195–197.
10. Subtelny JD, Mestre JC, Subtelny JD: Comparative study of normal and defective articulation of /s/ as related to malocclusion and deglutition. *JSHD* 1964; 29:269–285.
11. Rogers AP: Exercises for the development of the muscles in the face, with a view to increasing their functional activity. *Dent Cosmos* 1918; 60:857.
12. Truesdell B, Truesdell FB: Deglutition: With special reference to normal function and the diagnosis, analysis and correction of abnormalities. *Angle Orthod* 1937; 7:90.
13. Rix RE: Deglutition and the teeth. *Dental Record* 1946; 66:103.
14. Straub WJ: Malfunction of the tongue. Part II. *Am J Orthod* 1960; 46:404–424.
15. Hanson ML, Cohen MS: Effects of form and function on swallowing and the developing dentition. *Am J Orthod* 1973; 64:63–82.
16. American Speech-Language-Hearing Association: Position statement on tongue thrust. *ASHA* 1975; 17:331.
17. American Speech-Language-Hearing Association: The role of the speech–language pathologist in management of oral myofunctional disorders. *ASHA* 1991; 33(suppl 5):7.
18. American Speech-Language-Hearing Association: Orofacial myofunctional disorders; knowledge and skills. *ASHA* 1993; 35(suppl 10):21–23.
19. Rogers JH: Swallowing patterns of a normal population sample compared to those patients from an orthodontic practice. *Am J Orthod* 1961; 47:674.
20. Lowe AA, Johnston WE: Tongue and jaw muscle activity in response to mandibular rotations in a sample of normal and anterior open-bite subjects. *Am J Orthod* 1979; 76:565–576.
21. Lowe AA: Correlations between orofacial muscle activity and craniofacial morphology in a sample of control and anterior open-bite subjects. *Am J Orthod* 1980; 78:89–98.
22. Lamberton CM, Riechart PA, Trirtananimit P: Bimaxillary protrusion as a pathologic problem in the Thai. *Am J Orthod* 1980; 77:320–329.
23. Larsson E, Konnerman H: Clinical crown length in 9-, 11-, and 13-year-old children with and without finger sucking habit. *Br J Orthod* 1981; 4:171–173.
24. Modeer T, Udenrich L, Lindner H: Sucking habits and their relation to posterior crossbite in 4-year-old children. *Scand J Dent Res* 1981; 90:323–328.
25. Bresolin D, Shapiro PA, Shapiro GG, Chapko JK, Dassel S: Mouth breathing in allergic children: Its relationship to dentofacial development. *Am J Orthod* 1983; 83:334–340.
26. Larsson E: Effect of dummy-sucking on the prevalence of posterior crossbite in the permanent dentition. *Swed Dent J* 1986; 10:97–101.
27. Hannuksela A, Vaananen A: Predisposing factors for malocclusion in 7-year-old children with special reference to atopic diseases. *Am J Orthod-Dentofac Orthoped* 1987; 92:299–303.
28. Lindner A, Modeer T: Relation between sucking habits and dental characteristics in preschool children with unilateral crossbite. *Scand J Dent Res* 1989; 97:278–283.
29. Hanson ML, Andrianopoulos MV: Tongue thrust and malocclusion. *Int J Orthod* 1982; 20:9–18.
30. Behlfelt K, Linder-Aronson S, McWilliam J, Neander P, Laage-Hellman J: Dentition in children with enlarged tonsils compared to control children. *Eur J Orthod* 1989; 11:416–429.
31. Melsen B, Attina L, Santuari M, Attina A: Relationships between swallowing pattern, mode of respiration, and malocclusion. *Angle Orthod* 1987; 57:113–120.
32. Negri PL, Croce G: Influence of the tongue on development of the dental arches. *Dent Abstr* 1965; 10:453.
33. Harvold EP, Vargervik K, Chierici G: Primate experiment on oral sensation and dental malocclusion. *Am J Orthod* 1973; 63:494.

34. Harvold EP, Tomer BS, Vargervik K, Chierici G: Primate experiments on oral respiration. *Am J Orthod* 1981; 79:359–372.
35. Miller AJ, Vargervik K, Chierici G: Sequential neuromuscular changes in rhesus monkeys during the initial adaptation to oral respiration. *Am J Orthod* 1982; 81:99–107.
36. Bernard CL, Simard-Savoie S: Self correction of anterior openbite after glossectomy in a young rhesus monkey. *Angle Orthod* 1987; 57:137–143.
37. Mowrer ED, Wahl P, Doolan SJ: Effect of lisping on audience evaluation of male speakers. *JSHD* 1978; 43:140–148.
38. Shaw WC: The influence of children's dento-facial appearance on their social attractiveness as judged by peers and by adults. *Am J Orthod* 1981; 76:399–415.
39. Helm S, Kreiborg S, Solow B: Psychosocial implications of malocclusion: A 15-year follow-up study in 30-year-old Danes. *Am J Orthod* 1985; 87:110–118.
40. Sperry TP: An evaluation of the relationship between rest position of the mandible and malocclusion. *Angle Orthod* 1989; 59:217–226.
41. Pizarro C, Honorato R: Alteraciones neuromusculares bucofaciales. *Rev Che Pediatr* 1981; 52:299–303.
42. Vaidergorn B: Oral Habits and Atypical Deglutition in Certain Sao Paulo Children. Master's degree thesis, Paulista School of Medicine, Sao Paulo, Brazil, 1990. Translation and article by Hanson ML: *Int J Orofac Myol* 1991; 17:11–15.
43. Holik F: Relation between habitual breathing through the mouth and muscular activity of the tongue in distoclusion. *Dent Abstr* 1958; 3:266.
44. Watson RM, Warren VW, Fisher ND: Nasal resistance, skeletal classification and mouth breathing in orthodontic patients. *Am J Orthod* 1968; 54:367.
45. Ringel RL: Oral sensation and perception: A selective review. ASHA Rep 1970; 5:188.
46. Silcox BL: *Oral Stereognosis in Tongue Thrust.* Unpublished doctoral dissertation, University of Utah, Salt Lake City, 1969.
47. Mason RM, Grandstaff HL: Vertical facial excess in children: A clinical perspective. *Int J Orofac Myol* 1990; 16:3–4.
48. Saboya B de AR: The importance of the axis in the study of oromyofunctional disorders: An integrated approach. *Int J Orofac Myol* 1985; 11:5–13.
49. Ingervall B, Schmoker R: Effect of surgical reduction of the tongue on oral stereognosis, oral motor ability, and the rest position of the tongue and mandible. *Am J Orthod-Dentofac Orthoped* 1990; 97:58–65.
50. Lynch JI: Tongue reduction surgery: Efficacy and relevance to the profession. *ASHA* 1990; 32:59–61.
51. Parsons CL, Iacono TA, Rozner L: Effect of tongue reduction on articulation in children with Down syndrome. *Am J Ment Defic* 1987; 91:328–332.
52. Margar-Bacal F, Witzel MA, Munro IR: Speech intelligibility after partial glossectomy in children with Down's syndrome. *Plast Reconstruct Surg* 1987; 79:44–49.
53. Ohkiba T, Hanada K: Adaptive functional changes in the swallowing pattern of the tongue following expansion of the maxillary dental arch in subjects with and without cleft palate. *Cleft Palate J* 1989; 26:21–30.
54. Huang GJ, Justus R, Kennedy D, Kokich V. Stability of anterior openbite treated with crib therapy. *Angle Orthod* 1990; 60:17–24.
55. Justus R: Treatment of anterior openbite: A cephalometric and clinical study. *ADM* 1976; 33:17–40.
56. Haryett RE, Hansen FC, Davidson PO: Chronic thumb-sucking: The psychologic effects and relative effectiveness of various methods of treatment. *Am J Orthod* 1967; 53:569–574.
57. Uhde MD: Long Term Stability of the Static Occlusion after Orthodontic Treatment. Unpublished thesis, University of Illinois, Chicago, 1981. Reviewed by Graber TM: *Am J Orthod* 1981; 80:228.
58. Lopez-Gavito GW, Little TR, Joondeph DR: Anterior open-bite malocclusion: A longitudinal 10-year postretention evaluation of orthodontically treated patients. *Am J Orthod* 1985; 87: 175–186.
59. Andrianopoulos MV, Hanson ML: Tongue thrust and the stability of overjet correction. *Angle Orthod* 1987; 57:121–135.
60. Pancherz H: The nature of class II relapse after Herbst appliance treatment: A cephalometric long-term investigation. *Am J Orthod-Dentofac Orthoped* 1991; 100:220–233.
61. Subtelny JD: Malocclusions, orthodontic corrections and orofacial muscle adaptation. *Angle Orthod* 1970; 40:170.
62. Robson JE: *Analytic Survey of the Deviate Swallow Therapy Program in Tucson, Arizona.* Unpublished thesis, University of San Francisco, San Francisco, 1963.
63. Stansell B: *Effects of Deglutition Training and Speech Training.* Unpublished doctoral dissertation, University of Southern California, Los Angeles, 1969.

64. Overstake CP: Electromyographic study of normal and deviant swallowing. *Int J Oral Myol* 1975; 1:29–60.

65. Cooper JS: A comparison of myofunctional therapy and crib appliance effects with a maturational guidance control group. *Am J Orthod* 1977; 72:333–334.

66. Christensen M, Hanson M: An investigation of the efficacy of oral myofunctional therapy as a precursor to articulation therapy for pre-first grade children. *JSHD* 1981; 46:160–167.

67. Bigenzahn W, Fischman L, Mayrhofer-Krammel U: Myofunctional therapy in patients with orofacial dysfunctions affecting speech. *Folia Phoniatrica* 1992; 44(5):235–242.

68. Hanson ML: *Articulation.* Philadelphia, W.B. Saunders Co., 1983.

69. Bernthal JE, Bankson NW: *Articulation and Phonological Disorders,* 3rd ed. Englewood Cliffs, NJ, Prentice Hall, 1993.

3

Characteristics of Speech in Speakers with Glossectomy and Other Oral/Oropharyngeal Ablation

Rebecca J. Leonard, Ph.D.

Introduction

Ablative procedures of the oral cavity and oropharynx can produce profound impairments in all oral functions, including speech. If a speaker's ability to appropriately constrict and occlude the vocal tract is disrupted, he may be unable to effect normal resonance changes of the vocal tract, to generate noise sources required for some consonant sounds, or to manipulate airflows and air pressures in accordance with normal speech requirements. In addition, changes in the overall size and shape of the vocal tract may alter those properties of speech by which listeners identify a speaker; differentiate him or her from other speakers; and make accurate judgments about age, sex, or other of the speaker's personal attributes.

Consistent with the potential for serious speech impairment secondary to ablative procedures are possible difficulties in protecting the airway, deficits in food management and swallowing, and altered cosmesis. For a patient undergoing such treatment, any one or all of these problems may present an emotional challenge that rivals the seriousness of his physical well-being. Indeed, the breadth and complexity of functional losses associated with resection of oral or pharyngeal structures may sometimes intimidate even the most intrepid clinician. Such challenges notwithstanding, speech therapy efforts with speakers who have undergone ablative procedures can, for clinician and patient, be both rewarding and efficacious.

Background/Pathophysiology

Treatments that involve removal of some portion of the oral cavity and/or oropharynx are necessitated most frequently by carcinomas that originate in structures of the vocal tract or that metastasize to these areas from primary tumors elsewhere in the body. Data from the American Cancer Society[1] indicate

54

that cancers of the oral cavity and pharynx account for 4% of all cancers in males and 2% of all cancers in females. Statistics from the National Cancer Institute[2] further suggest that more than 30,000 new cases of oral cavity and/or pharyngeal cancer are identified in this country each year, and that approximately 8000 deaths per year occur as a consequence of this disease.

Medical treatment modalities include surgery, radiation, chemotherapy, or some combination of these. A 3-year survival rate across all therapeuses is estimated at 70% for localized disease, but is reduced significantly if regional or distant metastases is also present.[1] Not surprisingly, survival statistics also vary according to a number of other variables, including age of the patient and type of cancer. Tobacco use is one of the etiologic factors heavily implicated in these cancers, but the disease is also identified in patients with no history of smoking or chewing.

For epidemiologic purposes, oral and pharyngeal cancers may be described by general location, as of the lip, tongue, mouth, and/or pharynx. Further specification in the medical/surgical literature may localize cancers to the tonsil, soft palate, floor of mouth, various parts of the tongue (base, tip, lateral), mandible, maxilla, pharynx, and other structures. Cancers may also be classified according to a staging system proposed by the American Academy of Otolaryngology–Head and Neck Surgery[3] and based on both the site and extent of a lesion. In this schema, an oral cavity lesion no greater than 2 cm in diameter, for example, is designated "T1"; a "T4" classification would denote a tumor larger than 4 cm in diameter with deep invasion of other structures. In the oropharynx, a "T1" classification would again describe a lesion less than 2 cm in diameter, while a "T4" lesion would be larger than 4 cm, with possible invasion of bone, soft tissues of the neck, or deep muscles of the tongue root.

Tumor staging is usually a part of the physician's pretreatment diagnostic evaluation of a patient. A more definitive classification may emerge as treatment is actually undertaken. Regardless of the descriptive scheme utilized, it is important to recognize that *treatment* of a cancer described as originating in the tongue, floor of mouth, tonsil, or any single structure may involve ablation of parts of many surrounding tissues.

For example, lesions that originate in the tonsil may require excision of neighboring mandibular, floor of mouth, and tongue tissue. A "partial glossectomy" may involve not only tongue, but floor of mouth, mandible and/or pharynx depending on the anterior-posterior extent of disease. On the other hand, examination of a patient with "total" glossectomy may reveal at least a small amount of residual tongue tissue. Resections referred to as "composite" extend across tongue and mandible and also involve dissection of lymph nodes and perhaps other soft tissue structures of the neck. A careful review of treatment records, comprehensive clinical examination, and consultation with physicians involved in the patient's care may all be required to understand both the extent of a patient's deficit and the functional status of remaining tissues.

Effects of Ablative Treatments

The goal of medical/surgical treatments of the patient with an oral or oropharyngeal cancer is eradication of disease that, as noted, may extend across a number of anatomic boundaries. It is useful, however, to consider the consequences of ablative effects on individual structures. In this section, both theoretical and reported implications for speech of the major types of oral cavity and oropharyngeal ablations will be reviewed.

Glossectomy/Floor of Mouth

The tongue plays a role in producing all vowel and many consonant sounds and is considered the premier articulatory structure of the vocal tract. The muscular complexity of the tongue is such that during speech the anterior and posterior portions of it appear to act almost independently. Ablation of some portion of the tongue has been reported to result in unusual compensatory placements for lingual consonants, altered grooving patterns for lingual fricatives, alterations in contact patterns and burst characteristics of stop consonants, difficulties in effecting vowel transitions, and aberrant vowel formants.[4–16] However, intelligibility may be retained to a fairly remarkable degree, even in patients with extensive amounts of missing tongue.[11,16–22]

Perspective on the dilemma of the glossectomized speaker can be gained from Stevens'[23] description of the "quantal" nature of speech. According to Stevens, there are areas of the vocal tract where even very small articulatory changes produce significant acoustic (and perceptual) changes. Conversely, there are other regions of the tract where large articulatory alterations are of little acoustic consequence. In terms of the speaker with glossectomy, at least three possibilities for "de-quantization" exist. The first is that residual tongue movements are relatively discrete and wide-ranging but do not take place in appropriately "sensitive" areas of the tract. For example, tongue movements that extend over a considerable range but cannot come within at least a centimeter or so of a critical location,[24] such as anterior or posterior sites along the palate, may be ineffective in producing acoustic differentiations appropriate for some vowels or consonants.

A second possibility is that residual tongue is present in acoustically sensitive areas but is not capable of making small, very precise adjustments within an area to produce a broad range of acoustic outcomes, such as the small differences among high-front or high-back vowels. In the worst case, there is not sufficient tongue or tongue function in any area to allow for shape changes of the vocal tract. Each of these conditions represents different problems for rehabilitation.

EFFECTS ON VOWELS

Preliminary observations from our own laboratory suggest that the effects of glossal resection are particularly apparent in the second formant (F2) frequencies of vowels, with first formants remaining relatively (not completely) impervious to resection. Formants, it will be recalled, are frequency locations in the output spectra of vowels that correspond very closely to the natural resonance characteristics of the vocal tract.[25] That is, formants reflect the resonances associated with a given shape, or three-dimensional configuration, of the vocal tract during the production of a vowel.

Locations of the lower (in frequency) three formants, F1, F2, and F3, differ across vowels and collectively appear to constitute the major perceptual clue to vowel identification. Because the second formant (F2) is also believed to be primarily determined by the position of the tongue, such as where and to what extent it constricts the vocal tract, it follows that glossectomy procedures can have serious consequences for F2 values and ultimately on the accurate identification of vowel sounds by listeners.

In a series of studies, Leonard and Gillis[9,26,27] determined that the major effect of glossectomy on F2 was a compression of its range across vowels, a phenomenon that is illustrated in Figure 3–1. Predictably, the resulting neutralization of F2 was found to have profound implications for vowel intelligibility, with listeners having difficulty perceiving both low-high and front-back vowel distinctions. That is, for example, a high-front vowel, such as /i/, was sometimes confused with a similar high-front vowel, such as /I/, but was in other instances perceived by listeners as a high-back vowel, such as /u/, which, as is apparent in Figure 3–1, has a similar F1 value.

EFFECTS ON CONSONANTS

An inability to effect finely graded constrictions and occlusions, in this instance for the generation of perceptually appropriate source characteristics, can pose an additional threat to consonant intelligibility. Imai and Michi[4] correlated linguapalatal contact patterns for /s/, /ch/, and /t/ with perceptual judgments regarding the accuracy of these productions in speakers with glossectomy. The authors found that a speaker's ability to occlude the vocal tract along the dental arch and to constrict it along the anterior hard palate was critical to the perception of these sounds as "less distorted." For plosives, rapid release of the constriction was also directly related to the perceptual integrity of the sound. Fletcher[5] observed that speakers with partial glossectomy shifted the place of articulation for consonant sounds to locations congruent with residual tissue but attempted nevertheless to maintain certain other properties of articulatory gestures, such as the width of the groove formed by tongue and palate for the production of sibilant sounds.

A study recently completed in our laboratory required listeners to evaluate consonants produced by 50 speakers with various types of glossectomy. The consonant stimuli appeared in reading passages at frequencies reflecting their occurrence in spoken English. Recordings of subjects were presented to listeners who were asked to make judgments about the accuracy of selected consonants within the passages. Results indicated that across the 50 speakers fricatives and plosives were most frequently judged to be inaccurate, while nasals and, interestingly, semivowels appeared more resistant to perceptual disruption.

Mandibulectomy/Floor of Mouth

Mandibular movements during speech typically encompass less than a centimeter.[28] Thus, mandibular excisions that permit some motion of the mandible at normal velocities may not interfere significantly with speech intelligibility. A more serious consequence for speech is presented by disruption of the structural continuity of the mandible, particularly if the disruption is complete and involves the middle portion of the mandibular body.

Bloomer and Hawk[29] reported that speech dysfunction may not occur even in hemimandibulectomy unless bone resection occurs across the midline symphysis

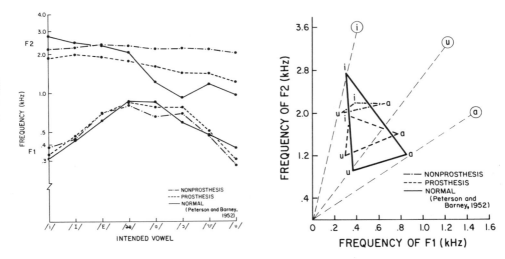

Figure 3–1.   Effects of glossectomy on first and second formants of vowels. Left: First (F1) and second (F2) formants for two speakers with glossectomy and for normal adult females.[73] Increased neutralization (unchanged across vowels) of F2 with increased degree of resection is apparent, as are resulting similarities between high-front and high-back vowels. Right: F1-F2 plot for /i/, /a/, and /u/ in normal speakers, a speaker with glossectomy, and the same speaker with a prosthetic appliance. Compression and neutralization of vowel space associated with glossectomy and improvement with prosthesis are features of interest.

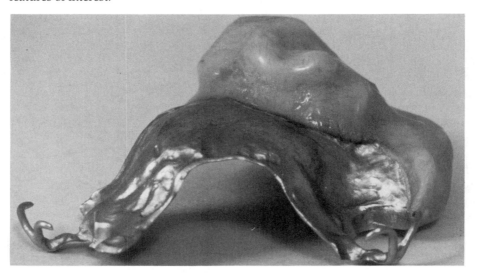

Figure 3–2.   Maxillary prosthesis. Stainless-steel clasps fit on upper teeth. Prosthesis base fits contour of the palate, with the elevated portion extending into the maxillary defect.

(bony midpoint of the mandible). Cantor and Curtis[30] described lateral resection of the mandible to the midline as producing the most serious consequences for speech, but felt this was primarily due to the missing tongue tip and genioglossus muscle that often accompany this procedure. Leonard, Goodrich, McMenamin, and Donald[31] noted that in patients with anterior resections involving tongue, floor of mouth, and mandible, speech deficits were worse when the mandibular resection crossed the midline, as compared with instances in which resections were more extensive and were also more lateral.

Maxillectomy/Palatectomy

Next to glossectomy, surgical excision of some portion of the palate presents perhaps the greatest deterrent to normal speech, at least in the immediate posttreatment period. In contrast to glossectomy, however, current capabilities for eventual restoration of palatal function via surgical or prosthetic approaches may markedly reduce residual impairment experienced by these speakers.[32,33] Effective separation of oral and nasal cavities during speech, of course, is critical to the production of all sounds except the nasals /m, n/ and /n/. If this separation is not maintained, as when some portion of the soft palate is resected, the nasal cavity is coupled with the tract and resonances change. Speech sounds are affected differentially, with those requiring the greatest amounts of intraoral pressure and flow (fricatives, stop consonants, and affricates) being most vulnerable to the lack of separation of valving between oral and nasal cavities and the subsequent difficulty in developing adequate intraoral air pressure for the obstruents.

Larger lesions, extending from the palate into other portions of the maxilla and perhaps involving sinuses, can produce marked deleterious effects on speech. Clinically, patients with such defects may demonstrate diminished intelligibility that goes beyond the effects of hypernasality. Speech may be labored as a patient struggles to generate appropriate air pressures and flows for speech. Changes in articulation, timing, and phrasing characteristics are likely sequelae.

Majid, Weinberg, and Chalian[32] reported speech intelligibility characteristics of a group of six patients who had undergone extensive partial maxillectomy and were subsequently obturated with a variety of maxillary prostheses. Without their prostheses, these patients demonstrated average intelligibility scores of 62% for consonant sounds and 58% for vowel sounds on the Consonant and Vowel Rhyme tests, respectively.[34,35] Articulation scores were improved with prosthetic treatment to as much as 96% for consonants and 94% for vowels. Fletcher, Sooudi, and Frost[36] reported diminished hypernasality with obturation, but also noted that only 50% of obturated subjects demonstrated nasality within normal limits. Plank, Weinberg, and Chalian[37] found that listeners could differentiate presurgical from final obturation speech samples in 50% of patients assessed before and after partial maxillectomy.

In our own laboratory, a number of speech measures were examined for 19 unilateral maxillectomy patients who were alternately wearing and then not wearing their maxillary prostheses (Fig. 3–2). One acoustic parameter examined, voice onset time, proved especially interesting. Without their prostheses, these patients tended to significantly lengthen both consonant closure time and vowel duration time (as in "It's a tIk," where closure for "t" and duration for "I" are calculated), as compared with data collected for normal speakers or to the subjects' own productions while wearing their prostheses. Typical burst plus aspiration characteristics of stop consonants were missing without a prosthesis, and often the consonant was indicated only by a cessation of voicing and/or glottal stop.

In other cases, such as "It's a tIk," no cessation of voice could be discerned to indicate the presence of voiceless plosives. We suggested that both the lengthening gestures and the failure to "turn off" the voice for voiceless consonants may be motivated by aerodynamic factors. That is, because of the enlarged supraglottal cavity that often accompanies maxillary resection, speakers may have difficulty in equalizing pressures across the larynx, a condition necessary to a cessation of voicing.

Changes in Residual/Reconstructed Tissues

In addition to a loss of tissues, ablative procedures can produce changes in residual tissues that may have implications for speech. For example, there is wide agreement that at least certain aspects of speech production are influenced or regulated by sensory capabilities of receptors in the skin, muscles, and joints of pertinent structures.[38] Certainly, touch-pressure, kinesthetic, and proprioceptive sensory receptors in oral/oropharyngeal structures might be expected to undergo temporary or permanent alteration as a consequence of ablative and reconstructive surgical procedures. Exactly what these changes might be and how they might contribute to the degree of speech impairment is not known.

Similarly, the effects of radiation therapy on oropharyngeal structures have not been extensively described. Mirza and Dikshit[39] reported short-term effects of radiation on oral tissues that include mucositis and mucosal soreness and lost or diminished sensations of taste or smell. Among the long-term effects noted by these authors were dryness of the mouth due to destruction of salivary glands, reduced blood supply to tissues, and increased connective tissue fibrosis. Such changes may alter sensory mechanisms in affected tissues as well, particularly those endings or receptors that lie close to the surface of oral structures. However, the possible influence of these factors—loss of sensation, diminished hydration, decreased blood supply, and fibrosis of at least some tissue components in the oral cavity or oropharynx—on speech is at this time primarily a matter of speculation. Determination of the precise relationship between any one of these variables and speech is further clouded by the speaker's ability to compensate or to reorganize in the face of alterations to structure and function. However rudimentary our understanding, an elaboration of speech characteristics related to ablative procedures must consider the consequences not only of loss of tissue, but also of alterations in residual and reconstructed tissues.

Speech Impairment Related to Type/Extent of Resection

In this section, the primary emphasis will be on speech characteristics associated with glossal and related resections. Evidence that speech may be differentially affected by location, extent, or other variables associated with glossal resection is not widely available. Intuitively, we would predict (and clinical experience would suggest) that smaller defects would produce less impairment, and there is experimental support for this speculation. Heller, Levy, and Sciubba[40] performed pretreatment and posttreatment speech evaluations on patients undergoing surgery for small carcinomas (< 3 cm in size) of the mobile tongue and found that by 6 months postsurgery recordings of all subjects were judged as "normal." Similarly, seven patients undergoing resection of T1 and T2 tumors were reported to have good intelligibility postoperatively by Pruszewicz and Kruk-Zagajewsky.[41]

Conversely, studies that have reported speech in patients with total or subtotal glossectomy have typically referred simply to the percentage of patients (figures ranging from 60 to 80% or higher) who regained "intelligible" speech and have elaborated very little on the details of residual speech impairment associated with these large-scale ablations.[40,42]

In a study that did consider differential effects of ablation on speech, Teichgraeber, Bowman and Goepfert[43] reported—in some contrast to our own observations—that patients with lesions involving retromolar trigone-anterior faucial pillar, anterior two-thirds of the tongue, and base of the tongue, respectively, demonstrated less speech impairment than patients with lesions of the buccal mucosa, alveolar ridge, or floor of mouth. Other authors[12,15,44,45] have speculated regarding the relative effects of extent versus mobility of residual tissues as indicators for residual speech function, with the edge typically given to mobility, but have generally not related these characteristics to specific types of ablation.

Our own interest in differential effects on speech of ablation was triggered by clinical observations of five speakers with glossectomy. Listeners' identifications of monosyllables produced by the speakers revealed that across the five speakers vowels were identified correctly 67% of the time (as the speaker intended); consonants were identified correctly 84% of the time. Subsequent research efforts have attempted to determine if findings for a small number of speakers could be generalized to others and if effects on speech could be differentially related to other variables, including, in particular, location and extent of resection.

In a study recently completed,[31] 50 speakers with oral/oropharyngeal resections were assigned to groups according to similarities in resection. Assignments were based on reviews of patients' operative records, surgeons' reports (oral and written), and clinical examination. This effort resulted in the tentative identification of five major categories of glossectomy (and associated oral/oropharyngeal) resections, including *unilateral limited, unilateral extensive, anterior-anterior, posterior-posterior, and bilateral extensive (with two subgroups, subtotal and total)* (Fig. 3–3). Speech measures examined for the 50 subjects included F2 range across vowels, severity ratings based on connected speech productions, and a measure of consonant accuracy.

Results of statistical analyses confirmed that subjects in four of the major resection categories differed significantly from each other on the three speech parameters and on an "overall speech rank" determined from subject rankings on the three measures. (The fifth category, posterior-posterior, included only two subjects and was not considered in the statistical analysis.) Comparison of the resection categories across all speech measures revealed that unilateral limited speakers

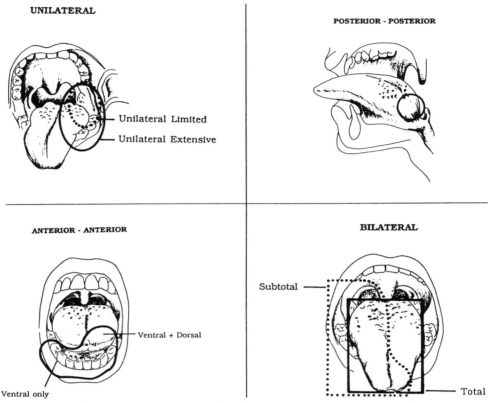

Figure 3–3. Major categories of glossal and related resection are shown, with approximate site and extent of ablation for each indicated in marked areas.

were typically least impaired, followed by posterior-posterior, anterior-anterior, unilateral extensive, bilateral (total), and bilateral (subtotal) speakers.

Two findings of particular interest included evidence that anterior–anterior speakers were the most variable in terms of impairment. Speakers in this category who had undergone resections affecting primarily the epithelial undersurface of tongue with little involvement of the muscular dorsum were minimally impaired, while speakers with resections involving dorsal musculature, and/or anterior mandible experienced substantial impairment. The second, somewhat surprising, finding was that in the bilateral extensive category, speakers with total glossectomy (no more than 25% residual tongue) were less impaired than subtotal speakers who had greater amounts of residual tongue. Scrutiny of the data suggested this may be related to the fact that, while patients with total glossectomy had lost huge amounts of tongue, they had experienced only minimal involvement of other structures, such as mandible and palate. Subtotal speakers, on the other hand, had more residual tongue but tended to have extensive resections of other oral/oropharyngeal structures. The integrity of these other structures thus appears important to residual speech integrity but also, we suspect, to the development of compensatory articulatory strategies.

Of further interest was evidence that speech appeared to be differentially influenced depending on location of resection, as well as, in a general way, on extent of resection. For example, patients with posterior resections tended to have smaller F2 ranges, indicative of disrupted vowel integrity, than did patients with anterior resections. Conversely, speakers with anterior resections typically had a larger number of impaired consonants than speakers with more posterior involvement. Other observations suggested that, depending on the group, factors such as edentulousness and hypernasality were variably contributory to speech impairment. Mild hypernasality (patients with moderate or severe hypernasality were excluded from the study) appeared to be a significant detriment to speech in the unilateral limited group for example, but less of a factor in unilateral extensive and bilateral extensive patients, who typically had many factors contributing to speech impairment.

In short, our preliminary efforts to acquire a data base that may eventually allow the quantification and prediction of speech impairment in this patient population have been promising and underscore the need for further research. The influence of location and extent of resection are just beginning to be elucidated, as is type of reconstruction. Other structures involved in resection, residual innervation, preoperative or postoperative radiation, and repeated surgeries (each with attendant scarring) represent just a few of the variables for which speech effects are still generally unknown.

Preassessment/Treatment Considerations

Assessment directed at phonological rehabilitation may be delayed until medical/surgical therapies have been completed and the patient's recovery has stabilized. This is not to say, however, that clinician involvement should be postponed until this time. In fact, an *ongoing assessment of the patient's communication needs* and *intervention strategies that change to meet immediate needs* and *maximize future potential* may require considerable clinician involvement before the patient is ever seen for articulation therapy.

Intervention Tailored to Stage of Treatment/Recovery

Many patients with oral and/or oropharyngeal cancer undergo a series of treatments involving multiple therapeutic modalities. Ideally, intervention should reflect the patient's changing status and needs at each of these stages. If the patient has just undergone surgery and is recovering in the hospital, management may be directed at meeting the patient's immediate communication difficulties, via handwriting, a language board, or perhaps other alternatives. More extensive intervention will need to wait until structures have sufficiently healed, and until the patient's recovery has sufficiently stabilized—determinations that are the responsibility of the patient's surgeon/physician.

If radiation therapy is being used as a primary or secondary treatment modality, patients may benefit from a daily regimen of oral exercises tailored to fit their specific deficits. For example, tongue exercises that require the patient to: (1) elevate and lower (front and back portions); (2) protrude and retract; (3) shadow a visual target that is moving at different rates in different planes; (4)

effect constrictions and occlusions at various locations along the palate; (5) work against resistance, as by pushing on a tongue blade held firmly in place; (6) tense and then relax tissues in different postures; and, finally, (7) attempt isolated speech sound targets or move from one target to another, as in the production of utterances such as "aka" and "ata," can be encouraged—again, assuming that the patient has been cleared for such activity. These exercises are designed to improve range of motion, strength, and accuracy of residual tissues and may even result in some increase in their bulk.

Tongue blades stacked together and then held between the patient's teeth, first in small numbers and then in successively larger numbers, may help to maintain or increase mandibular opening. A device called "Therabite" (Therabite Corp., Bryn Mawr, PA) is excellent for this purpose. Tongue exercises repeated for varying degrees of mandibular opening will assure independence of tongue-jaw activity and exercise the jaw at the same time. Lip rounding and spreading gestures can also be incorporated in the exercise repertoire, if appropriate.

An exercise program may constitute the speech clinician's primary focus during radiation therapy, which can extend over several weeks and considerably tax the patient's energy reserves. Our own clinical experience suggests that if such exercises can be practiced daily (preferably for a few minutes at a time, several times per day) during this period, mobility and function of residual structures may be maximized, particularly as compared with patients in whom any intervention is deferred until after radiation is completed.

Some contradiction to this clinical observation has recently been offered by Hamlet, Mathog, Patterson, and Fleming.[46] These researchers investigated tongue mobility relative to jaw movements in five patients with partial glossectomy. Jaw range of motion and tongue contour changes were assessed by videofluoroscopy at presurgery, postsurgery, and postradiotherapy intervals. The authors found that tongue mobility decreased following surgery, but had increased by the time of the postradiation assessment. Although based on a small number of subjects, these findings suggest that radiation may not preclude continued recovery of tongue function following surgery. However, it is not clear whether tongue function would have increased even further had subjects engaged in oral exercises during their radiotherapy.

Ancillary Interventions with Significant Speech Implications

Once primary surgical and/or radiation treatments have been completed, an additional issue can be addressed. That is, whether secondary interventions are planned for the patient that could result in large gains for speech function. Restoration of dentition or rehabilitation of palatal function by means of a prosthetic appliance are good examples of such procedures. Certainly, if a patient has a large maxillary or palatal defect that results in severe, pervasive hypernasality and nasal emission, any assessment of articulation capabilities is likely to be of limited use in planning long-term therapy goals for the speaker. To a lesser extent, the absence of teeth can also have a deleterious effect on speech production. If there are plans for restoration of these or other oral or pharyngeal structures or functions, they will need to be considered in the timing and ordering of treatment objectives.

Consultation with appropriate professionals by the speech clinician may serve to underscore the potential value of such interventions for speech (and perhaps swallowing) and may also help to assure the maximum benefit of each intervention. For example, analyses of speech before and after the introduction of appliances (as well as any further surgeries that might be planned to improve oral or pharyngeal function) can be helpful not only in quantifying the specific effects of each but also in providing insights into revisions that may result in further improvements.

Assessment

Patients may continue to undergo changes, particularly in tissues, for many months posttreatment so that assessment is perhaps best viewed as a process that continues throughout rehabilitation. However, with medical/surgical therapies completed more comprehensive assessments of phonological integrity directed toward speech rehabilitation can be considered. Most speakers with impairments related to ablative procedures have, presumably, had normal speech skills—have mastered the phonological system and engaged in intelligible speech for many years. Obviously, this phonologic knowledge remains intact following an ablative procedure. It is, rather, the speaker's ability to actually produce and manipulate phonetic segments, perhaps in isolation, but also in words, sentences, and larger utterances, that has been disrupted by ablation of vocal tract structures. Meaningful assessment of these capabilities may require special considerations and nonconventional approaches.

One of the particular challenges of assessment stems from the possibility that the redundancy or multiplicity of perceptual cues typically present in conversational speech may be missing or ambiguous in speech produced by a speaker with glossectomy who demonstrates multiple articulation errors. That is, when large numbers of phonetic segments are affected by ablation, it becomes difficult to determine to what extent perception of an individual sound as inaccurate is related to inappropriate features of the sound itself or to its embedding in a context composed of other sounds that are inaccurately produced. This characteristic of impairment is perhaps more prevalent in this patient population than in other groups of disordered speakers and must be given serious consideration when selecting assessment and treatment strategies.

Objectives of Assessment

The thrust of speech therapy for speakers with glossectomy is to some extent directed at *restoring articulatory targets,* in part by *maximizing the structure/movement capabilities of residual tissues* that compose and effect these targets. But, in addition, it may also be necessary to establish new targets, that is, to *develop compensatory methods* of producing speech sounds that approximate the characteristics of the originals sufficiently closely that listeners will perceive them as such. Thus, assessment procedures need to be directed at *identifying those phonetic segments or targets that are "in error," elaborating specific causes for the deficits,* and, at *exploring possibilities for new or modified ways of producing sounds* that are typically perceived as aberrant.

Phonetic Sampling/Test Stimuli

Conventional articulation tests that sample speech in words or sentences may be useful in identifying specific sounds affected by ablation in some speakers. As noted, however, if impairment is severe, it may be necessary to sample sound productions in very structured, uniform contexts, that is, in environments that minimize the possibility that a particular sound will be judged as in error because it is surrounded by other sounds that are defective. Further, because both vowel and consonant errors are a likely consequence of ablation, both must be carefully sampled. In our own experience, syllable contexts that sample vowels such as h/V/d, or h/V/p (V for vowel), perhaps in a carrier phrase, provide the clinician with at least a cursory impression of the speaker's vowel repertoire. The clinician should seek to determine how many perceptually distinct vowels are present, and where there may be perceptual ambiguities, that is, which vowels sound similar.

Consonants that share place or manner characteristics can be grouped and then sampled in environments that include sounds likely to be intact, such as the neutral vowel, /ə/, and perhaps a labial /p/ or /b/. Thus, a group of consonant stimuli sampling place characteristics might include "ətʌp," "əsʌp," "əshʌp," "əchʌp," and so on. Again, the emphasis is on identification of errors and also on how many perceptually distinct consonants are present and on perceptual ambiguities.

Sets of single-word utterances that vary by only one phonetic segment, vowel or consonant, may be particularly useful for the error identification task. In these tests, the speaker produces one of several stimuli that vary by only one segment, for example, "cup," "coop," "keep," "cope," "cap," and "cop." A listener must then select which of the items the speaker intended. Results provide information into which sounds are in error and further insights into the types of confusions that listeners experience as a consequence. The Consonant and Vowel Rhyme Tests[34,35] are good examples of this type of instrument. Due to the need for multiple listeners unfamiliar with the speaker and the time required for analysis, this kind of testing may not be easily or expediently accomplished in a clinical setting. However, the benefits may in some cases be worth the effort required.

An especially important assessment measure to consider is the speaker's overall level of *intelligibility*. This can be accomplished with a standardized test of intelligibility that requires listeners to make judgments about a speaker's productions of single word utterances and produces a percentage score. Somewhat similarly, listeners' ratings of speakers' connected speech passages using some type of severity scale, for example, a one to five scale in which one indicates normal speech, and five indicates intelligibility severely impaired can be used. It is also useful and insightful to include some index of a patient's own appraisal of his/her *communicative effectiveness* in different situations, with various types of listeners, and with and without repetition. In whatever combinations, intelligibility and/or severity measures are particularly valuable in allowing the clinician, other professionals involved in the patient's care, and the speaker, to stay apprised of speech function and communicative effectiveness across treatment and posttreatment stages.

Correlating Perceptual and Physical Characteristics

A speaker's sound production capabilities are more effectively investigated if perceptual and acoustic data and perhaps other characteristics of speech sounds are examined for the same sample of utterances. For example, speakers' productions of vowels in the context "It's a h/V/d" previously presented to listeners can be subjected to spectrographic analysis so that formant, durational, or other characteristics of the intended vowels can be determined. Analysis of the acoustic data provides insights into the perceptual errors observed.

Aeromechanic test batteries that sample the speaker's ability to differentially manipulate airflows and pressures appropriate for various classes of speech sounds can provide similar insights, achieving the second objective of assessment, which is elaborating specific causes of deficits. Similarly, acoustic and aerodynamic instrumentation can be a valuable adjunct to the ear when the clinician is exploring the speaker's potential for an expanded range of acoustic differentiation in the vocal tract. Admittedly, time and cost factors increase when acoustic, aerodynamic, or additional analyses are included in the assessment battery. Again, the information gained may be well worth the effort.

Other Investigations

In addition to phonological assessment, evaluations that provide information about function of oral and pharyngeal structures need to be considered. In our own clinical setting, patients with glossectomy who are undergoing dynamic videofluoroscopic x-ray studies as a part of swallowing evaluations are also routinely asked to produce the vowels, /i, a/, and /u/; the utterances, "aka" and "ata"; and perhaps other stimuli. (Alternatively, cephalometric still x-rays can be used to obtain information for isolated vowel productions.) From the videotaped recordings it is possible to determine the tongue's range of motion for vowel sounds (Fig. 3–4) and to ascertain how closely the tongue approximates the palate for /t/ and /k/ sounds. Examination of the radiographic study can also reveal locations in the oral cavity and pharynx, such as anterior, mid, and posterior, where tongue movements may be more or less extensive. Similarly, insights into the independence of tongue and jaw movements, as well as the movement capabilities of velar, pharyngeal, and other structures, may also be available. Such information can be very useful in planning therapy objectives and is particularly valuable if a prosthetic appliance to improve speech is being considered.

Speech Rehabilitation

Objectives of Therapy

The thrust of restorative therapy in speakers with oral/oropharyngeal ablation is articulation skill that affords intelligible speech. But the clinician should be aware that voice and speech characteristics are unique and reflect our individuality as much as facial or bodily characteristics do. The patient who undergoes surgical excision of highly visible oropharyngeal structures can suffer devastating changes to both speech and appearance, features that signal our unique identities as individuals. Ideally, restoration of speech and speaker identity would be the

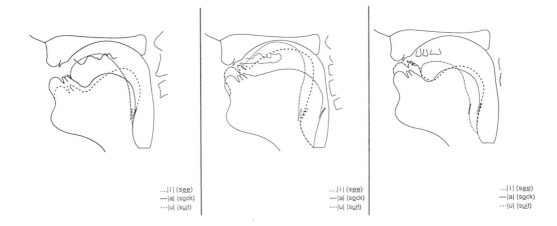

Figure 3–4. Drawings of oral cavity and oropharynx in lateral view indicate (in the *middle*) tongue positions for vowels /i/, /a/, and /u/ produced by normal speaker. Left: Vowels of speaker with glossectomy reveal decreased range of motion, with posterior mobility particularly reduced. Right: Vowel positions of a speaker with more extensive resection illustrate markedly reduced range of glossal mobility across vowels.

combined objectives of communicative rehabilitation in this patient population. Even when accomplishment of either poses a major challenge, both aims should be reflected in intervention efforts.

Restoration of speech in a speaker with glossectomy is dependent on the development of "compensated speech," that is, the ability of the speaker to compensate for physiological constraints (in normal speakers, see references 47–50). The production of a speech sound requires that a number of targets, including spatial, acoustic, and aerodynamic[51] be met. This "target-complex" may consist of both static and dynamic components. In the case of the tongue, for example, production of a sound may require assumption of a fixed position, as in a vowel, or a trajectory, for example, a path or pattern of movements, as in a diphthong, or both, as in the production of a stop consonant.

If this situation is complex for a sound in isolation, it becomes much more so when the sound is produced in connected speech where there are few truly static targets, but rather many dynamic ones that are subject to change depending on context. The normal tongue, in fact, appears supremely able to effect gestures that produce appropriate perceptual consequences for a given sound and to simultaneously accommodate whatever requirements may be demanded by the particular phonetic context within which the sound is embedded. Shaffer[52] has referred to this kind of phenomenon as evidence that speech movements are formulated at some speech control level to achieve compound trajectories, that is, patterns of movements that accomplish two (or possibly more) goals. If so, we would expect the speaker with glossectomy, whose formulation capacity for speech motor movements is presumably intact, to continue to attempt this kind of accommodation. How it may actually be realized, however, and how the clinician may facilitate and elaborate it, is not clear. The therapy process represents an exploration of, and hopefully, the realization of at least some of these possibilities.

Speech Therapy

The efficacy of speech therapy for speakers with glossectomy will remain unclear until appropriate research findings are available. In the absence of such data, a discussion of what our own clinical experience suggests as reasonable therapy goals will hopefully suffice. With reference to Stevens' description of the quantal nature of speech,[23] these goals involve (1) establishing or reestablishing acoustically "sensitive" areas of the vocal tract and (2) maximizing acoustic differentiations that can be effected within these areas. In general, specific efforts to improve articulation skill have focused on three major areas.

1. *Maximizing mobility and function in residual tissues* throughout therapy. Patients are asked to continue practice of oral exercises begun earlier. Every effort is made to provide graphic and quantitative evidence of any improvements to the patient. Our experience with oral exercise has generally been a positive one, with evidence in some cases not only of improved tissue function but also hypertrophy of tissues, that is, an apparent increase in volume of residual tissue.

2. *Restoring articulatory targets* consistent with the movement capabilities of the structures. In some cases, maxillary prostheses that replace or restore palate and dentures that can be fitted to the patient may help accomplish this goal. Palatal appliances designed to reshape the palate by lowering it in certain locations or a mandibular prosthesis that can act as a pseudotongue may deserve consideration when it is clear that movement capabilities have been maximized and deficits still remain in target restoration. Prosthetic appliances will be discussed in more detail in the next section. However, these strategies all have, in common, the purpose of improving the speaker's ability to shape the oral cavity and oropharynx to form constrictions and occlusions to critical extents and in critical locations, in an approximation of the normal vocal tract.

3. *Improving the speaker's ability to effect acoustic differentiation* in the vocal tract. Perceptual ambiguity or other perceptual failure comes about because of a speaker's inability to make distinctions critical to the acoustic differentiation of phonetic segments. For example, perceptual distinction between the high, front vowels, /i/ and /I/, may be obscured by the speaker's inability to make the subtle adjustments in place of articulation that account for their acoustic differentiation. Restoration of movements or structures may resolve some difficulties, but there are other strategies to be considered. Perception of the intended sound in the case of /i/ versus /I/ may be enhanced by emphasizing durational differences between the two segments, that is, by making the "long" vowel, /i/, slightly longer and the "short" vowel, /I/, slightly shorter. In other instances, alterations in degree of mandibular open-

ing or lip rounding may enable acoustic characteristics to more closely approximate normal vowels or enhance acoustic distinctions among them that will aid the listener.

Production of consonants requiring similar tongue dynamics and articulatory placements may be especially challenging. However, differentiation may be enhanced by concentrating on those aspects of each sound's production that *are* within the speaker's capabilities. For example, /t/ and /s/ both require tongue tip elevation and share a similar place of articulation. If a speaker with glossectomy is unable to clearly differentiate these sounds, perception of the intended sound may be enhanced by associating /t/ with a rapid offset of airflow effected by occluding the teeth or vocal folds, increasing voice onset time (decreasing it for /d/), and generating very brief turbulence at the release of the stop. Stated simply, a sufficiently short fricative may be perceived as a stop. In contrast, a focus on maintenance or lengthening of the same audible, turbulent airflow for the fricative /s/, even if comprised of an acoustic spectra different from normal, may serve to persuade the listener that a fricative was produced.

In another instance, a back consonant that requires tongue-palate contact, such as /k/ or /g/, may be simulated in some contexts by base of tongue-pharyngeal contact. Initially, the focus can be on production of a pharyngeal fricative in context with low vowels. If acceptable frication can be produced in this manner, reducing its duration and associating it with other, back vowels, may lead to reasonable substitutes for /k/ and /g/, at least in some environments. Instrumentation that provides the speaker with visual or amplified auditory information regarding these objectives can be very useful. A simple device such as "Tok-bak" may not only provide enhanced auditory feedback, but may also sensitize the speaker to airflow characteristics associated with sound productions.

A critical underpinning of this therapy is the premise that, when you cannot give a listener the "real" thing, that is, a normal speech sound, you may still be able to give him something both unique and functional—a gestalt of acoustic and aeromechanic variables (perhaps visual, as well)—that represents for a given speaker, a particular phonetic segment that is different enough from other segments to be perceptually distinctive, and close enough to the real thing that a listener will perceive it as such. Obviously, great weight is placed on the listener's role in the communicative process. That is, we assume that a listener comes to a communication event with a set of expectations, one of which concerns the phonetic segments that the speaker will manipulate to form words and sentences. Whatever the particulars of this expectation, it seems reasonable to assume that it is a closed set, that is, one in which the listener expects to hear "speech" sounds, not noises or hisses, or some other set of auditory stimuli. If the listener expects to hear speech, and we present him with auditory segments that are similar enough to the phonetic segments with which he is familiar, the listener will perceive them as speech sounds and even make judgments about which particular speech sounds they are. One measure of success in therapy is how frequently the listener's perceptions match the speaker's intentions.

The particular order in which treatment objectives are attempted should reflect a balance between (1) changes that are likely to result in the greatest, most immediate, improvements in the patient's intelligibility and (2) changes that can realistically be expected. For example, if vowel intelligibility appears impaired, perhaps more impaired than consonant intelligibility, work on vowels seems a reasonable initial priority for therapy. Vowels are pervasive in connected speech; require less in terms of vocal tract constrictions than most consonants; can be acoustically altered by manipulating structures that may be more intact, such as lips or jaw; and can be significantly influenced by factors such as duration, which the speaker can manipulate with ease.

Prosthetic Appliances in Speech Rehabilitation

The use of prosthetic appliances to improve speech (and swallowing) in speakers with glossectomy has been reported by numerous authors.[9,26,27,53–66] While providing strong evidence for the value of glossal prostheses in individual patients, these studies have generally not attempted to systemize approaches to glossal prosthesis design that could be applied to any treatment candidate. Nor have these investigators considered evaluation procedures that would provide insights into which speech and speaker variables influence the success of prosthetic reconstruction. If the value of prostheses is to be maximized in this patient population, such approaches must be forthcoming.

A primary objective of prosthetic approaches to speech rehabilitation is the modification of the vocal tract in a manner that enables the speaker to use residual tongue to effect constrictions, occlusions, and changes in orifice shapes, that allow for more appropriate production of speech. As noted previously, there are two major types of appliances. The first is a palatal reshaping prosthesis,[60,63] which has wide application, and the second is a mandibular, or "glossal" prosthesis,[9,62] which has been developed primarily for patients with extensive resections. A palatal reshaping prosthesis may enable residual tongue to approximate constrictions and occlusions in selected areas of the vocal tract (Fig. 3–5). When most of the tongue has been excised, an optimally shaped mandibular prosthesis

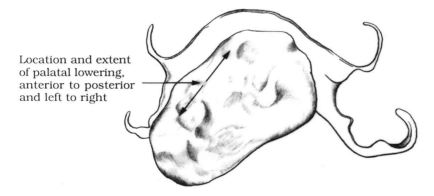

Location and extent of palatal lowering, anterior to posterior and left to right

Figure 3–5. Palatal reshaping appliance. Parameters that can be varied in attempts to improve speech are indicated.

that rides passively on the mandible may allow the speaker to achieve constrictions in anterior and posterior locations of the oral cavity that otherwise would be impossible to achieve (Fig. 3–6).

Our initial interest in this area was piqued by a patient with serious speech and swallowing problems subsequent to a total glossectomy, with no residual tongue to the lingual surface of the epiglottis. A mandibular prosthesis designed for the patient was able to improve speech significantly, as well as to eliminate the need for orogastric tube feeding.

Preliminary attempts to design the "ideal" prosthesis for this patient were completed largely on a trial-and-error basis. That is, a silicone base that would fit in the patient's floor of mouth (attached to the lower teeth by means of stainless-steel clasps) was fabricated with buttons on its superior portion to accommodate the top, or "tongue" portion of the prosthesis. A number of different top portions, reflecting differences in location and extent of elevations and different tip shapes, were then made and worn by the speaker while producing selected speech stimuli. Acoustic and perceptual analyses of recordings made with the different prostheses led to further revisions and, finally, a completed prosthesis that was believed to reflect the optimum shape for speech.

Palatal reshaping prostheses are typically fabricated for patients in a similar manner. The palate is modified in ways that allow it to interact with residual tongue. Analyses of speech produced with the protocol prosthesis leads to further revisions and, eventually, to an optimal design. (Details of our own experience with prosthesis design and construction and speech analyses have been described elsewhere.[9,26,27,54])

More recent efforts[65] have convinced us that a priori computerized approaches to prosthesis design offer potentially greater economy and effectiveness to the

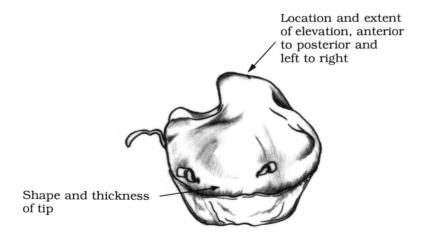

Location and extent of elevation, anterior to posterior and left to right

Shape and thickness of tip

Figure 3–6. Mandibular "glossal" prosthesis. Parameters that can be varied in attempts to improve speech are illustrated.

remediation process. We believe it will be possible in the near future to first acquire information regarding a particular patient's vocal tract, as from radiographic or other imaging data, and then use it to generate a simulated tract that can be prosthetically modified on the computer. Particular objectives for a given prosthesis would of course be determined and prioritized from previous speech "needs" assessments (acoustic, perceptual, and dynamic). For example, a mandibular prosthesis could be designed with the location and extent of elevations consistent with the speaker's observed constriction/occlusion deficits.

Tests on resulting speech "output" would then be used to direct further modifications. Effects of altered palatal contours or of jaw position on tongue constriction could be similarly modeled. Ultimately, an optimum prosthesis design could be determined on this a priori basis and then fabricated for the patient. Accomplishment of this objective could contribute significantly to the development of fundamentally sound, systematic and expedient approaches to prosthetic treatment of speakers with glossectomy.

A second issue in prosthesis design, one that remains largely unexplored, concerns materials currently used in the fabrication of oral prosthetic appliances. It is clear that the manufacturers of such materials (usually silicone) can specify many properties, including compressibility/elasticity factors, associated with particular compounds. However, the effects on speech of appliances made with various materials or compounds of a particular material have not generally been examined.

Surgical Factors in Speech Rehabilitation

Secondary surgeries that may be done to improve speech and other functions in the patient with oral/oropharyngeal ablation include pharyngeal flap procedures designed to minimize residual hypernasality and nasal emission of air, and tongue-release procedures[44] intended to improve glossal mobility. Decisions regarding a patient's candidacy for one of these procedures are based on a number of factors, including the likely benefit to speech and perhaps other functions, and the patient's appropriateness as a recipient of further surgery. In addition to these secondary procedures, there are some aspects of primary surgeries, beyond site and extent of resection, that appear to have implications for postoperative speech. Obviously, site and extent of resection, as described earlier, are dictated by the need to eradicate disease and afford the surgeon few, if any, choices. But there do appear to be options in terms of the reconstruction of defects caused by resection, and there is increasing evidence that at least some of these may be significant for speech.

One reconstruction option, for example, concerns the use of "flaps," or tissue moved into the defect site from a neighboring area. Michiwaki, Ohno, Imai, et al[17] described the use of both pectoralis major musculocutaneous flaps and microvascular free flaps in patients with similar lesions and reported that patients in the latter group had fewer complications and better speech intelligibility than patients in the first group. Stern, Keller, and Wenig[66] compared patients with T3 and T4 tumors who had undergone oropharyngeal reconstruction with either a pectoralis major musculocutaneous flap or a microvascular free flap and found fewer complications, better deglutition, and improved speech in the latter group. Similar results for free forearm flaps have been reported by

Kuroda, Tahara, Amatsu, et al[67] and Matloub, Larson, Kuhn, et al,[68] and for free groin flaps by Salibian, Allison, Rappaport, et al.[18] These authors suggested the capability to tailor the shape of "free" flaps, as opposed to flaps that remain pedicled to their site of origin, and the potential for some functions in free flaps may account for the improvements.

Another aspect of reconstruction that has been considered experimentally, if not extensively, is that of residual mobility in glossal tissue. Schramm, Johnson, and Myers[69] found reductions in length of hospitalization and complications and a quicker return to oral alimentation with skin graft reconstructions, as opposed to pectoralis myocutaneous and deltopectoral flap reconstructions. McConnell et al[70] reported that patients reconstructed with split thickness skin grafts had better oral function, including better speech, than patients with myocutaneous or hemitongue flaps. Zieske et al[71] have also described good results with the use of split thickness grafts, particularly in instances of composite reconstructions in which the defect was not massive and did not involve anterior mandible.

Clinically, it also appears that patients who have graft reconstructions, as opposed to primary closures, retain better oral function. In a primary closure, remaining tongue might be sewn on itself or into a floor of mouth defect to close the excision site. A graft in which tissue is taken from one site to "resurface" the tongue and perhaps the floor of the mouth defect maintains the independence of each structure and appears to minimize the kind of tethering that results from primary closure. Michi et al[44] provided further support for this observation in patients who had undergone secondary skin graft procedures to relieve tethering and mobilization of residual tongue. In the four patients investigated, intelligibility scores were higher following the tongue release procedure, with greatest improvement observed for plosive and affricate productions.

Katstantonis[72] described in animals an attempt to provide some innervation to a pectoralis major flap by means of either a hypoglossal nerve pedicle or hypoglossal-genioglossus muscle neuromuscular pedicle. There was some function noted postoperatively in half of the subjects. Though highly experimental at this point, neurotized flaps that offer the possibility of providing neural function to reconstructed tissues is obviously an attractive alternative.

Summary and Final Comments

It is difficult to imagine pathology that affects more functions critical to life and the quality of life than those that require ablation of oral and/or oropharyngeal structures. Speech, and more basically, eating and swallowing, airway maintenance and cosmesis, may all be altered as a consequence of ablative procedures. As noted previously, the challenge to speech restoration, as with the challenge to restoration of other functions, is large and fraught with complex questions and many difficulties. The lack of information regarding speech characteristics in this population, particularly as these relate to treatment variables, is significant.

Information that would enable the clinician to predict both the degree and nature of speech impairment associated with ablative treatments would be useful in counseling patients about their impairment, as well as their potential for improvement. Similarly, generalizations extracted from data regarding an entire population of impaired speakers would be a valuable resource for the clinician in formulating realistic treatment objectives, and in appropriately prioritizing and sequencing them for an individual speaker. As results of systematic inquiries addressing these issues become available, possibilities for improved rehabilitation strategies will also be elaborated.

Until then, it is useful to consider what we *do* know about speakers with oral/oropharyngeal ablation. Characteristics of these speakers include: (1) phonological errors that include both vowels and consonants that, in some cases, may be so pervasive that accurate assessment is difficult; (2) vowel errors that appear related, at least in part, to a compression and neutralization of the range of second formant frequencies across vowels, with the extent of compression directly related to degree of perceived impairment; (3) consonant errors, probably best described as distortions, most likely involving sounds requiring the greatest degrees of constriction/occlusion, that is, fricatives and plosives. Here again, impairment can be related to compression and neutralization of the speaker's ability to generate a wide range of perceptually distinct, acoustic/aerodynamic sound sources in one or more oral/oropharyngeal locations. Additional evidence suggests that impairment is further related to site and extent of glossal resection, as well as to other structures involved in ablation and to the integrity of residual tissues. Other treatment variables that impact this population have just begun to be examined.

Speech impairment experienced by the speaker with oral/oropharyngeal ablation is unique and may require novel approaches designed to restore or develop new articulatory patterns. The potential of the field of speech–language pathology to do this to the maximum extent possible via speech therapy, prosthetics, or surgical alternatives has yet to be realized. It is clear, however, that the challenge is one of major proportions. Clinical experience also suggests that a return of normal speech, not a choice for some patients with glossectomy at this point in time, is not the only acceptable or successful alternative for many patients.

We have found that patients who describe their communicative interactions as frequent failures (50% or below), typified by several repetitions, handwriting, or just "giving up," are patients who are likely to be psychologically isolated and socially reclusive. Conversely, patients who describe their efforts at oral communication as successful most of the time (70% or above), improving even more with an occasional repetition, are likely to be functioning better, socializing more, and adapting well to the resumption of their lives and work. There may be several interpretations of this observation, but one in particular is worth keeping in mind—the difference between success and failure (in this case, on the order of 20%) may be smaller than the difference between normal and disordered. Rehabilitation efforts that focus on maximizing a patient's potential rather than on restoring previous speech capabilities can be effective, and will become more so, as clinicians concentrate on what *can* be done now, and on what needs to be accomplished, to expand the possibilities in the future.

References

1. Boring C, Squires T, Tong T: Cancer statistics, 1991. *Ca—A Can J for Clin* 1991; 41:19–36.
2. Cancer Statistics Branch. Bethesda, MD, National Cancer Institute, 1991.

3. Robbins KT (ed): *Pocket Guide to Neck Dissection Classification and TNM Staging of Head and Neck Cancer.* Alexandria, VA, American Academy Otolaryngology-Head and Neck Surgery and Oncology Foundation, 1991.

4. Imai S, Michi K: Articulatory function after resection of the tongue and floor of the mouth: Palatometric and perceptual evaluation. *JSHR* 1992; 35:68–78.

5. Fletcher S: Speech production following partial glossectomy. *JSHD* 1988; 53:232–238.

6. McKinstry RE, Aramany MA, Beery QC, Sansone F: Speech considerations in prosthodontic rehabilitation of the glossectomy patient. *J Prosth Dent* 1985; 53:384–387.

7. Morrish L: Compensatory vowel articulation of the glossectomee. *Br J Disorders Commun* 1984; 19:125–134.

8. Allison G, Rappaport I, Salibian A: Adaptive mechanisms of speech and swallowing after combined jaw and tongue reconstruction. *Am J Surg* 1987; 154:419–422.

9. Leonard R, Gillis R: Effects of a prosthetic tongue on vowel intelligibility and food management in a patient with total glossectomy. *JSHD* 1982; 47:25–30.

10. Georgian D, Logemann J, Fisher H: Compensatory articulation patterns of a surgically treated oral cancer patient. *JSHD* 1982; 47:154–159.

11. LaRiviere C, Seilo M, Dimmick K: Report on the speech intelligibility of a glossectomee: Perceptual and acoustic observations. *Folia Phoniatr* 1975; 27:201–214.

12. Bradley P, Hoover L, Stell P: Assessment of articulation after surgery in the tongue. *Folia Phoniatr* 1980; 32:334–341.

13. Amerman J, Laminack K: Evaluation and rehabilitation of glossectomy speech behavior. *J Commun Disorders* 1974; 7:365–374.

14. Skelly M, Spector D, Donaldson R, Brodeur A, Paletta F: Compensatory physiologic phonetics for glossectomee. *JSHD* 1971; 36:101–114.

15. Massengill R, Maxwell S, Pickrell K: An analysis of articulation following partial and total glossectomy. *JSHD* 1970; 55:170–173.

16. Weber RS, Ohlms L, Bowman J, Jacob R, Goepfert H: Functional results after total or near total glossectomy with laryngeal preservation. *Arch Otolaryngol Head Neck Surg* 1991; 117:512–515.

17. Michiwaki Y, Ohno K, Imai S, Yamashita Y, Suzuki N, Yoshida H, Michi K: Functional effects of intraoral reconstruction with a free radial forearm flap. *J Cranio-Maxillofac Surg* 1990; 28:164–168.

18. Salibian AH, Allison GR, Rappaport I, Krugman ME, McMicken BL, Etchepare TL: Total and subtotal glossectomy: Function after microvascular reconstruction. *Plast Reconstruct Surg* 1990; 55:513–524.

19. Keyserlingk JR, de Francesco J, Breach N, Rhys-Evans P, Stafford N, Mott A: Recent experience with reconstructive surgery following major glossectomy. *Arch Otolaryngol Head Neck Surg* 1989; 115:331–338.

20. Sultan MR, Coleman JJ: Oncologic and functional considerations of total glossectomy. *Am J Surg* 1989; 158:297–302.

21. Mitrani M, Krespi YP: Functional restoration after subtotal glossectomy and laryngectomy. *Otolaryngol Head Neck Surg* 1988; 98:5–9.

22. Duguay M: Speech after glossectomy. *NY State J Med* 1964; 64:1836–1838.

23. Stevens K: The quantal nature of speech: Evidence from articulatory-acoustic data, in Penes P, David E (eds): *Human Communication, A Unified View.* New York, McGraw-Hill, 1972, pp 51–65.

24. Stevens K, House A: An acoustical theory of vowel production and some of its implications. *JASA* 1961; 33:1725–1736.

25. Lieberman P: *Speech Physiology and Acoustic Phonetics.* New York, Macmillan Publishing Co., 1977, pp 65–67.

26. Leonard R, Gillis R: Differential effects of prostheses in glossectomized patients. *J Prosthet Dent* 1990; 64:701–708.

27. Leonard R, Gillis R: Effects of a prosthetic tongue on vowel formants and isovowel lines in a patient with total glossectomy. *JSHD* 1983; 48:423–426.

28. Sussman H, MacNeilage P, Hanson R: Labial and mandibular dynamics during the production of bilabial consonants: Preliminary investigation. *JSHR* 1973; 16:397–420.

29. Bloomer H, Hawk H: Speech considerations: Speech disorders associated with ablative surgery of the face, mouth and pharynx—Ablative approaches to learning. *ASHA Rep* 1972; 8:42–61.

30. Cantor R, Curtis T: Prosthetic management of edentulous mandibulectomy patients. Part I. Anatomic, physiologic and psychologic considerations. *J Prosthet Dent* 1971; 25:446–457.

31. Leonard R, Goodrich S, McMenamin P, Donald P: Differentiation of speakers with glossectomies by acoustic and perceptual measures. *Am J Speech Lang Pathol* 1992; 1:56–63.

32. Majid A, Weinberg B, Chalian B: Speech intelligibility following prosthetic obturation of surgically acquired maxillary defects. *J Prosthet Dent* 1974; 32:87–96.

33. Masuda M, Kida Y, Ohtani T: Oral rehabilitation by prosthetic restoration after maxillectomy for malignant tumors. *Int J Oral Surg* 1979; 8:356–362.
34. House A, Williams C, Hecker M, Kryter K: Articulation testing methods: Consonantal differentiation with a closed response set. *J Acoust Soc Am* 1965; 37:158–166.
35. Horii Y: *Specifying the Speech-to-Noise Ratio: Development and Evaluation of a Noise with Speech-Envelope Characteristics.* Unpublished doctoral dissertation, Purdue University, West Lafayette, IN, 1969.
36. Fletcher S, Soodi I, Frost SD: Quantitative and graphic analysis of prosthetic treatment for "nasalance" in speech. *J Prosthet Dent* 1974; 32:284–291.
37. Plank D, Weinberg B, Chalian V: Evaluation of speech following prosthetic obturation of surgically acquired maxillary defects. *J Prosthet Dent* 1981; 45:626–638.
38. Abbs JH, Eilenberg GR: Peripheral mechanisms in speech motor control, in Lass NJ (ed): *Contemporary Issues in Experimental Phonetics.* New York, Academic Press, 1976, pp 139–170.
39. Mirza F, Dikshit J: Use of implant prostheses following radiation therapy. *J Prosthet Dent* 1978; 40:663–667.
40. Heller KS, Levy J, Sciubba JJ: Speech patterns following partial glossectomy for small tumors of the tongue. *Head Neck* 1991; 13:340–343.
41. Pruszewica A, Kruk-Zagajewska A: Phoniatric disturbances in patients after partial tongue resection for malignant neoplasms. *Folia Phoniatr* 1984; 36:84–92.
42. Salibian AH, Allison GR, Rappaport I, Krugman ME, McMicken BL, Etchepare TL: Total and subtotal glossectomy: Function after microvascular reconstruction. *Plast Reconstruct Surg* 1990; 85:513–524.
43. Teichgraeber J, Bowman J, Goepfert H: New test series for the functional evaluation of oral cavity cancer. *Head Neck Surg* 1985; 109:9–20.
44. Michi K, Imai S, Yamashita Y, Suzuki N: Improvement of speech intelligibility by a secondary operation to mobilize the tongue after glossectomy. *J Cranio-Maxillofac Surg* 1989; 17:162–166.
45. Rentschler G, Mann M: The effects of glossectomy on intelligibility of speech and oral perceptual discrimination. *J Oral Surg* 1980; 38:348–350.
46. Hamlet SL, Mathog RH, Patterson RL, Fleming SM: Tongue mobility in speech after partial glossectomy. *Head Neck* 1990; 12:210–217.
47. Kent R, Minifie F: Coarticulation in recent speech production models. J Phonet 1977; 5:115–133.
48. Folkins J, Abbs J: Lip and jaw motor control during speech: Responses to resistive loading. *JSHR* 1975; 18:207–225.
49. Lindblom B, Sundberg J: Acoustical consequences of lip, tongue, jaw and larynx. *J Acoust Soc Am* 1971; 50:1166–1179.
50. Kawamura J: Neuromuscular mechanisms of jaw and tongue movement. *J Am Dent Assoc* 1965; 62:545–555.
51. Daniloff R: Articulation: dynamics, in Daniloff R, Shuckers G, Feth L (ed): *The Physiology of Speech and Hearing.* Englewood Cliffs, NJ, Prentice-Hall, 1980, pp 286–366.
52. Shaffer L: Rhythm and timing in skill. *Psychol Rev* 1982; 89:109–122.
53. Christensen JM, Hutton JE, Fletcher SG: Evaluation of the effects of palatal augmentation on partial glossectomy. *J Prosthet Dent* 1982; 50:539–542.
54. Gillis R, Leonard R: Prosthetic treatment for speech and swallowing in a patient with total glossectomy. *J Prosthet Dent* 1983; 50:808–814.
55. Davis J, Lazarus C, Logemann J, Hurst P: Effect of a maxillary glossectomy prosthesis on articulation and swallowing. *J Prosthet Dent* 1987; 57:715–719.
56. Izdebski K, Ross J, Roberts W, deBoie R: An interim prosthesis for the glossectomy patient. *J Prosthet Dent* 1987; 57:608–611.
57. Robbins K, Bowman J, Jacob R: Post-glossectomy deglutitory and articulatory rehabilitation with palatal augmentation prostheses. *Arch Otolaryngol Head Neck Surg* 1987; 113:1214–1218.
58. Knowles J, Chalian V, Shanks J: A functional speech impression used to fabricate a maxillary speech prosthesis for a partial glossectomy patient. *J Prosthet Dent* 1984; 51:232–237.
59. Lauciello F, Vergo T, Schaaf N, Zimmerman R: Prosthodontic and speech rehabilitation after partial and complete glossectomy. *J Prosthet Dent* 1980; 43:204–207.
60. Wheeler R, Logemann J, Rosen J: A maxillary reshaping prosthesis: Its effectiveness in improving the speech and swallowing of postsurgical oral cancer patients. *J Prosthet Dent* 1980; 43:491–495.
61. Hufnagle J, Pullon P, Hufnagle K: Speech considerations in oral surgery: II. Speech characteristics of patients following surgery for oral malignancies. *Oral Surg Oral Med Oral Pathol* 1978; 46: 354–361.
62. Moore D: Glossectomy rehabilitation by mandibular tongue prosthesis. *J Prosthet Dent* 1972; 28: 429–433.
63. Cantor R, Curtis T, Shipp T, Beumer J, Vogel B: Maxillary speech prostheses for mandibular sur-

gical defects. *J Prosthet Dent* 1969; 21:253–256.

64. Lehman W, Hulicka I, Mehringer E: Prosthetic treatment following complete glossectomy. *J Prosthet Dent* 1964; 16:244–246.
65. Leonard R: Computerized design of speech prostheses. J Prosthet Dent 1991; 66:214–230.
66. Stern JR, Keller AJ, Wenig BL: Evaluation of reconstructive techniques of oropharyngeal defects. *Ann Plast Surg* 1989; 22:332–336.
67. Kuroda H, Tahara S, Amatsu M, Inoue K: Articulatory evaluation after mesopharyngeal reconstruction with the radial forearm flap. *J Oto-Rhino-Laryngol Soc Jpn* 1991; 94:1727–1732.
68. Matloub HS, Larson DL, Kuhn JC, Yousif NJ, Sanger JR: Lateral arm free flap in oral cavity reconstruction: A functional evaluation. *Head Neck* 1989; 11:205–211.
69. Schramm V, Johnson JT, Myers EN: Skin grafts and flaps in oral cavity reconstruction. *Arch Otolaryngol* 1985; 109:175–177.
70. McConnell F, Teichgraeber J, Adler R: A comparison of three methods of oral reconstruction. *Arch Otolaryngol Head Neck Surg* 1987; 113:496–500.
71. Zieske LA, Johnson JT, Myers EN, Schramm VL, Wagner R: Composite resection reconstruction: Split-thickness skin graft—a preferred option. *Otolaryngol Head Neck Surg* 1988; 98:170–173.
72. Katsantonis GP: Neurotization of pectoralis major myocutaneous flap by the hypoglossal nerve in tongue reconstruction: Clinical and experimental observations. *Laryngoscope* 1988; 98:1313–1323.
73. Peterson G, Barney H: Control methods used in a study of the vowels. *J Acoust Soc Am* 1952; 24: 175–184.

Part II
Neurological Factors

4

Toddlers with Medical Needs

KEN M. BLEILE, PH.D., AND
SHARI A. MILLER, M.S.

There are several reasons to include a discussion of toddlers in a book on articulation and phonology in special populations, even though many of these children either are too young to speak or are only in the earliest stages of using speech for purposes of communication. The primary reason for their inclusion is that a delay in phonological or articulatory development has a significant impact on toddler's well being. Through its effect on the child's use of sound for communication, articulatory and phonological delay limit the child's ability to express thoughts and needs and may influence bonding between child and caregiver, and through its impact on the development of the child's expressive vocabulary, may lead to future disorders in language and learning.[1,2]

Another reason to discuss toddlers in the present book is that the presence of articulatory and phonological difficulties are relatively common among selected subpopulations of young children. It is estimated that at least 89 syndromes affecting infants and toddlers are likely to result in articulatory and phonological delay.[3,4] Two interrelated factors are likely to increase the number of children with medical needs in the future, and, thus, might be expected to give rise to additional populations of young children with articulatory and phonological problems. First, due to advances in medical care, neonatologists are saving ever younger and more medically fragile infants. Second, the number of children with medical needs is growing as a result of the spreading acquired immunodeficiency syndrome (AIDS) epidemic, the increasing number of children born into poverty, and the escalating use of drugs and alcohol among pregnant woman. The effects of these new morbidities on society and the health care system are just now beginning to be felt.

The primary goal of this chapter is to explore what articulation and phonological treatment offers. Although the principles and procedures described in this chapter are applicable to any young child at risk for articulatory or phonological delay, the chapter is directed to providing speech–language services to the increasing number of children with moderate to severe medical disorders arising from such circumstances and conditions as prematurity, neurological conditions and insults, and physical disabilities.

The chapter describes concepts and methods to facilitate the use of sound for purposes of expression and communication. Because of the importance of expressive vocabulary in communication development, special attention is given to articulatory and phonological aspects of facilitating word acquisition.[1,2,5,6] While family counseling and training of professional caregivers are critical aspects of providing speech–language services to children, this chapter will focus primarily on direct care provision, because that aspect of articulatory and phonological treatment is most unique from other aspects of professional practice in our field.

The chapter is divided into the following topical sections: the rationale for providing articulatory and phonological services to toddlers, assessment issues, and treatment issues. The chapter concludes with a discussion of special concerns that arise in providing care to children with long-term tracheostomies. This population was chosen for special consideration because of the unique challenges that the tracheostomy presents to communication development.

Why Provide Treatment?

Perhaps the most fundamental question encountered by those who provide articulation and phonological services (henceforth called speech services) to toddlers is why should treatment be provided at such a young age?

Conceptually, the motivation for early speech intervention for toddlers is to provide developmental services proactively. The goal of therapy is to address developmental problems either in their first stages or even before they appear. The desired result in providing such service during this sensitive period of development is that speech problems can be "nipped in the bud." In this way, the many well-recognized sequelae of developmental disabilities—reduced income, poorer educational outcome, diminished self-image—may be avoided.[7-13]

Communication services to toddlers is a new clinical endeavor and still lacks a strong research foundation. Although data are not yet available regarding the effectiveness of speech intervention with young children with medical needs, several studies have shown the benefit of early intervention programs on future development.[12,14-17] Most pertinent to the present concerns, the Infant Health and Development Program[14] evaluated the developmental outcomes of preterm at-risk infants (birthweight less than 2500 grams) at eight different clinical centers. The study found that the children who received early intervention had intelligence quotients (IQs) from 6.6 to 13.2 points higher than those preterm infants who received only routine follow-up. The lower IQ difference (IQ 6.6 higher than for those who received only routine follow-up) was reported for the subgroup of children with birthweights less than 2000 grams, and the higher IQ difference (IQ 13.2 higher than for those who received only routine follow-up) was reported for the subgroup of children with birthweights between 2000 to 2499 grams. Low birthweight children who did not attend early intervention were 2.7 times more likely to have IQ scores in the mentally retarded range at 3 years of age.

From a legal perspective, the basis for providing early speech intervention is

Public Law 99–457. Public Law 99–457 mandates intervention services to two classes of children aged 0 to 2 years: (1) those with documented developmental delays in speech, language, and other major areas of development; and (2) children with diagnosed physical or mental conditions that have a high probability of resulting in developmental delays. Relatively common diagnoses included in this category are fetal alcohol syndrome, seizure disorders, and chromosome disorders such as Down's Syndrome. Public Law 99–457 also gives individual states the option of providing intervention services to a third class of children aged 0 to 2 years. These are children who, while not developmentally delayed, are at risk for such delays in the future. Commonly encountered "at-risk" conditions include low birthweight, asphyxia, and respiratory distress.

Developmentally, the first years of life is an active period in both speech acquisition and neurological maturation, suggesting that children are highly receptive to new learning during this time. The foundations for the speech system are acquired during the first 2 years of life. To illustrate, during the first year of life the infant appears to learn through sound play how to orchestrate the laryngeal, respiratory, and articulatory systems, which serve as the basis for oral communication.[18–20] Toward the end of the first year and into the second year, the toddler learns how to use "sound to mean."[21] The magnitude of this accomplishment is seen in the growth of the toddler's expressive vocabulary between 12 to 24 months. By 12 months, a toddler typically speaks from 0 to 5 words. Yet, by 24 months many children speak 100 different words or more.[22]

Lastly, neurological development during the first years of life proceeds on many fronts. Myelination, for example, occurs largely during this period, permitting the rapid transmission of signals both within the brain and to the other parts of the body, including the speech musculature. Neurological development also affects the number of dendritic connections between brain cells. Children under approximately 2 years old possess many more connections between neurons than older children and adults. These "extra" connections are pruned near the beginning of the third year of life. Researchers speculate that neurons are pruned because learning has not established connections between them and other brain cells.[23]

Evaluation

It is easy enough to feel overwhelmed at the prospect of providing a speech evaluation to a healthy toddler, let alone to a child with significant and, possibly, at times life-threatening health problems. The speech evaluation can be a particularly daunting task if the child is tethered to a formidable array of beeping and flashing machinery. Fortunately, with experience the speech evaluation of a child with medical needs seems to become more challenging and exciting than daunting and intimidating.

This section describes issues encountered in performing the speech evaluation. The following topics are addressed: assessment goals, the role of the speech–language clinician on the health care team, medical factors affecting the speech evaluation, standardized and nonstandardized assessments, and the steps in reaching a diagnosis. The discussion includes infants and toddlers because both populations are assessed similarly.

Assessment Goals

The goal of the speech evaluation is to determine how the child uses sound for purposes of interaction and communication. The evaluation results are used to: (1) provide information to caregivers and health care professionals regarding the child's current speech development and the child's prognosis for future development; (2) determine if treatment is needed; and (3) provide information useful in planning treatment, if it is found to be warranted.

The Health Care Team

The speech–language clinician seeing young children with medical needs is likely to be a part of a health care team. The team approach is necessary because the needs of children with medical involvement generally are too complex and varied to be understood and cared for by a single discipline. Team efforts may be multidisciplinary, interdisciplinary, or transdisciplinary.[24] Multidisciplinary teams are groups of professionals who perform related tasks independently of each other. Interdisciplinary teams are groups of professionals who, while performing related tasks independently, interact with each other and share information to reach common goals. Transdisciplinary teams are groups of professionals who perform related tasks interactively by sharing both information and professional roles. Multidisciplinary and interdisciplinary teams are typically found in hospital settings, and interdisciplinary and transdisciplinary teams are typically found in community settings.

Members of the health care team are likely to include the child's caregivers; professionals from nursing, medicine, audiology, recreational therapy, occupational and physical therapy; and social workers. As a member of the health care team, the speech–language clinician learns to rely on other team members to inform her on a wide variety of issues, including the child's visual and hearing status, fine and gross motor abilities, and the child's medical readiness for speech evaluation and therapy. Similarly, the other members of the team rely on the speech–language clinician regarding the child's status and progress in the areas of speech, language, and oral motor development. Increasingly, the speech–language clinician (often in conjunction with the occupational therapist) is also called on to evaluate and treat feeding disorders.

Medical Factors That Can Affect the Speech Evaluation

There are several factors that should be considered when performing the speech evaluation of a child with medical needs. Most fundamentally, the evaluator needs to observe common sense health precautions. This includes hand washing before and after evaluating the child, wearing gloves if the evaluator plans to place fingers in the child's mouth or if oral secretions are excessive, and observing any health precautions posted at the child's bedside. Toys, too, can be a source of transmission of infection, and the evaluator should clean all toys at the completion of each evaluation session.

If the evaluation is to be performed, the child should appear calm and alert. The child's muscles should be relaxed and it should be possible for the evaluator to make some eye contact with the child, if cognitive development permits, unless medical or physical conditions interfere. If the child is receiving supplementary oxygen, the evaluator should determine if the child is well oxygenated. A sign of good oxygenation is a slightly pink skin color. Signs of poor oxygenation may include increased irritability, sweating, blue color around the lips and fingernails, chest retractions, and nasal flaring.

The evaluation area should be quiet and clean. In general, extraneous auditory and visual stimuli should be minimized. The room should be well lit, but not so bright as to cause discomfort to a young child's sensitive eyes. A well-controlled environment is particularly important if the child has a neurological condition that may make it difficult for her to manage stimulation. For some babies born prematurely, even an animated expression accompanied by a loud voice can cause the child to become agitated. Overstimulation can also result from too many new toys and persons in the child's environment. Indications of overstimulation and distress include back arching, yawning, splaying of fingers, hiccoughs, avoidance of eye contact, and general agitation. Physiological signs of distress may include increased respiration and heart rate. To counteract overstimulation, frequent breaks during the evaluation should be provided when they appear to be needed. If the child continues to appear distressed, the speech–language clinician should discontinue the session and inform the child's nurse, physician, caregiver, or teacher.

The positioning of a child is often critical to the success of the evaluation session. In general, both the child and the speech–language clinician should be comfortably positioned in such a manner that eye contact between the two is easily achieved and maintained. If a child has physical limitations or special motoric needs, positioning should be undertaken with guidance from occupational or physical therapy. If necessary, the child should either be cradled by the caregiver or the speech–language clinician, propped on the lap, or positioned with adequate support in an infant seat. Some premature or previously drug-addicted children can only tolerate minimal handling, and these children may need to be swaddled or bundled to reduce agitation and irritability. Children may also be seated in a chair with adequate support for the upper body. A chair with an attached tray is optimal.

If the child is evaluated as a hospital inpatient, she is likely to interact with the evaluator relatively easily because the child has become accustomed to unfamiliar persons. However, if a child appears reluctant to interact, the speech–language clinician should proceed slowly rather than attempting to force the interaction. The speech–language clinician could play silently alongside the child, occasionally passing the child toys that appear to interest her, waiting for the child to initiate communication. Alternately, if a familiar adult is present, the evaluator might use that person to help elicit speech from the child. An adult familiar with the child can also serve as an informant for speech behaviors that may occur outside the evaluation session.

Typically children with medical needs are more passive communication partners than other children, as feeling sick can reduce the desire or ability to communicate. Additionally, if the child is relatively immobile or dependent on stationary equipment, she likely has become conditioned to other persons initiating interactions. Lastly, a child living in a busy hospital may appear more passive because she has learned that others set the times of the interactions. The speech–language clinician should expect the assessment to take longer than for children with less medical involvement. For this reason, the initial evaluation is often performed over several short sessions rather than having the child become fatigued.

The Assessment

LANGUAGE ASSESSMENT

The speech evaluation of young children with medical needs begins not with the assessment of the speech system, but with the assessment of the child's cognitive development and her knowledge and use of language. This "top-down" approach allows the speech–language clinician to discover the "big picture" before examining the smaller pieces that make up the speech system. Information on language reception is also used to help determine if the child's speech development is commensurate or delayed relative to her language skills.

SPEECH ASSESSMENT

Providing speech services to toddlers is still a relatively new clinical enterprise, and, as such, few formal assessment instruments are available to assist the speech–language clinician. The assessment tool that addresses the most questions in speech development is the *Sequenced Inventory of Communication Development*.[25] The *Clinical Linguistic and Auditory Milestone Scale*[26] contains items on expressive vocabulary. At present, lacking formal tests many speech–language clinicians rely on nonstandardized testing. Results of nonstandardized testing are typically expressed in terms of a developmental age that best corresponds to the child's speech abilities. For example, a child whose major speech abilities approximates those of a child near 1:6 (years:months) would have 1:6 as her developmental speech level. If some speech skills more closely approximated a child 1:2, that judgment would also be stated.

The developmental milestones and definitions presented in this section and summarized in Table 4–1 are offered to help orient the reader to the types of questions that the speech–language clinician attempts to answer in the speech

Table 4–1.   Assessment Questions

Populations of Children	Questions
All children	1. How does the child communicate her thoughts and needs?
0–12 mo	2. Does the infant engage in reciprocal communication? 3. What is the child's capacity to vocalize?
12–24 mo	4. What is the child's ability to produce words? 5. What is the child's capacity to produce sounds and syllables? 6. What co-occurrence restrictions exist in the child's speech? 7. What are the organizing principles in the child's speech?

assessment. The reader is referred to the citations for complete discussions of the topics presented below. In the subsection that follows, when sufficient information on a developmental milestone or a concept exists, the information is presented in a table along with any data on standard deviations, if available. When insufficient information exists to justify inclusion of a table, the information is presented in the text.

ASSESSMENT QUESTIONS

Some assessment questions are asked of all children, while others are asked of children at certain periods of development.

This question is asked of all children:

1. How does the child communicate her thoughts and needs? This question serves to determine the extent to which the child relies on speech as a means to communicate. Considered in conjunction with information from the language section of the evaluation, answers to this question provide insights into the functional role of speech in the child's communication system. Children typically begin to use sound accompanied by gestures to obtain objects near the latter part of the first year of life. During the first months of the second year of life, children typically communicate using a combination of facial expression, gestures, words, and vocalizations. By the middle of the second year of life, children begin using words to express their wants and needs. By 20 months, children are able to use words to relate experiences.[25]

The following two questions are asked of children who only use speech as an occasional means of communication:

2. Does the child engage in reciprocal communication? The question serves to identify the extent to which the child is able to interact in highly routinized communication activities with family or professional caregivers. Research indicates that communication development is facilitated in such highly familiar, reciprocal contexts as meal time, diaper changing, and bedtime.[27,28] Sound-gesture games such as peek-a-boo are hypothesized to perform similar functions. The familiarity of the contexts is thought to permit the child to focus attention on the linguistic characteristics of the interaction, while the reciprocal aspect of the settings is thought to promote the active acquisition of speech and language skills.

The acquisition of sound-gesture schemes provides an illustration of how children gradually learn to interact in a communicative context. Children typically begin to take turns with sound near the end of the first half of the first year of life. By 5 or 6 months of age, children begin to participate in adult-initiated sound-gesture games. Research indicates that by 9 months of age most children readily play such games.[26] By the end of the first year of life, the child covers his own eyes in peek-a-boo and will initiate this and other sound-gesture games.

3. What is the child's capacity to vocalize? The motivation for asking this question is that prespeech vocalizations are thought to provide the motoric basis for oral communication beginning near the second year of life.[18,29,30] Stated

differently, the child who babbles learns how to "get her mouth to go where she wants it to go." At the same time, the child's babbling creates a loop between production and perception. The child who babbles "ba-ba" learns that the movements of her articulators that produce sounds corresponds to the perception of these same sounds. The major milestones in the development of vocalizations during the first year of life are listed in Table 4–2.

The following three questions are asked of children who are using speech as a primary means of communication:

4. What is the child's ability to produce words? The reason for wanting information on the child's expressive vocabulary is that vocabulary size reflects the child's growing ability to use oral communication to express her ideas and feelings. Equally important, researchers hypothesize that children learn the rules of language through the words in their own vocabulary rather than simply by hearing speech. Thus, increasing the child's expressive vocabulary offers more opportunities to "discover" the rules of the speech system. The approximate size of children's expressive vocabulary at various ages are presented in Table 4–3.

5. What is the child's capacity to produce sounds and syllables? This topic is important because sounds and syllables constitute building blocks of oral communication. Thus, knowing the child's phonetic productions allows the evaluator to better understand the limitations the child will experience in using words to communicate. Information on the development of vowels, consonant clusters, syllables and word shapes at 14 to 16 months and 24 months is listed in Table 4–4 (Part A), and information on consonant acquisition at 15, 18, 21, and 24 months is provided in Table 4–4 (Part B).

Table 4–2. Approximate Ages of Acquisition for the question: What is the Child's Capacity to Vocalize Speech-Type Sounds?

Average Age	Behavior
Birth to 2 mo	Vegetative sounds
2–3 mo	Begins to produce cooing behaviors
2–4 mo	Begins to produce pleasure sounds such as "mmmm"
3–4 mo	Cooing behavior is well established, babbling behavior (repetition or consonants and vowels) begins to appear
4 mo	Produces some intonation during sound making and may engage in vocal play when playing with toys; vocalizations begin to be dominated by sounds produced at the front of the mouth, including raspberries and trills
6 mo	Reduplicated babbling (repetitions of the same syllable) begins to appear
7–8 mo	Reduplicated babbling well established
9 mo	Produces short exclamations such as "ooh!"
10 mo	Produces nonreduplicative babbling (changes of consonants and vowels within syllables)

Sources: References 19, 20, and 26.

Table 4–3. Approximate Ages of Acquisition for the Question:
What is the Child's Ability to Produce Words?

Average Age (Mo)	Standard Deviation	Behavior
11	(0:2)	First word
12–13	(0:2)	2–3 words
14–15	(0:2)	4–6 words
16–17	(0:3)	7–20 words
20–21	(0:3)	50 words

Source: Ref. 26.

6. What co-occurrence restrictions exist in the child's speech? This question is asked to determine which elements can occur together in the child's speech. The reason for this line of inquiry is that the child's speech in addition to containing a limited number of sounds and syllables also contains restrictions on which units can occur together. The co-occurrence restrictions most commonly encountered in children under 2 years old are listed in Table 4–5.

7. What are the organizing principles in the child's speech? This question is asked to identify the organizing principles that underlie the child's use of speech. These principles include favorite sounds, selectivity, word recipes, homonym avoiding and seeking strategies, word-based organizations, and phrase-length units. Each of these principles is normal and expected in normally developing children who are under 2 years old. Knowledge of these principles provides better understanding of why a medically involved child might find certain sounds and words easier or harder to pronounce. The persistence of some organizing principles in children developmentally over 2 years old may signify the presence of a speech disorder. The major organizing principles encountered in the speech of children under 2 years old are listed in Table 4–6.

DIAGNOSIS AND PROGNOSIS

An important outcome of the evaluation is a diagnosis of the child's speech problem if one is found to exist. An important aspect of conveying a diagnosis to a child's family or another professional is offering the most informed judgment possible regarding the child's prognosis for future speech development. The diagnosis and prognosis are obtained through the following steps.

ACROSS-CHILD COMPARISONS

The first step in the diagnostic process is to determine if the child is delayed in speech acquisition relative to other children. Individual differences in the rate of acquisition are frequent and expected. Relatively well-standardized assessment instruments report standard deviations (SD) of between 2 to 4 months for most speech behaviors for children from 0 to 2 years old.[25,26] For example, a skill listed as being acquired at 1:6 might be acquired by some children as early as 1:2 to 1:4 and by other children as late as 1:8 to 1:10.

When standard deviations are not provided, the speech–language clinician must make the intellectually unsatisfying but necessary estimation of variation.

Table 4–4. Approximate Ages of Acquisition for the question:
What is the Child's Capacity to Produce Sounds and Syllables?

A. Vowels, Consonant Clusters, Syllables, and Word Shapes

Average Age (Mo)	Behavior
14–16	Consonant clusters rarely occur Most frequent syllable shapes: CV and VC Most common word shapes: CV and CVCV, although VC and CVC may also occur Few or any words contain more than 2 syllables Vowel errors are likely to occur, although not as commonly as consonant errors
24	The child is likely to have several words containing consonant clusters Approximately 4 to 9% of words are longer than two syllables Vowel errors are relatively infrequent, although some errors may still occur (the most frequent vowel patterns: vocalization of syllabic consonants and epenthesis [insertion of a vowel between consonants])

B. Average Number and Most Commonly Occurring Consonants

	Word-Initial Consonants		Word-Final Consonants	
Age (Mo)	Mean (Range)	Sounds Produced by 50% of Children	Mean (Range)	Sounds Produced by 50% of Children
15*	3.4 (2–5)	b d h	0.6 (0–2)	(none)
18	6.3 (2–10)	b d m n h w	2.8 (0–6)	t
21	6.7 (2–13)	b t d m n h	3.6 (0–7)	t n
24†	9.5 (4–16)	b t d k g m n h w f s	5.7 (0–11)	p t k n r s

*Near 14 to 16 months, the speech of children typically consists of voiced stops, nasals, one or two glides, and sometimes a voiceless fricative. The predominant place of articulation is anterior (labial and alveolar). A large number of the child's consonants are in error relative to the adult language.

†Compared to 14 to 16 months, by 24 months the child's speech has expanded to include voiceless anterior stops, voiced and voicelss velar stops, and voiceless fricatives. Approximately 70% of the child's consonants are correct relative to the adult language. The most common consonant patterns are stopping, final consonant deletion, and gliding.

Sources: Refs. 42, 49, and 50.

Using a 4-month standard deviation, the evaluator will likely "miss" infants and toddlers who should be diagnosed as having a speech disorder (false-negatives). Similarly, standard deviations of 2 or 3 months are likely to lead evaluators to diagnose children as having speech delays when their speech development is within the normal limits (false-positives). Many speech–language clinicians utilize a 2- or 3-month standard deviation criterion when statistical information is lacking because the consequences of "missing" (false-negative) children with medical needs having speech disorders outweigh the consequences of providing

Table 4–5.   Acquisition Data for the Question: What Co-Occurrence Restrictions Exist in the Child's Speech?

Co-occurrence Restriction	Description
Voiced words	Some children appear to experience difficulty "turning voicing on and off" within a syllable or word. For these children, many words are either entirely voiced or entirely voiceless. This restriction is most commonly found in children under 1:6.
Consonant to vowel assimilations	Vowels can affect the place of articulation of adjacent consonants. For example, velar and bilabial consonants may become alveolar before a front vowel. To illustrate, while a child might pronounce "go" as [goU], she may pronounce "gay" as [deI]. In like manner, a child might pronounce "boo" as [bu], but pronounce "bee" as [di]. Clinical experience suggests that velar consonants are more likely to assimilate to vowels than bilabial consonants, and that high front vowels are more likely to induce assimilation than other front vowels. Consonant to vowel assimilation patterns are most commonly found in children under 1:6.
Consonant to consonant assimilations	The place of articulation of a consonant in one part of a word can affect the place of articulation of consonants elsewhere in the word. Two common consonant assimilation patterns are labial assimilation and velar assimilation. In labial assimilation, nonlabial consonants (especially alveolar consonants) assimilate to the place of articulation of a labial consonant elsewhere in the word. Examples: "Beat" may be pronounced [bip], but "tip" may be pronounced [pIp]. In velar assimilation, nonvelar consonants (again, especially alveolar consonants) assimilate to the place of articulation of a velar consonant elsewhere in the word. Examples: "Kit" may be pronounced [kIk], but "dig" may be pronounced [gIg]. These patterns are both relatively common in the speech of children under 2 years old.

Sources: Refs. 5, 32, 52, and 53.

speech services to children with medical needs whose speech would likely improve without speech intervention (false-positives).

WITHIN-CHILD COMPARISONS

The next step in the diagnostic process is to compare the child's speech development with her chronologic age and her language reception abilities. If the child was born prematurely, her adjusted age is used as her chronologic age. Adjusted age is determined using the formula: chronologic age – weeks premature = adjusted age. To illustrate, a baby who was born at 30 weeks gestation would

Table 4–6. Acquisition Data for the Question: What are the
Organizing Principles in the Child's Speech?

Organizing Principle	Description
Favorite sounds	Some children have "favorite" sounds. For example, a toddler might produce a syllabic fricative such as [s] to pronounce all words that in the adult language begin with fricatives, stops, or affricates.
Selectivity	It appears that some children "pick and choose" the sounds and sequences of sounds that they will attempt to pronounce. In general, children appear to choose to pronounce words that contain sounds already in their expressive vocabularies. To illustrate, a child may have an expressive vocabulary containing words beginning with [t] and [k] and may only be willing to attempt to pronounce new words that begin with the same sounds. Selectivity has been documented in children under 20 months old.
Word recipes	Some children pronounce words the way some inexperienced cooks make dinner: using a very few recipes over and over again. For example, such a child might have a CV word recipe and another CVCV word recipe. The child's CV recipe might be: "All monosyllabic words in the adult language will be pronounced as CV and the consonant will be [d]." Similarly, the child's CVCV recipe might be: "All multisyllabic words in the adult language will be pronounced CVCV and both consonants will be identic in place of articulation." Typically, word recipes are found in the speech of children with small expressive vocabularies. This may be because as the child's vocabulary grows the child must develop more flexible ways to pronounce words if she is to avoid being extremely unintelligible.
Homonym	Children appear to differ in the amount of homonym they permit in their speech. Some children appear to pronounce words in such a way as to increase homonyms. Other children appear to follow the opposite approach and may produce unusual pronunciations to avoid having too many homophonous words.
Word-based organization	It appears that many children learn speech "word by word." For such children, how a sound is pronounced is dependent on the word in which it occurs. For example, a word beginning with [p] in the adult language may be pronounced by the child as [b] in one word, as [t] in another word, and as [p] or [s] in other words. This type of word-based organization of speech appears to occur most commonly in children with relatively small expressive vocabularies (typically, less than 50 words).
Phrase-length units	It appears that some children learn "the tune before the words." Such children may accurately produce the intonation of a sentence, although the speech sounds in the sentence may be inaccurate relative to the adult language. Sometimes children who pronounce the intonation of sentences better than the sounds in the sentence are called "gestalt learners." Another word for this type of speech behavior is "jargoning."

Sources: Refs. 30 and 53–61.

have her chronologic age reduced 8 weeks (38 weeks is considered fullterm) to arrive at her adjusted age. For example, at 3 months old (12 weeks) the child would have an adjusted age of 1 month (4 weeks).

The child's (adjusted) chronologic age is used to compare the child's development with her chronologic peers, and the developmental level of the child's language reception abilities is used to establish the expected level of the child's speech development. To illustrate, if a child has an adjusted chronologic age of 1:10 and language reception abilities of a child 1:6 (1:4 to 1:8 with a SD of 2 months), a child without a speech delay would be expected to have speech abilities commensurate with the child's language reception abilities (1:4 to 1:8 with a SD of 2 months). The child's speech abilities typically do not exceed the child's language reception skills.

DEGREE OF DELAY

After the child's speech development has been compared with her adjusted chronologic age and her language reception abilities, the child's speech is assigned a degree of delay. The designations of mild, moderate, or severe delay are often used for this purpose. Degree of delay is determined relative both to the child's adjusted chronologic age and the language reception abilities. For example, a child's speech might be mildly delayed relative to her language reception abilities and moderately delayed relative to chronologic age. The number of months that correspond to mild, moderate, and severe delay are typically established by district, county, or state agencies. To illustrate, the following would be degrees of delay for a child aged 1 year or older based on a standard deviation of 2 months: 0 to 2 months = no delay, 2 to 4 months = mild delay, 4 to 6 months = moderate delay, and 6 or more months = severe delay.

PROGNOSIS

After establishing the child's degree of delay, the speech–language clinician makes a prognosis of the child's future speech development. Unfortunately, it is far easier to establish a child's current level of speech development than her future speech development. A prognosis is established chiefly by comparing an individual child to a group of similar children. The limitation of this approach is that the performance of a group does not define the potential of an individual. Every clinician can cite examples of children who achieved far beyond what similar children achieved. Alternately, all clinicians can describe children whose development was far more delayed than was expected.

Children with medical needs have associated risk factors that may negatively influence the prognosis for development. In general, risk factors arise from three major sources: the environment (for example, low socioeconomic scale, or parental neglect), neurology (for example, conditions that are likely to result in neurological impairments, such as bleeding in the brain or episodes of asphyxia), and physical difficulties (for example, impairments of hearing, the oral-motor system, or supportive structures).

EXAMPLES

The following examples illustrate how diagnostic and prognostic statements might be presented to another professional in the summary section of a clinical report. The examples use a 2-month interval between degrees of speech delay. For the first example, the child was born prematurely and has an adjusted chronologic age of 1:5. The child's language reception and speech abilities approximate 1:3. The diagnosis for this child might be the following: "Speech is within expected limits compared with her adjusted chronologic age and speech is commensurate with receptive language. The child is at risk for future speech disorders due to prematurity."

The second child was born at term and is 1:11. Her language reception abilities approximate a child 1:4 and her speech abilities approximate a child 0:11. The child's diagnosis might be as follows: "The child's language is delayed relative to her chronologic age. Speech is severely delayed relative to chronologic age and moderately delayed compared with the child's language reception abilities. The child does not evidence prognostic indicators that place her at greater risk for speech delays in the future."

Treatment

This section addresses issues arising in speech treatment. The following topics are addressed: treatment goals, treatment options, treatment activities to facilitate oral communication, and speech techniques to facilitate the acquisition of expressive vocabulary.

Treatment Goals

The primary goal of speech treatment is to facilitate the child's use of sound to interact and communicate to the maximum extent permitted by her cognitive, social, and medical status. In general, if the child's speech and receptive language development are similar, the goal of therapy is to keep speech development from falling behind receptive language. However, if the child's speech development lags behind her language reception abilities, the goal is to bring speech up to the developmental age of the child's language reception abilities. The therapy activities to promote speech development also facilitate the acquisition of language and social skills.

Treatment Options

There are four therapy options that the speech–language clinician can offer a child with medical needs. The first option is not to provide speech services. This is an option in theory but because all children with medical needs are at risk for future developmental difficulties they are all candidates for speech services. In practice, the only children who would not receive speech services are those who are either too medically fragile or are dying. Further, even dying and medically fragile children are frequently monitored and contact with the child's family frequently maintained.

The second option is to provide parent counseling without other speech services. This option is offered only when (1) a child's speech and receptive language development are commensurate and both are within normal limits for the child's (adjusted) chronologic age and (2) the child carries no risk factors beyond prematurity. In such situations, re-evaluations at 6-month or yearly intervals are offered along with parent counseling and suggestions to facilitate speech and language development.

The third option is to provide speech therapy without providing the child any other language services. Although this option is possible, it is seldom selected because the vast majority of medically involved children also have both language and speech difficulties. Thus, children benefit from a full program in which speech and language stimulation co-exist throughout the day.

The fourth option is to provide speech therapy as part of an early developmental intervention program. This is the therapy option of choice in the majority of children.

Treatment Activities

An outside observer is likely to mistake therapy for play when therapy is done well with young children. This is because what the observer may see, for example, is a small child and an adult rolling a ball back and forth, or an adult clapping her hands while a child stands up in her crib and babbles. Speech–language clinicians perform therapy activities as well as helping to train families and staff. Whether direct care or parent training is being provided, there are three primary criteria to consider in choosing therapy activities for any toddler: (1) the child's play preferences; (2) the child's level of cognitive development; and (3) the child's motor skills. A child's play preferences are determined based on observation and interviews with the child's family. The child's level of cognitive development typically is the developmental age of her language reception abilities.

Illustrative examples of speech facilitation activities organized according to the developmental level of the child are provided in Table 4–7. The developmental age ranges depicted in the table are the approximate ages during which the activity is introduced. In many cases, the activity is continued in a more sophisticated form during later stages in development. For example, a music box that is introduced when the child is developmentally between 0 to 6 months may continue to be utilized as the infant grows into a toddler and a preschooler.

Looking at picture books, playing musical instruments, and riding on toys constitute good speech activities for children whose cognitive development approximates children aged 12 to 18 months. Picture books facilitate the use of speech through naming and labeling while facilitating attention to task and reciprocal interactions. While looking at picture books is particularly useful in facilitating the acquisition of the sounds in names of objects, acquisition of the sounds in action words are facilitated through playing music instruments and riding toys. These activities provide excellent opportunities to facilitate the acquisition of such functionally important words as go, more, stop, up, down, soft, and loud.

In addition to the activities listed above, speech therapy for children whose cognitive development approximates that of children aged 18 to 24 months may include play with dolls and putting together big-piece puzzles. Playing with dolls can serve to facilitate both reciprocal communication and the child's pronunciation of the names of body parts and clothing. Through the use of pretend games, dolls can also be used to introduce sounds in the names and activities

Table 4–7. Therapy Activities for Toddlers with Medical Needs

Developmental Age Range (Mo)	Activities
0–6	Shaking rattle Listening to music box Watching mobile Grasping hand-held toy Shaking noise-making toy Exploring busy box
6–12	Looking in mirror Participating in daily living activities Blowing bubbles Playing with pop-up toy Singing gestural song Exploring manipulable toy Banging toy drum Rolling toy car
12–18	Riding in wagon or on tricycle Looking at picture book Sorting shapes Playing music instrument Building Mr. and Mrs. Potato Head
18–24	Playing see 'n say Playing with doll Building blocks Making big-piece puzzle

associated with countless other objects and activities. Big-piece puzzles offer therapeutic functions similar to dolls. Additionally, puzzles are particularly valuable in promoting attention as well as facilitating the acquisition of the sounds in names of the persons, objects, and actions depicted in the puzzle.

Lastly, it should be emphasized that speech development can proceed even if the child is unable to vocalize. A child who is temporarily unable to vocalize due to medical or physical reasons may still learn about the communicative use of sound from interacting with others. The child's contribution to such dialogues may include eye widening, smiling, movement of the extremities, or imitative oral motor movements. If the child does not have the ability to ever vocalize, engaging in reciprocal communication is still valuable in promoting social and language development.

Facilitating Speech in the Child's Expressive Vocabulary

Perhaps the most unique role of the provider of speech services lies in the use of knowledge of phonetics and speech development to facilitate the development of the child's expressive vocabulary. As indicated several places in this chapter, expressive vocabulary is important because it affords the child a linguistically based means to communicate and because of the crucial role that words play as an interface between the speech and language systems.

ANALYSIS OF PHONETIC INVENTORY

The following is an overview of the steps used to facilitate the speech development in a child's expressive vocabulary. Data from the child's expressive vocabulary depicted in Table 4–8 serve to illustrate this process.[31,32]

The first step in facilitating speech development in a child's expressive vocabulary is a careful analysis of the child's phonetic inventory, including her ability to produce and combine word shapes, syllables, stress patterns, consonants, and vowels.[32] Special note should be made of any potential co-occurrence restrictions or organizing principles that might either assist or interfere with the child's ability to pronounce new words. Analysis of the data in Table 4–8 indicates that the most frequent words in the child's expressive vocabulary are composed of CV and CVCV syllables. Further, the CVCV words are all reduplicated syllables. The only CVCCVC word also is reduplicated. Turning from the word to the syllable level, the most prevalent syllable shape is CV (12 instances), followed distantly by CVC (2 instances) and V (1 instance). Turning to the level of sounds, the consonant inventory includes [b d g p t k m n h w]. The vowel system includes [i eI u a aU]. There do not appear to be any obvious consonant-to-consonant or consonant-to-vowel assimilation patterns, although this cannot be fully determined until word probes are performed (see below).

Based on the information contained in Table 4–3, the size of the child's expressive vocabulary described above approximates that of a child near 16 to 17 months. Based on the information in Table 4–4, the child's phonetic inventory appears to approximate that of a child between 14 months to approximately 18 months. The child's phonetic repertoire of vowels, consonant clusters (none), syllables, and word shapes approximates that of a child near 14 to 16 months. The child's consonant inventory (10) contains a greater number of consonants than typically found in a child near 14 to 16 months, although her speech does not contain the classes of sounds (fricatives) that you might expect in the speech of a child near 24 months. The number of consonants in word-final position (1) is compatible with that of a child near 18 months.

Table 4–8.   A Child's Expressive Vocabulary

Word	Pronunciation
Eye	eI
Goose	gu
Hi	ha
Bye	ba
Kitty	ki
Button	bʌ
Mouth	maU
Clock	taʔ
Dog	wuwu
No-no	nunu
Popcorn	pap pap

Source: Ref. 31.

The standard deviation of the information in Table 4–4 is 3 months, so the child's phonetic inventory appears appropriate for the size of her expressive vocabulary. For the purposes of this illustration, it will be assumed that the child's language reception abilities approximate that of a child 28 months old, thus indicating the need for speech services.

SELECTION OF TREATMENT TARGETS

The next step is to identify possible treatment targets. Because speech treatment usually focuses on those aspects of speech development in which the child is most delayed, the first question to ask is: Is the child more delayed in any particular aspect of speech? The inventory of segments of the child depicted in Table 4–8 does not appear unusual compared with children near 14 to 18 months. Consideration of the child's inventory of syllables and word shapes also does not yield an obvious therapy target.

The second question in deciding on a therapy target is: Is the child's phonetic inventory incomplete when analyzed in terms of place, manner, and voicing? The child depicted in Table 4–8 has a complete set of oral stops, nasal stops produced at two places of articulation, a glottal fricative, and a glide. Although not necessarily a signal of delay, the most obvious omission in this inventory is the absence of a supraglottic fricative.

The third question to ask is: Are there distributional gaps in the child's phonetic inventory? The most obvious gap in the child's segment, syllable, and word shape inventory is the virtual absence (except for "pat-pat") of words ending in consonants. It should be noted that the word-final [p] is a reduplication of the initial consonant. For the purpose of this example, the treatment target will be to facilitate the child's acquisition of words ending in consonants.

PHONETIC ENVIRONMENTS

The next step is to review phonetic principles to identify possible environments within which to introduce word-final consonants. Phonetic environments that may assist in aspects of speech production are listed in Table 4–9. This table suggests that the ends of words may be a facilitating environment for voiceless consonants (context 3) and velar consonants (context 5). Lastly, the place of articulation of a word-final consonant may be facilitated if it shares the place of articulation of another consonant in the word (context 4).

WORD PROBES

Word probes are designed to discover which of the therapy targets can be achieved by the child, as well as serving to determine if the child has constraints or strategies that might interfere with the success of therapy. Nonsense words might also be used for this purpose. Naming games are helpful word probe activities. To illustrate, the child might be shown a book or a toy and told that "his name is [n n]" (to help establish if the child is able to produce word-final [n] when both consonants in the word are identical—context 4), or that "his name is [d t]" (to help establish if the child is able to produce word-final [t] when both consonants agree in place of articulation—context 4). Another probe might be, "his name is [f] (to help establish if the child is able to produce a word-final

Table 4–9.   List of Facilitating Speech Contexts

Number	Facilitating Phonetic Contexts
1	The production of consonants and vowels tends to be facilitated in stressed syllables
2	The production of voiced consonants may be facilitated (a) between vowels and (b) at the beginning of syllables and words
3	The production of voiceless consonants may be facilitated at the end of syllables and words
4	The place of articulation of a consonant may be facilitated if another consonant in the same syllable or word is identical to the consonant or shares the same place of articulation
5	The production of velar consonants may be facilitated (a) at the end of syllables and (b) when preceding a back vowel occurring in the same syllable
6	The production of alveolar consonants may be facilitated when preceding a front vowel occurring in the same syllable
7	The production of fricatives may be facilitated between vowels

Source: Ref. 32.

voiceless fricative—context 3). When performing word probes, it is convenient to write all possible targets on a piece of paper that is brought to the therapy session. A check is placed next to a word that a child pronounces correctly, and a minus is placed next to words that the child "misses."

WORD SELECTION

Lastly, two or three therapy targets are selected from the list of words that the child produced correctly during the probes. The final step is placing the sound target in words of high functional value to the child. These words may be obtained through interviews with family members and the professional staff and from observing the child during play and daily activities. To illustrate, if a therapy target were word-final [p], the word "top" (for the toy) might be introduced in therapy, if that activity were enjoyable to the child. It is helpful to keep a master list of words that you organize by therapy targets to avoid having to develop new words for each new client. To illustrate, the master list should contain words ending in voiceless consonants, words beginning with voiced consonants, etc.

Clinical Alternatives

The above techniques are successful with most children. Some special procedures, however, are useful when the child either appears "stalled" in speech development or whose speech contains a great many homonyms.

CHILDREN WHO ARE "STALLED"

Some children appear to experience temporary "stalls" in speech development. If the above approach does not lead to developmental gains, an alternative is to augment the child's increased use of her existing phonetic inventory. In such a situation, the goal is not to teach the child new sounds and syllables; rather, the goal is to teach new words using the phonetic material she already produces. For example, because the child depicted in Table 4–8 possesses [k] and [aU], the clinician might attempt to teach her "cow." An alternative goal might be to teach the child the word "bee" because she already possesses [b] and [i]. Still another goal might be to teach the child to pronounce "me" because she possesses both an [m] and [i]. Lastly, the clinician might attempt to teach the child to say "wawa" for "water" because she already produces [wuwu] ("dog") and [a].

CHILDREN WHOSE SPEECH CONTAINS MANY HOMONYMS

Some children have vocabularies with many homonyms (words that sound alike, but have different meanings). To illustrate, if the child depicted in Table 4–8 had a vocabulary with a great deal of homonym, seven or more of her words might be produced as [b]. While many children with a great deal of homonym respond well to the vocabulary-building techniques described above, others show few or no developmental gains. An alternative or adjunct to the approach described above is to "flood" the child's speech with new words that phonetic analysis suggests will be pronounced in the same way as the old words. "Flooding" appears to temporarily increase communicative breakdown and frustration, inducing change in the child's pronunciations as she attempts new pronunciations to communicate her intent. For example, "flooding" might increase the percentage of homonyms in a child's expressive vocabulary from 50 to 75% and thus increase the likelihood that the child will experience frustration when she attempts to communicate. The increased frustration appears to be the impetus for the child's attempt to find new speech patterns.

Children with Long-term Tracheostomies

The principles and procedures described in previous sections are applicable for facilitating the speech development of a wide variety of populations of toddlers, including those with in-place tracheostomies. As with a number of specific subpopulations of children with medical needs, providing speech services to children with in-place tracheostomies requires specialized knowledge beyond that described above. This section provides an overview of the special concepts, terminology, and special evaluation and therapy techniques encountered in providing speech services to children with tracheostomies. Because of the complexity of the medical and developmental issues that arise in caring for these children, the procedures listed in this section should not be attempted without thorough training and appropriate supervision.[33]

Basic Terminology

A tracheostomy is an artificial opening between the cervical trachea and the neck.[34] A tube (cannula) is placed in the opening to provide a means for the air to enter and exit the lungs. When the cannula is in place, the child breathes through the opening in her throat. When the cannula is removed (decannulation), the child reverts to breathing through the mouth and nose.

Many children with tracheostomies also receive mechanical ventilation at some point during the course of their illness. A mechanical ventilator is a device that assists or supports the child's lungs in breathing.[35] The most common mechanical ventilators (positive pressure ventilators) operate by forcing air into the lungs through the tracheostomy tube. The elastic recoil of the lungs provides the expiration. The length of time during which mechanical ventilation is received can range from hours to years, depending on the nature of the child's medical disability. Chronic respiratory failure is said to be present in the diagnosed condition when mechanical ventilation is required for 28 days or longer.

Many children with tracheostomies are born prematurely. Birthweight is an important issue when considering prematurity. Birthweight refers to the baby's weight at the time of delivery. "Low birthweight" is defined as birthweight of less than 2500 grams and "very low birthweight" is defined as birthweight less 1500 grams (about 3.3 lb). "Extremely low birthweight" is defined as birthweight of less than 800 grams. Birthweight serves as an index of a neonate's development in the womb. The lower the birthweight, the more likely less development of the baby occurred before birth. Further, lower birthweights often signify more difficult deliveries.

Prevalence and Mortality Rate

It is estimated that 884 to 2600 children undergo a tracheostomy annually.[36] Approximately 70% of these children also breathe through the assistance of mechanical ventilation.[37] Common medical indicators for tracheostomies and ventilatory assistance include bronchopulmonary dysplasia (a lung disease associated with prematurity that results initially from respiratory distress shortly after birth), subglottic stenosis (narrowing of the airway below the glottis), and a variety of other congenital anomalies and neuromuscular disorders.

The mortality rate for children receiving tracheostomies or ventilatory assistance is between 22 to 30%.[38,39] Approximately 70 to 85% of these deaths occur during the first year after the surgical procedure is performed. The primary cause of death during this period is the original medical condition for which the tracheostomy was performed. After the first year of cannulation, the most frequent cause of death is related to mechanical failure resulting in accidental asphyxia.

Developmental Outcome and Risk Factors

For the first several years after decannulation, receptive language tends to be in advance of speech development, especially if the child was unable to vocalize around the cannula while the tracheostomy was in place.[40–43] The use of sign language, which may have been introduced to reduce communicative frustration while the child was tracheotomized, fades as the oral modality gradually becomes the predominate form of communication.

Research is only beginning to document the long-term developmental outcomes of previously tracheotomized children. At present, the most complete information is for children about 5 years of age who were decannulated near 2 years of age.[37,44,45] The verbal and nonverbal intelligence of these children almost always is commensurate.[44] Approximately 50% of these children have normal intelligence, although IQs tend to be low-average. The other 50% are developmentally delayed (mentally retarded). The lowered IQs are thought to reflect the child's initial medical condition and episodes of asphyxia while tracheotomized. Approximately one half of the children with normal intelligence and an even a higher percentage of the children with mental retardation experience behavior problems or social isolation. Such difficulties are thought to result from a combination of factors, including the illness, lengthy hospitalizations, and the family's reaction to the child's disability.

Approximately 13 to 17% of children who have been tracheotomized reflect significant speech delay at 5 years of age relative to other areas of development. Investigators do not have adequate explanations about why certain previously tracheotomized children have speech difficulties at 5 years while the majority of such children are free of such problems. Nor can investigators predict with certainty that the previously tracheotomized child will experience speech and language difficulties at older ages. However, certain risk factors are known to increase the likelihood of a child having a less successful developmental outcome. Some risk factors are associated with the tracheostomy itself, while others are associated with the conditions giving rise to the need for tracheostomy, and still others are associated with environmental situations that are known to adversely influence speech development. Table 4–10 lists the major risk factors associated with children with tracheostomies.

Special Issues in the Speech Evaluation

Some children with tracheostomies are able to vocalize by an air leak around the tracheostomy tube. Such a leak develops either because the size of the tube is

Table 4–10. Risk Factors for Children with Tracheostomies

Risk Factors	Causes of Disability
Prematurity and low birthweight	Increased risk of neurologic damage
Respiratory Distress Syndrome (RDS)	Increased opportunities for oxygen deprivation (RDS may also indicate a more serious underlying condition)
Intraventricular hemorrhage	Increased risk of neurologic damage
Birth outside of a hospital	More severe illness and birth trauma
Mechanical ventilation	Increased opportunities for oxygen deprivation (longer ventilation time may also reflect a more serious underlying condition)
Lower socioeconomic status	Poorer developmental outcome due to either lack of available developmental services or lack of knowledge regarding how to obtain developmental services
Family history of speech disorders	Possible genetic predisposition for speech problems

decreased or the child grows and is not fitted with a larger tube. Typically, a smaller tube is allowed if the reason for the tracheostomy was to bypass an obstruction. In such circumstances, air leakage around or through the stoma may not be critical, and the tube can be smaller. Most often, air leakages develop near the end of the first year of life. If an air leak around the tracheostomy tube does not develop, no amount of therapy will permit the child to vocalize.

PRELIMINARY CONSIDERATIONS

Prior to the evaluation, the nursing staff—or the child's caregiver, if the child is in the community—should be consulted to determine that no medical complications exist that would inhibit the assessment. In most cases, the nurse will suction the secretions from the child's tracheostomy tube prior to the evaluation to reduce secretions that might hinder breathing and vocalization. Signs indicating that suctioning is required include coughing, production of wet gurgly sounds, changes in skin color, gagging, and the presence of secretions in the tracheostomy tube. If the child is being evaluated outside her room, all emergency equipment should accompany her. At the conclusion of the evaluation, the emergency equipment should be returned with the child, and the appropriate monitors set to "on." Lastly, nursing or the child's caregiver should be informed that the child has been returned.

ASSESSMENT

The assessment of voicing potential is one of the most unique aspects of the speech assessment of a child with an in-place tracheostomy. Potential for vocalization can be assessed in several ways. To help guide the speech–language clinician, parents and health care providers can be asked if the child ever "makes any sounds." The speech–language clinician should remember that the vocalizations may be intermittent and that not all caregivers recognize such vocalizations when they occur. If the informant answers affirmatively, the evaluator should ask the person to describe the sounds and to tell where, when, and how often they occur.

Direct evidence comes from observing the child vocalize. It often is easiest to elicit vocalizations by having the child either sit or stand as erect as possible to keep the diaphragm from collapsing. Next, the evaluator and the child might play together, attempting to make the child excited and induce deeper breathing. If a child can vocalize, she will often do so under such conditions. Another (though much less pleasant) circumstance under that a child may vocalize is when crying or coughing.

In addition to assessing whether the child can vocalize, the evaluator should also determine the child's ability to produce sound using other sources of vibration. The most common source of nonlaryngeal vibration is air trapped inside the cheeks. Vocalizations produced in this fashion are called buccal speech. Typically, buccal speech only permits single words and short utterances.

Special Issues in Treatment

Special problems arise in providing speech services to a child who lacks the capacity to vocalize. Most importantly, because no amount of training can help a child to vocalize if sufficient air does not enter the oral tract to set the vocal folds in vibration, therapy for children who cannot vocalize consists of working around the disability.

The therapeutic options that are used to provide communication services to children with in-place tracheostomies are listed in Table 4–11. The oral communication therapy options are speaking valves, cannula occlusion, fenestrated cannulas, the electrolarynx, buccal speech, and esophageal speech. For the reasons given below, buccal speech, esophageal speech, and fenestrated cannulas are used far less often than the other therapy options. Many children with in-place tracheostomies receive therapy to facilitate nonoral communication. Nonoral communication options include sign language and alternative communication systems (communication boards and electronic communication devices).[46,47]

The above therapeutic options are not exclusive choices. For example, a child can be taught to use both sign language and an electrolarynx. Alternately, a child might use a combination of sign language, cannula occlusion, and an electronic communication device. The major benefits and limitations of each oral therapeutic option are outlined below; the nonoral therapy options are described as they relate to speech development. None of the therapy options described below should be provided without a thorough understanding of the selection criteria, contraindication, and procedures involved.[46]

SPEAKING VALVES

Speaking valves permit air to enter the cannula and then block the air from exiting so that the air must exit through the mouth. The obvious and most important advantage of a speaking valve is that it permits the child to vocalize. If the child's cognitive development does not yet support the use of speech, she can still exercise her vocal system. If the child is more developed cognitively, she can learn to use spoken language to communicate. A disadvantage of this option is that the child's tolerance of a speaking valve must be strictly monitored. Any signs of respiratory compromise, including decreased oxygen saturation, can also be a complication. Signs of decreased oxygen saturation include blue coloration of the skin, breathing difficulties, coughing, gagging, sweating, irritability, and increased heart rate. Typically, the decision to use a speaking valve is made on

Table 4–11.   Therapy Options to Facilitate Expressive Communication in Children with In-Place Tracheostomies

Category	Therapy Options
Facilitates oral communication	Speaking valve Cannula occlusion Electrolarynx Buccal speech Esophageal speech Fenestrated cannula
Facilitates nonoral communication	Manual communication Alternative communication systems

the recommendation of the speech–language clinician and members of the medical team. The medical team is likely to advise against using a speaking valve if the child's respiratory system is not strong enough.

CANNULA OCCLUSION

Cannula occlusion involves placing the child's hand, finger, or chin over the opening of the tracheal tube. This technique blocks the air from exiting the through the tracheostomy and allows it to pass up through the larynx. The principle advantages of cannula occlusion are (1) it permits phonation and (2) its use requires no mechanical devices. A disadvantage of this option is that it requires careful monitoring to guard the respiratory status of the child. Cannula occlusion cannot be used if the child is receiving mechanical ventilation.

ELECTROLARYNX

An electrolarynx serves as a source of vibration for sound production. The electrolarynx is placed on the side of the child's neck and slightly forward and is used to produce words or, if the child is younger, simply to promote vocalizations. The electrolarynx can be used with infants as young as 9 to 10 months. A principle limitation of the electrolarynx is that its use sometimes requires a lengthy training procedure before the child will accept the devise or proper placement can be obtained. Because children can find the devise to be "scary," the clinician should engage in modeling, demonstrating the use of the devise on herself and on the child's hand.

BUCCAL SPEECH, ESOPHAGEAL SPEECH, AND FENESTRATED CANNULAE

Buccal speech uses air trapped in the cheeks to produce speech. It provides articulatory practice and helps the child express her most basic needs. Some children are able with practice to use buccal speech to produce short phrases. Many caregivers dislike buccal speech because they perceive that it gives their child a "Donald Duck" voice.

Esophageal speech is produced by swallowing air and then releasing it into the throat again. Esophageal speech provides practice in articulation. It is typically used with children who have permanent tracheostomies, are cognitively 3 years or older, and who do not have dysarthria. Esophageal speech is not used with children receiving mechanical ventilation because of the complex coordination required to both breathe and inject air into the esophagus.

A fenestrated cannula is a tracheostomy tube with an opening that allows air to flow across the vocal cords. Fenestrated cannulae are seldom attempted with infants and toddlers because the material of the cannula deteriorates, causing weakening of the tracheal walls and placing the child at risk for developing tracheal granulomas.

SIGN LANGUAGE

Sign language provides the child a means of communication, and, therefore, reduces possible frustration resulting from a child being unable to express her needs and thoughts.[48] Some parents are reluctant to introduce sign language because they fear that it will inhibit the child's speech development after decannulation. However, as discussed above, clinical experience does not support this concern. In all known cases, after decannulation the child's use of sign language decreases as her ability to use speech for purposes of communication increases. A more worrisome concern is that sign language limits the population to whom the child can communicate. This population is likely to be even more restricted if the child uses idiosyncratic signs or if the child's motor limitations adversely affects her ability to produce standard signs. Nonetheless, despite these problems, sign language remains an important therapeutic option.

ALTERNATIVE COMMUNICATION SYSTEMS

Alternative communication systems exist in a wide variety of forms, from simple communication boards to very elaborate and relatively expensive electronic communication devices. Decisions about which device to use are made by an augmentative communication specialist, who may or may not also be the speech–language clinician providing services to the tracheotomized child. In general, manual communication boards can be used long or short term with any child with the prerequisite cognitive development and physical skills. Electronic communication devices are more likely to be used with children who are predicted to have in-place tracheostomies for several years. Use of an assistive communication system is not intended to preclude speech. Instead, as with sign language, the major goals of assistive communication systems are to facilitate communication development and to provide the child a method to express her immediate needs, thoughts, and feelings.

Conclusions

The study of speech intervention for toddlers with medical needs is scarcely older than the children being studied. Many basic issues in the care of these clients remain to be explored. Particular need exists for better empirical data on long-term speech outcome, for determining the efficacy of specific therapy programs, and for establishing that delays in the acquisition of early speech behaviors best predict future speech and language difficulties. While resolution of these issues will require a great deal of time, energy, and financial resources, the costs would seem to be easily offset by the benefits that accrue to these youngest of all speaking clients.

Acknowledgments

The authors thank Michael Robb for reading and commenting on an earlier draft of this chapter.

Suggested Readings

Batshaw ML, Perret YM: *Children with Handicaps: A Medical Primer*. Baltimore, Paul H. Brookes, 1992.

Bernbaum JC, Hoffman-Williamson M: *Primary Care of the Preterm Infant*. Philadelphia, Mosby Year Book, 1991.

Billeaud F: *Communication Disorders in Infants and Toddlers: Assessment and Intervention*. Boston, Andover Medical Publishers, 1993.

Bleile K (ed): *The Care of Children with Long-Term Tracheostomies*. San Diego, Singular Publishing Group, 1993.

Butler K (ed): Early intervention: Infants, toddlers, and families. *Topics Lang Disorders* 1989; 10:1–96.

Goldberg B: How soon should intervention start? *ASHA* 1991; April:40.

Long T, Katz K, Pokorni J: Developmental intervention with the chronically ill infant. *Infants Young Child* 1989; 1:78–88.

MacDonald J, Carrroll J: A partnership model for communicating with infants at risk. *Infants Young Child* 1992; 4:20–30.

Meisels FJ, Shankoff JP: *Handbook of Early Childhood Intervention*. Cambridge, UK, Cambridge University Press, 1990.

Stark RE: Early language intervention: When, why, how? *Infants Young Child* 1989; 1:44–53.

References

1. Paul R: Profiles of toddlers with slow expressive language. Topics Lang Disorders 1991; 11:1–13.
2. Thal D, Bates E: Language and gesture in late talkers. *JSHR* 1988; 31:115–123.
3. Siegel-Sadewitz V, Shprintzen, R: The relationship of communication disorders to syndrome identification. *JSHD* 1982; 47:338–354.
4. Billeaud F: *Communication Disorders in Infants and Toddlers: Assessment and Intervention*. Boston, Andover Medical Publishers, 1993.
5. Locke J: The sound shape of early lexical representations, in Smith MD, Locke JL (eds): *The Emergent Lexicon: The Child's Development of a Linguistic Vocabulary*. New York, Academic Press, 1988, pp 3–22.
6. Rescorla L, Goossens M: Symbolic play development in toddlers with expressive language impairment. *JSHR* 1992; 35:1290–1302.
7. Hall PK, Tomblin JB: A follow-up study of children with articulation and language disorders. *JSHD* 1978; 43:227–241.
8. Kenworthy O, Bess F, Stahlman M, Lindotrom D: Hearing, speech, and language outcome in infants with extreme immaturity. *Am J Otol* 1987; 8:419–425.
9. Aram D, Nation J: Preschoolers with language disorders: 10 years later. JSHR 1984; 13:159–170.
10. Garvey M, Gordon N: A follow-up study of children with disorders of speech development. *Br J Disorders Commun* 1973; 8:17–28.
11. King RR, Jones C, Lasky E: In retrospect: A fifteen year follow-up report of speech-language disordered children. *Lang Speech Hear Serv Schools* 1982; 15:24–32.
12. Ramey CT, Campbell FA: Preventive education for high-risk children: Cognitive consequences of the Caroline Abecedarian Project. *Am J Mental Defic* 1984; 88:515.
13. Gerber PJ, Schneiders CA, Paradise LV, Reiff HB, Ginsberg RJ, Popp PA: Persisting problems of adults with learning disabilities: Self-reported comparisons from their school-age and adult years. *J Learn Disab* 1990; 23:570–573.
14. Infant Health and Development Program: Enhancing the outcomes of low birthweight, premature infants: A multisite, randomized trial. *JAMA* 1990; 263:3035–3042.
15. Bricker P, Bailey E, Bruder M: The efficacy of early intervention and the handicapped infant: A wise or wasted resource, in Wolraich M, Routh D (eds): *Advances in Developmental and Behavioral Pediatrics*. Greenwich, CT, JAI Press, 1984, pp 373–424.
16. White KR, Mastrapierl M, Casto G: An analysis of special education early childhood projects approved by the joint dissemination review panel. *J Div Early Child* 1984; 9:11.
17. Mantovani J, Powers J: Brain injury in premature infants; Patterns on cranial ultrasound, their relationship to outcome, and the role of developmental intervention in the NICU. *Infants Young Child* 1991; 4:20–32.
18. Locke J: *Phonological Acquisition and Change*. New York, Academic Press, 1983.
19. Stark RE: Stages of speech development in the first year of life, in Yeni-Komshian G, Kavanagh J, Ferguson C (eds): *Child Phonology: Production*. New York, Academic Press, 1980, pp 73–92.
20. Oller D: The emergence of sounds of speech in infancy, vol. 1, in Yeni-Komshian G, Kavanagh J, Ferguson C (eds): *Child Phonology: Production*. New York, Academic Press, 1980, pp 93–112.
21. Ferguson C, Macken M: The role of play in phonological development, in Nelson K (ed): *Child Language IV*. Hillsdale, NJ, Erlbaum, 1983, pp 262–282.
22. Rescorla L: The language development survey: A screening tool for delayed language in toddlers. *JSHD* 1989; 54:587–599.
23. Geschwind N, Galaburda AM: *Cerebral Lateralization*. Cambridge, MA, MIT Press, 1987.
24. Kitley D, Buzby-Hadden J: Legal rights to education services, in Bleile K (ed): *The Care of Children with Long-Term Tracheostomies*. San Diego, Singular Publishing Group, 1993, pp 187–202.

25. Hedrick D, Prather E, Tobin A: *Sequenced Inventory of Communication Development*. Seattle, University of Washington Press, 1984.
26. Capute AJ, Palmer FB, Shapiro Bk, Wachtel RC, Schmidt S, Ross A: Clinical linguistic and auditory milestone scale: Prediction of cognition in infancy. *Dev Med Child Neurol* 1986; 28:762–771.
27. Bruner J: *Child's Talk: Learning to Use Language*. New York, Norton, 1983.
28. Snow CE, Goldfield BA: Turn the page please: Situation-specific language acquisition. *J Child Lang* 1983; 10:551–569.
29. Locke J, Pearson D: vocal learning and the emergence of phonological capacity: A neurobiological approach, in Ferguson C, Menn L, Stoel-Gammon C (eds): *Phonological Development: Models, Research, Implications*. Timonium, MD, York Press, 1992, pp 91–130.
30. Vihman MM, Miller R: Words and babble at the threshold of language acquisition, in Smith MD, Locke JL (eds): *The Emergent Lexicon: The Child's Development of a Linguistic Vocabulary*. New York, Academic Press, 1988, pp 151–184.
31. Branigan G: Syllabic structure and the acquisition of consonants: The great conspiracy in word formation. *J Psycholinguist Res* 1976; 5:117–133.
32. Bleile KM: *Child Phonology: A Book of Exercises for Students*. San Diego, Singular Publishing Group, 1991.
33. Bleile K (ed): *The Care of Children with Long-Term Trachestomies*. San Diego, Singular Publishing Group, 1993a.
34. Handler S: Surgical management of the tracheostomy, in Bleile K (ed): *The Care of Children with Long-Term Tracheostomies*. San Diego, Singular Publishing Group, 1993, pp 23–40.
35. Metz S: Medical management of the ventilator, in Bleile K (ed): *The Care of Children with Long-Term Tracheostomies*. San Diego, Singular Publishing Group, 1993, pp 41–55.
36. United States Congress, Office of Technology Assessment: *Technology-Dependent Children: Hospital v. Home Care—A Technical Memorandum*. OTA-TM-H-38. Washington, DC, US Government Printing Office, May 1987.
37. Singer L, Kercsmer C, Legris G, Orlowski J, Hill B, Doershuk C: Developmental sequelae of long-term infant tracheostomy. *Dev Med Child Neurol* 1989; 31:224–230.
38. Line WS, Hawkins D, Kahlstrom EJ, McLaughlin E, Ensley J: Tracheotomy in infants and young children: The changing perspective. *Laryngoscope* 1986; 96:510–515.
39. Schreiner M, Downes J, Kettrick R, Ise C, Volt R: Chronic respiratory failure in infants with prolonged ventilator dependency. *JAMA* 1989; 258:3398–3404.
40. Locke J, Pearson D: Linguistic significance of babbling: Evidence from a tracheostomized child. *J Child Lang* 1990; 17:1–16.
41. Bleile KM: Children with long-term tracheostomies, in Bleile K (ed): *The Care of Children with Long-Term Tracheostomies*. San Diego, Singular Publishing Group, 1993b, pp 3–19.
42. Bleile KM, Stark RE, Silverman McGowan J: *Evidence for the relationship between babbling and later speech development*. London, International Symposium on Clinical Linguistics and Phonetics, July 1992.
43. Saletsky Kamen R, Watson B: Effects of long-term tracheostomy on spectral characteristics of vowel production. *JSHR* 1991; 34:1057–1066.
44. Hill B, Singer L: Speech and language development after infant tracheostomy. *JSHD* 1990; 55:15–20.
45. Simon B, Fowler S, Handler S: Communication development in young children with long-term tracheostomies: A preliminary report. *Int J Pediatr Otorhinolaryngol* 1983; 6:37–50.
46. Silverman McGowan J, Bleile K, Fus L, Barnas E: Communication disorders, in Bleile K (ed): *The Care of Children with Long-Term Tracheostomies*. San Diego, Singular Publishing Group, 1993, pp 113–140.
47. Simon B, Silverman McGowan S: Tracheostomy in young children: Implications for assessment and treatment of communication and feeding disorders. *Infants Young Child* 1989; 1:1–9.
48. Hall SS, Weatherly K: Using sign language with tracheostomized infants and children. *Pediatr Nurs* 1989; 15:362–367.
49. Stoel-Gammon C. Phonetic inventories, 15–24 months: A longitudinal study. *JSHR* 1985; 28:505–512.
50. Stoel-Gammon C: Phonological skills in 2-year-olds. *Lang Speech Hear Serv Schools* 1987; 18:323–329.
51. Bernthal J, Bankson N: *Articulation and Phonological Disorders*. Englewood Cliffs, NJ, Prentice-Hall, 1993.
52. Stoel-Gammon C, Dunn C: *Normal and Disordered Phonology in Children*. Baltimore, University Park Press, 1985.
53. Waterson N: Child phonology: A prosodic view. *J Linguist* 1971; 7:179–221.
54. Schwartz R, Leonard L: Do children pick and choose: An examination of phonological selection and avoidance in early lexical acquisition. *J Child Lang* 1982; 9:319–336.
55. Schwartz RG: Phonological factors in early lexical acquisition, in Smith MD, Locke JL (eds): The

Emergent Lexicon: *The Child's Development of a Linguistic Vocabulary.* New York, Academic Press, 1988, pp 185–222.

56. Menn L: *Pattern, Control and Contrast in Beginning Speech: A Case Study in the Development of Word Form and Word Function.* Unpublished doctoral dissertation, University of Illinois, Urbana, IL, 1976.

57. Scollon R: *Conversations with a One Year Old: A Case Study of the Developmental Foundation of Syntax.* Honolulu, The University Press of Hawaii, 1976.

58. Peters A: *The Units of Language Acquisition.* New York, Cambridge University Press, 1983.

59. Ingram D: Surface contrast in children's speech. *J Child Lang* 1975; 2:287–292.

60. Vihman M: Phonology and the development of the lexicon: Evidence from children's errors. *J Child Lang* 1981; 8:239–264.

61. Ferguson C, Farwell C: Words and sounds in early language acquisition: English initial consonants in the first fifty words. *Language* 1975; 51:419–439.

5

Developmental Verbal Dyspraxia

SHELLEY L. VELLEMAN, PH.D., AND
KRISTINE STRAND, ED.D.

Overview

Apraxia of speech is not an easy diagnostic entity for clinicians or researchers, whether it occurs in adults or children as the result of a known cerebral insult or for unknown reasons. Developmental verbal dyspraxia (DVD), a disorder associated with children, was named after adult-onset apraxia of speech by researchers who noted similar struggle behaviors in individuals with both disorders.[1] Yet, there are as many differences as similarities between acquired and developmental apraxia, and attempts to draw parallels between the two have often exacerbated the difficulties inherent in the differential diagnosis and treatment of DVD.[2]

Much discussion centers around the characterization of DVD as a purely motoric disorder with some linguistic symptoms versus a linguistic disorder affecting motor speech.[2,3] The existence of a subgroup of children with phonological disorders who demonstrate multiple articulation errors, effortful speech, and slow progress in remediation is rarely questioned,[1] but the nature, etiology, prognosis, and remediation of this disorder have been the subject of debate for a century[2]

In this chapter, we will attempt to characterize DVD from both theoretical and clinical perspectives. Our focus will be on the fundamental nature of this disorder, with implications for differential diagnosis, assessment, and treatment.

What is Dyspraxia?

Praxis refers to the generation of volitional movement patterns for the performance of a particular action.[4] The actual motor pattern is secondary; it is the ability to select, plan, organize, and initiate the motor pattern that is the foundation of praxis. Ayres[4] suggested that our superior praxis is one trait that differentiates us from subhuman species. Thus, a cat may be able to raise her hind leg to scratch her head, but cannot conceive of implementing the same action to remove a piece of yarn from her head; she lacks the *praxic* ability to do so. Ayres stressed that a motor plan includes a series of different movements that must be smoothly sequenced into one complex act. Importantly, this sequencing includes not only ordering the individual gestures that make up the whole, but coordinating them with each other and moving quickly and smoothly from one to the other. To do this, one must have appropriate temporo-spatial goals and be able to use tactile, kinesthetic (sense of position and movement), vestibular (balance), and other proprioceptive information about the body's current state and its location in space in planning those goals.

The terms *"apraxia"* and *"dyspraxia"* refer to deficits in praxic abilities. Strub and Black[5] defined *apraxia* as "a disorder in carrying out or learning complex movements that cannot be accounted for by elementary disturbances of strength, coordination, sensation, comprehension, or attention." Apraxia can affect all aspects of motor coordination or be specific to one or more limbs, to oral motor movements, or to speech. Often automatic actions such as brushing one's teeth, which are so overlearned that they no longer require planning, are unimpaired, but the same person may be unable to mime the same action upon request. When an action is explicitly elicited outside of its habitual context, the activity is brought to conscious consideration and the automatized plan for carrying it out is no longer readily available. Similarly, a well-learned motor plan may not be applicable to a very slightly different situation. The effects of different types of apraxia range from an inability to perform unpracticed sequences of fine-motor movements smoothly to an inability to even conceptualize a routine action plan. Strub and Black[5] described one patient who demonstrated symptoms at the conceptual level:

> We watched one woman carefully unwrap a lump of sugar for her coffee only to be completely baffled about what to do thereafter. She had the sugar in one hand, wrapper in the other, and after painful deliberation, she put the paper in the coffee and threw away the sugar.

Such examples demonstrate the abstract ideational levels of impairment that can be observed despite the definition of apraxia as a motor disorder. Motor planning encompasses a wide range of skills, from knowing the function of a spoon to being able to competently use some other unfamiliar tool to stir something when a spoon is not available.

The left hemisphere plays a major role in praxis in most people and therefore apraxia often results from left hemisphere lesions. Regardless of the system affected, the transition from one position or one movement to the next may be more difficult than achieving the individual body postures or movements themselves. For example, Kimura and Archibald[6] found that patients with left hemisphere damage had no more difficulty copying static hand postures than did patients with right hemisphere damage. However, the left hemisphere (presumably apraxic) patients were significantly more impaired on copying hand movements that required them to transition from one hand position to another.

Apraxia of Speech in Adults

Given the association of apraxia with left hemisphere damage and the location of the speech and language areas of the brain on the left, it is not surprising that some patients with left hemisphere injuries exhibit the specific characteristics of "apraxia of speech" (AOS), which may be accompanied by some other form of apraxia. This syndrome is differentiated from dysarthria in that there is no impairment of muscle function and automatic speech (eg, counting, singing) may often be spared; articulation is typically the only speech production system affected (ie, the patient has normal resonance and phonation), and phonological additions, repetitions, unrelated substitutions, and prolongations are more common than are simplification errors.[7] Also, apraxics may respect the suprasegmental rules of their language, such as vowel reduction in longer words, despite prolonged durations overall.[8] AOS is also differentiated from aphasia in that comprehension, formulation, word retrieval, reading, and writing are typically unimpaired in adult apraxics. Furthermore, treatment that is effective for aphasia is far less so for AOS.[7]

Despite the fact that this complex of symptoms is reported by numerous sources, there continues to be some dispute in the field of adult neurolinguistics about whether adult-onset apraxia is in fact a distinct disorder. (See Martin,[9] Lebrun,[10] and Rosenbek, Kent, and LaPointe[11] for discussion of these issues).

Dyspraxia in Children

Introduction

The existence and nature of a distinct praxic disorder in children, commonly referred to as "developmental verbal dyspraxia" (DVD) or "developmental apraxia of speech" (DAS),* also continues to be the source of some controversy. Some of the issues include:

1. Is DVD really a separate entity from severe phonological disorder?
2. Is DVD a pure motor planning disorder (as the term "developmental apraxia of speech" implies) or a linguistic disorder (as our preferred term, "developmental verbal dyspraxia" implies) or are both symptoms of some more comprehensive disability?

The answers to these questions have important implications for our choice of treatments.

DVD differs from adult AOS in three important ways. First, children with DVD have never talked so they have no automatic speech to fall back on. Often, their histories indicate that they did little or no babbling as infants, so they may have limited experience in nonmeaningful syllable production as well. Second, their errors may be either inconsistent (as are adults') or consistent. Each child's level of consistency may also vary from sound to sound, word to word, sentence to sentence, day to day, and listener to listener.[12] Finally, accompanying difficulties with syntax, morphology, and spelling may also be observed.

Diagnostic protocols for identifying DVD usually focus on exclusionary and articulatory/motoric features of the disorder. Exclusionary features that are cited

---

*As there is growing evidence of concomitant language-learning impairments as well as articulatory difficulties (as we shall see), we will use the term "developmental verbal dyspraxia" or "DVD" here.

include no apparent organic conditions, no muscle weakness, hearing and IQ within normal limits, and receptive language within normal limits (Bridgeman and Snowling[13]; Pollock and Hall[14]; Bashir and Strand[15]; Byrd and Cooper[16]; le Normand and Chevrie-Muller[17]; Ekelman and Aram[18]; Crary, Landess, and Towne[19]; Robin[3]; Snowling and Stackhouse[20]; and Williams, Ingham, and Rosenthal[21]).

Articulatory/motoric features that are most diagnostic include the following:

1. Persistent speech difficulty and/or unintelligibility, including vowel misarticulations, poor or reduced production of consonants, increase in errors as length or complexity of utterance increases, and two and three phoneme features in error.

2. Inconsistent errors with some awareness of errors as they occur.

3. Difficulty sequencing phonemes, especially in diadochokinesis tasks.

4. Groping/silent posturing and difficulties in performing volitional oral movements and sequences of movements.

5. Inconsistent timing and control of nasality and prosody.

In addition, slow progress in remediation and identification by a speech–language pathologist have also been mentioned as diagnostic features (Hall[22]; Aplin[23]; Henry[24]; Bridgeman and Snowling[13]; Pollock and Hall[14]; Crary, Landess, and Towne[19]; Bashir and Strand[15]; le Normand and Chevrie-Muller[17]; Ekelman and Aram[18]; Snowling and Stackhouse[20]; Byrd and Cooper[16]; Robin[3]; and Williams, Ingham, and Rosenthal[21]) as have articulatory prolongations, syllable segregation, and increased sentence durations.[25]

Difficulty with volitional speech manifests itself in adults with AOS in relatively better production of automatic or over-learned verbal routines. In children with DVD there is comparatively better production of more iconic, less semantically loaded verbalizations, such as environmental noises ("vroom", "beep", "woof-woof", etc.), emotional responses ("ow", "uh-oh", etc.), and rote-learned productions such as songs and poems when compared with more volitional speech. In addition, there may be occasional clear productions that cannot be repeated. It may seem that the child is refusing to say words upon request that he or she has previously demonstrated the ability to produce.

Etiology

No specific neurological basis for DVD or any other type of developmental apraxia has been identified, with the exception of a few specific syndromes that are associated with particular types of nonverbal developmental apraxia. For example, Developmental Gerstmann's syndrome (a specific learning disability composed of finger agnosia, right-left disorientation, and dyscalculia) is often associated with constructional apraxia,[26] an inability to assemble parts to form a single whole structure resulting in difficulty conceptualizing and planning motor activities that are highly dependent on visual space perception.[4]

Research has shown that children with "articulation disorders" generally tend to have more motor coordination problems and soft neurological signs than do children whose speech skills are developing normally. However, as a group these children with "articulation disorders" do not necessarily show typical signs of apraxia (such as those listed above) either in their speech or in their motor skills.[27] Apraxia is often associated with left hemisphere parietal or temporal lobe lesions in adults,[28] but even in adults there is some difficulty localizing praxis. It may be dependent on a complex network of subcortical and cortical structures.[4] Certainly, many children with various forms of the disorder appear to be otherwise neurologically quite intact, although some relationships have been identified between praxis skills and tactile sensory processing, visual perception,[28] and learning disabilities.[29] Similarly, there is no known association with any particular perinatal risk factors. Although some studies have reported associations with problem pregnancies and deliveries, low birth weight, or asphyxia, others have failed to replicate these findings.[30]

Differential Diagnosis

The results of studies intended to differentiate children with DVD from children with (other) phonological disorders have been mixed and confusing. One factor that has added to this confusion is the fact that the degree of impairment in DVD can range from mild to profound. Some children with DVD may only show one consistent phoneme substitution pattern that persists into school age.[22] Clusters of characteristics that might differentiate children with DVD from children with "functional articulation disorders" in one study[31] may not facilitate the identification of any clear "apraxic-like" subgroup in a similar study.[21] Nonspeech oral apraxia and language deficits tend to co-occur with DVD, but neither is always seen in children who show signs of the disorder.

The fact that there has been little agreement on the symptoms or the theoretical constructs that are important to the diagnosis of DVD has led reviewers like Guyette and Deidrich[32] to claim that no necessary and sufficient characteristics have been described to indicate a unitary disorder. Yet, speech–language pathologists continue to encounter this subgroup of children with phonological disorders who demonstrate multiple articulation errors, effortful speech, and slow progress in remediation. Problems of etiology, characteristics, and definition raise many questions about the fundamental nature of DVD: is it a more generalized linguistic disorder, or are accompanying linguistic deficits merely the symptoms of neurological damage or differences in neighboring areas of the brain? Is it a fundamentally motoric disorder, the symptoms of which are more evident for complex motoric tasks such as speech than for simpler oral motor tasks? Even the strongest proponents of the motor view acknowledge that language deficits often accompany DVD, and they describe this disorder as an impairment of the analysis, organization, and integration of knowledge for problem-solving and adaptive behavior in the face of specific task requirements and components.[3] However, just such an impairment could be responsible for the language symptoms that often accompany DVD as well as for speech and other motor features of the disorder. Could the speech, language, and motor characteristics of DVD all be symptoms of some deeper core disability affecting both linguistic and motor development?

From both theoretical and clinical perspectives, attempting to define DVD as a unitary disorder may be akin to using a telephoto lens to photograph and understand the Grand Canyon. A wide angle lens is needed to encompass the entire scope and depth of the problem. There is growing agreement that the big picture of DVD may best be considered as a symptom complex. For example, in 1984 Aram[33] stated that "viewed as a syndrome . . . developmental verbal apraxia might be defined as a severe and persistent phonological disorder coupled with an expressive syntactic disorder with variable neurological and articulatory findings". If this is the case, then we would not necessarily expect that every child would exhibit every characteristic of the syndrome, nor that any one child's symptoms would remain static over time.[2]

If DVD is a symptom complex, what are its defining symptoms? Studies indicate that the most important areas for differential diagnosis are likely to be: motor and motor-speech skills, sequencing, suprasegmentals, vowels, voicing, and other linguistic deficits. We will consider these possible differentiating characteristics individually, including the evidence that is available for each.

MOTOR AND MOTOR-SPEECH SKILLS

Children with congenital ocular motor apraxia, which is characterized by impaired voluntary coordination of eye movements, tend also to exhibit more pervasive motor organization deficits, including oral-motor apraxia.[34] Dewey, Roy, Square-Storer, and Hayden[35] also reported that limb and oral apraxia tend to co-occur with verbal apraxia. They stated that children with verbal sequencing deficits tended to show a more generalized praxis problem, including limb apraxia. These authors indicated that children with DVD have particular difficulty in making transitions between different actions within the same motor sequence (eg, pull a knob, then turn it); repetition of the same action (such as finger-tapping) does not appear to be impaired. The children they studied also had more difficulty miming object use either on command or in imitation than demonstrating the action when they held the actual object in their hands.

Crary and Anderson[36] also investigated hand, facial (ie, nonspeech oral), and speech praxic abilities of children with and without diagnoses of DVD. They asked their subjects to perform single movements, repeated movements, and sequences of two to three movements in each domain. They found children with DVD to be slower and less accurate on sequences of movements in all domains. Their errors did not represent a breakdown in sequencing per se, but rather a breakdown in execution when sequencing made the task more of a challenge. Crary and Anderson also reported a stronger relationship between nonspeech oral skills and speech skills than between either of these and hand praxis.

Henry[24] also reported significant differences between children with probable DVD and children with normal speech and language on measures of "nonlinguistic rhythm" and diadochokinetic rate. The "speech disordered" group showed particular difficulties with more complex sequencing tasks (eg, diadochokinesis with sequences of three different syllables). Similarly, Byrd and Cooper[16] reported significant differences between groups of children who were apraxic versus those who were normal-speaking on the oral-motor movement subtest of the Screening Test for Developmental Apraxia of Speech (STDAS).[37] Interestingly, however, the performance of children with DVD did not differ significantly from that of children who stutter on this subtest.

All of these studies highlight the difficulties that *transitions between postures* pose for children with any form of apraxia. These children can often achieve the absolutes—the static articulatory, oral, or manual postures. Unfortunately, the rapid movement patterns of connected speech entail constant approximations of articulatory targets as there are no absolute or static postures. The problem for children with DVD, then, is the relativity in the organization of sequential motor-speech elements.

SEQUENCING

Sequencing difficulties—or other speech production difficulties (such as decreased accuracy or rate) that are noted when sequencing taxes the speech planning system—have been implicated in many studies, some of which have been described above. Aram and Horwitz'[38] subjects with DVD did not have difficulty with single oral movements, but demonstrated difficulty with sequences of nonspeech volitional oral movements. Byrd and Cooper[16] also found significant differences between apraxic and normal-speaking groups of children on the verbal sequencing and "transpositions" subtests of the STDAS,[37] but again the performance of the children with apraxia did not differ significantly from that of children who stutter on these subtests.

Crary, Landess, and Towne[19] reported, based on process analysis, that children with DVD exhibit high incidences of omission and voicing errors. They hypothesized that the occurrence of these sequence-dependent processes reflects spatial-temporal incoordination of the multiple components of the speech production mechanism, and that this incoordination reflects a central motor planning deficit. However, they did not compare the occurrence of these processes among children with DVD to their occurrence among other children with phonological delay/disorder.

Velleman, Huntley, and Lasker[39] found children's "phonological deviancy scores" on the Assessment of Phonological Processes-Revised[40] (APP-R) to be significantly correlated to the frequency of singleton omissions and to the number of other phonemic sequencing errors (syllable reduction, epenthesis, metathesis, migration, reduplication, coalescence, and assimilation) that occurred, but these error types were not significantly associated with apraxic characteristics when the effects of severity were controlled. That is, the frequency of occurrence of such errors appeared to be based on the severity rather than the nature of the child's phonological disorder (ie, DVD versus "functional" phonological disorder).

Thus, although sequencing does appear to be an important factor in the speech performance of children with DVD, sequencing difficulties may not manifest themselves in **phonemic** sequencing errors per se. The sequencing errors may be more evident at the articulatory level, affecting the relative timing of glottal and articulatory gestures. Errors of sequencing at this level would result in perceived errors of voicing and vowel production (especially for diphthongs); such errors are, in fact, associated with DVD (see above and below).

SUPRASEGMENTALS

Henry's[24] findings indicate that children with severe articulation problems have great difficulty reproducing modeled stress patterns on a "nonlinguistic rhythm" syllable repetition task.[†] This result is in keeping with Shriberg, Kwiatkowski, and Rasmussen's[41] suggestion that children with suspected DVD are likely to have questionable phrasing, stress, and voice quality. Byrd and Cooper[16] also reported differences between children with and without DVD on the prosody subtest of the STDAS,[37] but once again the performance of the children with DVD did not differ significantly from that of children who stutter on the subtest. This issue is reported in more depth by Robin, Hall, Jordan, and Gordan,[42] who compared the sentence stress production of six children with DVD between the ages of 7 and 10 years and six age-matched controls. They found that children with DVD were far less successful than their peers (as measured by listener identification as well as acoustically) at using fundamental frequency, duration, and intensity to mark the stressed word in a sentence.

Shuster, Ruscello, and Haines[25] replicated Kent and Rosenbek's[43] acoustic findings of prolonged segments, syllables, and sentences among adults with AOS with a 15-year-old subject with DVD. Robin et al[42] also found increased sentence durations among 7 to 10 year olds with DVD. Velleman et al[39] did not find significant duration differences in children with "functional" phonological delays versus children with DVD. However, their 29 subjects were far younger (ages 2;5 to 6;8) and therefore subject to much more temporal variability than are older children and adults (Kent and Forner[44] and Smith[45]).

VOWELS

Vowel production requires ongoing control of several muscles of the tongue and lips, with very brief static portions and no contact (eg, on the alveolar ridge) to provide tactile feedback. Vowel production errors have been reported in the DVD literature from as early as 1891.[14] Pollock and Hall[14] studied the vowel misarticulations of five children between the ages of 8 and 11 years who were diagnosed with DVD. They identified rhotic vowel errors, diphthong reduction, tense/lax neutralizations, and backing of vowels as the most common vowel errors in this group. These patterns were verified acoustically.[46]

Pollock and Hall's findings were confirmed in part for younger children (ages 2;5 to 6;8) with DVD by Velleman et al.[39] Approximately 50% of their subjects' vowel errors involved diphthongs; another 23% affected rhotic vowels. Simple vowel feature changes were also common but quite varied, without a clear dominance of tense/lax or backing errors. Although a very similar pattern of errors was noted for control subjects with other phonological delays/disorders, the frequency of vowel errors was lower among the controls even when severity levels were statistically controlled. There was a significant relationship between the number of vowel errors a child made on the APP-R[40] and the number of characteristics of DVD that child displayed (eg, deficits in initiation and imitation, rhythmic irregularities, prolongations and transpositions of sounds and syllables, possible oral dyspraxia, history of limited babbling, and slow DDK rates) according to his primary speech–language pathologist. In other words, children with

---

[†]Her "nonlinguistic rhythm" task involves repeating the syllable [ma] using modeled suprasegmental patterns, and so it is not actually speech-free.

DVD made more frequent vowel errors, but their errors did not differ **in kind** from those of other children with phonological delay or disorder.

VOICING

Voicing requires coordination and precise timing of laryngeal musculature with oral articulators. Voicing errors have been suggested as a common characteristic of adult AOS (Trost and Canter[47] and Odell et al[48]) and of DVD.[15] Crary et al[19] reported frequent use of voicing and devoicing processes among children with DVD. Of course, voicing errors are also common among children with other phonological delays/disorders and among young children whose phonologies are developing normally.[49] However, Velleman et al[39] found voicing errors to be more common among children with DVD than among children with other phonological delays/disorders, regardless of their severity.

OTHER LINGUISTIC DEFICITS

A few studies have highlighted other linguistic deficits. Such deficits are not typically reported for adults with pure adult-onset AOS, but they may accompany DVD. Marion, Sussman, and Marquardt,[50] for example, have demonstrated deficits in rhyming skills among children with DVD. Stackhouse[51] showed that children with DVD have difficulty with nonsense-word matching tasks that require use of grapheme-phoneme relationships, whereas children with cleft palate, who also have articulation difficulties, have far fewer difficulties with such metaphonological tasks. Snowling and Stackhouse[20] reported that children with DVD performed significantly worse when asked to orally imitate, spell, and read simple CVC words than did control subjects matched for reading age. Interestingly, there was not a direct correspondence between the children's pronunciation and spelling errors. Furthermore, the children with DVD did try to segment the words orally before spelling them, but this often did not seem to help. The most striking example cited was of a child who correctly repeated 'Nick', attempted to segment it orally, saying, "[kə- kə- n- ɪ- tə]", then spelled it as *C-A-T*.

It is not surprising that children with articulation disorders such as DVD have difficulty with morphology, especially morphological markers such as the English plural, possessive, and third person singular -s, and the past tense -ed, which often require the speaker to produce a consonant cluster in final position (eg, cats, Bob's, asks, marched). However, these difficulties may not be solely phonological in origin. Ekelman and Aram[18] explored the syntactic skills of children with DVD and found errors on syntactic structures that are not phonologically difficult, such as misselection of pronouns and verbs and omissions and noninversions of auxiliaries and copulas in yes-no and wh-questions. These children's grammatical skills lagged well behind their mean lengths of utterance (MLUs).

Aram and Horwitz[38] found that nine of 10 children with DVD between the ages of 4 and 13 years scored lower than one standard deviation below the mean on the sequencing portion of the *Denver Auditory Phoneme Sequencing Test*.[52] However, this task requires a sequential pointing response, so the role of possible limb apraxia cannot be ruled out. More recently, Bridgeman and Snowling[13] studied the perception of phoneme sequences in children with DVD using a task with a nonsequential motor response (pushing a button once). Building on Stackhouse's[53] clinical observation that some children with DVD have more difficulty discriminating nonsense words that differ only in the sequence of phonemes (bikut-bituk) than in discriminating nonsense words that differ in the phonemes themselves (bikut-bikup), they tested children's ability to discriminate word final segment contrasts (eg, loss-lot) versus word-final sequence contrasts (eg, lost-lots) in monosyllabic real and nonsense words. They found that children with DVD have more difficulty than controls discriminating nonsense word sequence contrasts but not segment contrasts or real word sequence contrasts.

Henry[24] also studied input processing among children with probable DVD.‡ Her subjects were given the Auditory Sequential Memory subtest of the *Illinois Test of Psycholinguistic Abilities*,[54] which assesses digit repetition skills. They performed significantly worse than age-matched peers on this subtest. However, given that repetition is required in this task, it is not clear whether their reduced performance represents input or output difficulties.

In summary, children with DVD demonstrate deficits in transitions and sequencing for speech, oral-motor, and manual tasks. These difficulties manifest themselves in speech as errors in the production of suprasegmentals, vowels, and voicing. Parallel deficits have been reported in grapheme-phoneme tasks, speech perception, and syntax.

A Model of DVD

Is it possible to discover a set of underlying unifying characteristics common to this group of symptoms within the DVD symptom complex? Recent advances in theoretical phonology provide some tentative answers.

The theory of "nonlinear phonology" emphasizes the hierarchical nature of phonological organization: phrases within sentences, words within phrases, groups of sounds (syllables, clusters, etc) and/or morphemes within words, individual sounds within groups or morphemes; phrase stress and intonation within sentence stress and intonation, word stress within phrase stress, and so forth.[55] Another recent, more biologically based model of phonology suggests that phonology and syntax share a "frame-content" organization, with syllable structure as the frame for sound segments, and grammar (including function words) as the frame for content words in sentences.[56] These two models share the concept of linguistic units at different levels within a hierarchy that are organized for the processing and production of speech. The units are the content, and the organization provides the frame.

Using these models, children with DVD could be seen as impaired in their ability to generate and utilize frames, which would otherwise provide the mechanisms

---

‡Henry implies that these children have DVD by reviewing the literature on DVD and by comparing her results with those of others who have studied children with DVD. She also comments that many of these children have vowel errors, which may distinguish them from children with milder phonological disorders. However, she states that she uses the term "speech disordered" to avoid a terminology debate.

for analyzing, organizing, and utilizing information from their motor, sensory, and linguistic systems for the production of spoken language. This would account for the fact that children with DVD are often better able to produce sounds in isolation than in the context of a whole word, and that they are often better able to produce words in isolation than to assemble them into sentences. It would explain the inability of children who are severely apraxic to get beyond the very simple open CV syllables with which many children begin the acquisition of words. From a linguistic standpoint, children with DVD might "have" the appropriate phonological (or syntactic) elements but be unable to organize them into an appropriate cognitive hierarchy. Without the proper hierarchical representation of the action, an appropriate motor plan could not be devised. The lack of a hierarchical frame into which elements of action could be organized would account for the transition difficulties that are noted in reports of all forms of apraxia.

In this view, apraxia would be seen as a disorder of hierarchical organization that manifests itself in many ways, resulting in the variety of symptoms discussed above. Thus, one might propose that the underlying source of the symptoms manifested in DVD is difficulty with "on-line" planning or programming of elements of the language/speech system into larger organized patterns. Such a single underlying source viewed as an integral part of both a theoretical model and a corresponding clinical syndrome for DVD may result in a variety of motor, phonological, linguistic, or neurological signs or symptoms, and in fact inconsistency among symptoms may be expected as typical. If this is the case, the argued distinction of whether DVD is a motor movement disorder or a linguistic disorder is irrelevant because the difficulty with organizing elements into larger and larger wholes would affect both movement and linguistic aspects of development. Taken further, DVD should not be considered a problem of elements per se whether they be articulatory postures, phonemes, morphemes, words, or sentences, but a problem of **bridging among the various elements** that constitute language performance.

Assessment

As we have seen, DVD is a dynamic symptom complex; inconsistency both between and within identifying features is inherent to the disorder. For this reason, part of the difficulty in the evaluation of DVD is that the diagnosis of the disorder can vary with the methods used to assess it. In addition, with children we are always assessing a dynamic, developing system. As a result, the clinical picture of DVD at any time depends on when the child is evaluated during the developmental period and the procedures used in the assessment.

Given that DVD, like any other developmental disorder, involves a continuum from function to dysfunction and in addition, no mutually exclusive set of symptoms, it is more appropriate to discuss areas of ability or types of symptom to be addressed in the evaluation rather than specific tests to be administered. The areas that should be included in any protocol for the assessment of DVD are the following:

1. Early history
2. Hearing status

3. Play skills (for young children)
4. Language abilities/symptoms
5. Speech abilities/symptoms
6. Motor abilities/symptoms

Each of these areas will be discussed with comments about the characteristics that we or other specialists have found to be diagnostic for the DVD symptom complex. Unfortunately, the amount of clinical research that is available on DVD is very small. For this reason, much of this discussion will reflect our own clinical experiences and those that others have shared with us.

Early History

Table 5–1 lists characteristics found to be typical of the early developmental histories of children diagnosed with DVD. The most consistent characteristics reported by parents are the lack of or late onset of `canonical' (speech-like) babbling and/or minimal variety in babbling. These symptoms of DVD were also on the "top ten list" of diagnostic characteristics reported by Velleman et al.[39]

Oller[57] has delineated the following four aspects of the well-formed syllables that are the hallmark of "canonical" (speech-like) babbling:

1. Normal phonation (not cry or vegetative)
2. Articulatory movement during phonation, yielding phonetic changes in output
3. Full resonant vocalicness—vocal tract not at rest during phonation
4. Rapid, speech-like transitions between consonant-like and vowel-like elements in the syllable

---

Table 5–1. Characteristics of Early History

---

1. Poor coordination of sucking response.
2. *Very* quiet baby.
3. Little or no babbling but vowel-like vocalizations may be heard.
4. Limited differentiation of consonants and vowels in the babbling repertoire.
5. Little spontaneous imitation of syllables.
6. Excessive drooling in spite of adequate feeding skills.
7. Language comprehension within normal limits for age.
8. Early expressive language milestones may or may not be delayed.
9. Pointing accompanied by "vowel-like" vocalization or single syllable to request or comment.
10. Natural gesture or pantomime system.
11. Isolated productions: on rare occasions the child has said a word or phrase clearly that (s)he could not repeat upon request.
12. By 24 months, excessive frustration is noted; problems with behavior management may be present.
13. Often reported to be excessively dependent or shy, especially in unfamiliar social settings.
14. Family member often cited as interpreter.

Source: Ref. 15.

His research has shown that by 5 to 10 months of age typically developing children produce this canonical babbling ([babababa], [dididi], etc.). He concluded that if a child does not produce canonical babbling by 10 months, there is reason for concern. Late onset of babbling or minimal babbling may, for children with DVD, reflect very early difficulty with the organization of consonantal and vocalic elements to form a simple canonical syllable.

Paucity in syllable variation is another hallmark of the early history of children with DVD. Stoel-Gammon[58] studied phonetic syllable forms in natural conversational interactions with 2-year-old children. Her findings showed that the average consonant inventory of typically developing 2 year olds included nine to 10 consonants in open and closed syllables.[§] This variety of syllable shapes is rarely heard in young children with DVD. If children approach 2 years of age without a repertoire of syllable shapes, they have no phonetic foundation for word production,[59,60] and both they and their parents become increasingly frustrated. It is no surprise that it is at this point that parents often seek an initial speech and language evaluation.

Stoel-Gammon[58] also reported that 2-year-old children produce target consonants in words and syllables at a level of 70% correct. The young child with DVD often has extreme difficulty with consonant production and becomes frustrated when parents attempt to engage him or her in imitation tasks.

Thus, by 2 years of age children with DVD are often demonstrating frustration with communication attempts because of the gap between their relatively good comprehension skills and their extremely limited speech and expressive language abilities. Some children develop elaborate natural gesture systems and may even sequence gestures, indicating a developing knowledge of word order. Most children are reported by their parents to be very communicative and able to get their point across despite limited speech production skills. However, in new or pressure-filled situations many young children with DVD become excessively shy and will cling to a parent whom they often use as an interpreter.

Hearing Status

As with all speech and language evaluations of young children, an audiological assessment must be completed. Young children with DVD may sound like children with severe hearing impairments because of the difficulty they have with intonation patterns. By 8 to 10 months, children who are normally developing begin to exhibit the rhythmic and intonational properties of the languages to which they have been exposed.[61] Rising and falling intonation contours associated with certain communication functions have been documented in the prelinguistic vocalizations of children who are developing normally.[62,63] As noted by Henry[24]; Shriberg, Kwiatkowski, and Rasmussen[64]; Byrd and Cooper[16]; and Robin, Hall, Jordan, and Gordan,[42] children with DVD often have difficulty varying and modulating intonation patterns as well as intensity levels for speech despite normal hearing sensitivity.

[§]Initial position classes included stops, nasals, fricatives and glides; range: 4 to 16 phonemes. Final position classes included primarily stops with some nasals, fricatives and liquids; range: 0 to 11 phonemes.

Play Skills

Assessment of representational play skills is an important part of the assessment of the young child. It has been our observation that many young children with DVD may be able to complete single functional play elements (eg, comb a doll's hair, feed a doll) but have difficulty organizing a series of play elements into an integrated pretend play sequence (eg, cook food, feed the doll, then put the doll to bed). This inability to organize and sequence play elements, in our view, is one more outward manifestation of their underlying praxis "frame" deficit; it marks an underlying difficulty in nonverbal symbolic cognitive organization similar to that noted in speech and language.

Unfortunately, the performance of children with DVD on standardized measures of symbolic play (such as the *Communication and Symbolic Behavior Scales*[65] and *The Symbolic Play Test*[66]) has not been systematically compared with that of children who are developing normally. It seems possible that a distinctive profile would emerge if this were done.

Language Abilities/Symptoms

Although DVD may be found to coexist with other developmental delays, it is difficult to make a primary diagnosis of DVD in the young child unless receptive language abilities are found to be within the normal range for chronological age. However, an apraxic component may be identified in children with other primary diagnoses (such as developmental delay or autism) when other apraxic symptoms are present and a substantial gap is found between expressive and receptive skills that cannot be attributed to other physiological sources (such as cerebral palsy). In addition, it is important to remember that as children with mild-to-moderate DVD gain better control over lower-level speech-production skills through therapy, the primary symptoms of DVD in the elementary and middle-school years may begin to be manifested in on-line comprehension and metalinguistic deficits in academic settings despite a good language knowledge base.

The focus in evaluating expressive language skills of children with DVD should be on their knowledge and use of the language structure as a frame for content words. English syntax depends fundamentally on word order. Therefore, it is important to look for emerging expressions of order in young children, such as sequencing of gestures or sequencing of word+gesture combinations. For example, a child may say "dada" and pat the floor to communicate "Daddy, sit on the floor," indicating early use of syntax-based noun+locative ordering despite limited speech production capabilities. In contrast, variable use of word ordering, such as the child who randomly alternates in early two-word utterances, between for example, "boy hat" and "hat boy" (to express "the boy has a hat" or "the boy's hat"), may be indicative of limited ability to utilize the rudiments of English sentence frames.

In the preschool and school-age years it is rare (although not unknown) for children with DVD who have progressed to the sentence production level to have difficulty with word order. More typically, these children have difficulty in organizing and using the function-word and grammatical morpheme links between the sequenced content words. Such a child might say, "Me big me policeman" to express his desire to be a police officer when he grows up. This difficulty may be demonstrated first in spoken language and later in written language, with grammatical morphemes and function words of English omitted or used incorrectly. At first this linguistic behavior may appear to be secondary to speech production problems, but studies of language samples in children with DVD have shown that omissions of grammatical morphemes are not related to deletion of unstressed syllables.[18,67] One of the authors (KS) has conducted a series of unpublished longitudinal case studies of children who were diagnosed with DVD prior to 3 years of age. She has found continuing problems with the omission of grammatical morphemes in the written narratives of these children as they grow older, even when they have learned to include the same grammatical markers in their spoken language.

Speech Abilities/Symptoms

In evaluating speech production, the nature of DVD as a disorder in the hierarchical organization of speech and language elements, including movements, transitions, and timing, should be given primary consideration. Therefore, it is crucial that speech production be assessed in a variety of contexts. Semantic context (level of vocabulary and conceptual complexity), syntactic context (length, syntactic complexity), and phonetic/phonological context all contribute to the performance load for children with DVD and should be varied systematically in an assessment of their speech production capabilities. Although the STDAS[37] and the *Tests for Apraxia of Speech and Oral Apraxia-Children's Battery*[68] address systematic changes in the phonetic complexity of speech production tasks, these tests do not take into account the added complexity provided by semantic and syntactic contexts. Such systematic performance load changes are best accomplished through informal procedures (such as a play-based spontaneous speech sample) and/or based on information from the language assessment portion of the evaluation.

In assessing speech production abilities, it is important to analyze both segmental and suprasegmental speech characteristics.

SEGMENTAL SPEECH CHARACTERISTICS

Young children or children with severe DVD may be unwilling or unable to produce specific words or phrases upon request, especially in the presence of an unfamiliar examiner in an unfamiliar location exerting such communication pressure on the child. Indeed, they may be able to produce only a very small number of words in any context. For these children, a transcribed speech sample may be the only speech production data available to the examiner. In this case, a careful analysis of the child's phonetic (sound), phonotactic (word and syllable shape), and (if the sample size is large enough) phonemic repertoires should be carried out. Phonological process or rule analyses are inappropriate for children with very limited expressive vocabularies[69]; those portions of more in-depth analysis procedures (such as *Procedures for the Phonological Analysis of Children's Language*,[70] *Phonological Assessment of Child Speech (PACS)*,[71] and Bernhardt's suggestions for applying nonlinear phonological theory to disordered speech[72,73]) that specifically address phonetic and phonotactic repertoires are more appropriate. Variety within each of these repertoires, especially word and syllable shapes, is key to the assessment of severity. In our experience, the child who produces very few consonant and/or vowel sounds and/or has a highly restricted number of syllable/word shapes (eg, [ba], [da], [bʌ], [dʌ]) has a more guarded prognosis than an equally unintelligible child who produces more varied syllables and words. The former child has a more significant deficit in organizing frames and in filling these frames with appropriate content.

With children who are older or less impaired, an extended sample may be elicited. Although most articulation tests assess speech segments at the level of the phoneme, the basic element in the assessment of the speech production skills of children with DVD should be the syllable. Therefore, the contexts in which the phonemes are assessed must be taken into serious consideration. The variety of syllable and word shapes produced by the child is typically not addressed by traditional articulation tests and must be assessed informally by the examiner who uses these measures. Additionally, assessment tools that focus on both segmental and syllable/word-level phonological patterns, such as the *Bankson-Bernthal Test of Phonology* (BBTOP),[74] *The ALPHA Test of Phonology*,[75] and the *Khan-Lewis Phonological Analysis* procedure[76] are very helpful.

Even more critical is the production of the syllable within connected speech. In this regard, articulation tests such as the ALPHA[75] that assess target segments within a controlled phrase context are useful, as are more detailed phonological analysis procedures based on longer spontaneous speech samples, such as *Procedures for the Phonological Analysis of Children's Language*,[70] *PACS*,[71] and *Natural Process Analysis (NPA)*.[77]

Apparently inconsistent substitutions have been considered a hallmark of DVD. If we consider DVD to be a problem of organized movement within and between syllables, accurate production of segments would depend on the position of the phoneme in the syllable sequence and on any movement components within the phoneme itself far more than on the static properties of the particular articulatory posture for that phoneme. For example, deficits in controlling the precise timing requirements for appropriate voicing could affect any consonant depending on the voicing status of neighboring segments. Thus, the actual production of any one consonant would differ in differing phonetic contexts. Similarly, the movement components of all diphthongs (including rhotic vowels) would be expected to be troublesome, with the level of difficulty dependent in part on the positioning requirements of other portions of the word (eg, the back-to-front articulation of the diphthong [aɪ] could be facilitated by the parallel back-to-front articulatory pattern of the surrounding consonants in "kite"). As we saw above, errors of voicing and of diphthong and rhotic vowel production are endemic to DVD. For these reasons, it is vital that we use assessment tools such as those listed above that identify production patterns affecting whole **classes of sounds** (ie, processes or phonological rules) in addition to more traditional sound-by-sound analyses.

In children under 8 years of age, it is important to consider that two issues coexist: a developing phonological system, which may include appropriately immature phonological patterns or "processes"; and the child's attempts to compensate for phonetic performance difficulties, which may result in unusual phonological patterns ("deviant processes"). In older children with DVD, phonetic performance difficulties with phonemes that require complex coordinated articulatory adjustments often continue into the middle-school years, long after immature phonological processes are expected to have disappeared. These ongoing difficulties may appear to manifest themselves as either limited use of earlier processes (eg, simplification of more complex consonant clusters) or as articulatory distortions of particular sounds in particular contexts. Both types of patterns may result from attempts to simplify the required coordination of a complex articulatory gesture or sequence of gestures while aiming to retain critical features. For example, a lateralized production of /s/ is a frequent misarticulation produced by middle-school children with DVD. They maintain the critical feature of frication but cannot simultaneously coordinate the groove in the middle of the tongue with elevation of the sides of the tongue. Such distortions result not from muscle weakness as seen in dysarthria, but from an inability to organize several movement components at one time within the flow of speech.

Children with DVD often have difficulty maintaining control of a syllable shape for multiple repetitions. Therefore, on a test of diadochokinetic syllable rates, the syllable shape often becomes increasingly distorted with multiple repetitions unless the child slows the rate considerably to return to a neutral position after each syllable production. Intermittent pauses between syllables, words, and phrases are typically heard in the speech of children with DVD as they "buy time" for the organization and initiation of upcoming movement plans. Returning the oral musculature to a neutral position during the pause provides a familiar starting point for organizing upcoming motor plans.

At the word level, imitation of words that increase in number of syllables (eg, "please, pleasing, pleasingly") should be included in the assessment to look at the increasingly complex organization of syllables at the word level. Children with DVD often have less difficulty with the production of words composed of multiple morphemes (eg, doorkeeper) than with a single-word morpheme composed of multiple syllables (eg, decrepit), possibly because the shorter individual morphemes are familiar chunks with pre-existing motor plans, freeing the child to focus on transitions at the level of a larger organized pattern, the multisyllabic word.

SUPRASEGMENTAL SPEECH CHARACTERISTICS

Difficulty with dynamic organization is not only a problem in the articulation of segments and syllables but is also apparent at the suprasegmental level, as the child struggles to coordinate the laryngeal and respiratory systems with the oral motor mechanism. It is this coordination of the segmental with the suprasegmental organization that often distinguishes children with DVD from children with other types of articulatory/phonological problems.

Very young children with DVD often have difficulty varying intonation contours to appropriately communicate meaningful intent. Indeed many parents have reported that when listening to their child from another room, they cannot tell whether the child is laughing or crying because there is little change in the quality of the vocalizations. In addition, many very young children have been noted to have difficulty vocalizing exclusively on exhalation and will vocalize on inhalation long after such vocalization patterns have been eliminated by typically developing children (at about 6 months of age[78,79]).

Children with DVD often have difficulty modulating their loudness levels, resulting in speech that is either too loud or too soft. In addition, the voice quality of children with DVD often alternates between hyponasality and hypernasality as a result of difficulty with the automatic, precise, and rapid organization required for velopharyngeal valving and oral movements.

Prosody may be functionally characterized as the ability to maintain the rhythm and intonation of speech over time. Interruption of prosody is heard as dysfluency. As children with DVD show improvement in their segmental speech characteristics, they often suddenly become dysfluent. They may be heard to prolong vowels because by prolonging the steady state of the vowel they are "buying time" to organize the coordination of the next series of movements. Also, difficulty with initiation of speech is often noted in children with DVD as they are attempting to plan the shape of the syllable. These tendencies no doubt account for the similarities between children who are dysfluent and children with DVD reported by Byrd and Cooper.[16] Long pauses, slow rate, and articulatory prolongations in children with DVD must be assessed within the context of underlying phonetic organizational difficulties varying with semantic, syntactic, and phonological complexity and within the bigger picture of previous history, language, play, and nonverbal oral-motor skills to differentiate DVD from stuttering in such children.

Motor Abilities/Symptoms

As we have seen, the presence of oral dyspraxia in DVD is a source of controversy in the literature. Some sources say oral apraxia usually accompanies DVD, while others suggest incidences of 50% or less.[38] For this reason it is often useful to ask the parents about the child's feeding history and current status. Oral motor movement tasks as well as other motor coordination tasks (such as a thumb-finger opposition task or the fist-edge-palm test) should also be included in the assessment but do not bear directly in the actual diagnosis of DVD. As part of the syndrome some children may have additional praxis problems, while others do not. Also, some children with DVD exhibit mildly reduced tone, making them appear to be "floppy" overall. In these cases, referral for an occupational therapy evaluation may be helpful.[80]

For these reasons, it is important that the motor assessment of children with DVD include measures of strength, tone, and stability of the oral structures. The following questions should be addressed:

1A. What does the child have to do to stabilize the mandible for speech production? (eg, Does he thrust the mandible forward, thrust his head back?)

  B. What effect do those adjustments have on other body movements?

  2. Can the child move the tongue independently of the mandible?

Often excessive jaw movement is observed, which slows tongue movement. A bite block for jaw stabilization might be introduced to assess differences in the rate and precision of lingual movements.

For many children with DVD drooling is more excessive than normal during the early years and persists for a longer time. The drooling is often least problematic when the child is eating and increases when he or she is engaged in other motor activities, especially when speaking. For many older children, drooling may not be obvious but saliva pooling may be present and sometimes apparent during speech.

Finally, for many children oral motor or speech imitation abilities are poor,[39] particularly if they are provided only with an auditory model. It has often been noted that imitation improves with the introduction of visual and tactile feedback.[81] As we might expect, imitation difficulty may not be apparent for single articulatory positions. It is the relative temporal and spatial relationships and the constantly changing organizational patterns required in connected speech that are difficult. In addition, the task of imitating brings the motor planning process to a more conscious, less automated level, which we have seen exacerbates the praxis deficits in DVD and other forms of apraxia.

Prognosis

A commonly held notion among many speech–language pathologists is that a diagnosis of DVD suggests a poor prognosis, with an exceptionally long and slow course of treatment. Likewise, many clinicians have been known to use a child's rate of progress in treatment as a deciding factor in the diagnosis of DVD (ie, if he or she has a slow course of treatment, the diagnosis of DVD is confirmed and if perchance his or her progress in treatment is rapid, the diagnosis of DVD must have been incorrect). Unfortunately, objective data regarding predictive indicators for DVD are seriously lacking. However, it is clear that prognosis for DVD, as for any other primary developmental speech or language disorder, exists along a continuum and depends on many factors, not the least of which is matching the appropriate treatment approach to the diagnosis. It is our opinion that much of the history surrounding the poor prognosis and slow rate of progress for children with DVD has existed because the treatment methods were not appropriately matched to the areas of specific difficulty. As researchers and clinicians have progressed in understanding the disorder of DVD, it is to be hoped that a better match between diagnosis and treatment approaches will result in greater success in remediation.

Treatment

Any useful diagnostic category should have implications for treatment. In the case of DVD, in which the difficulty lies in the organization of elements into wholes, any effective treatment program must have the overall goal of habituating rapid and precise planning or programming of segments of the language/speech system into larger organized patterns. Treatment becomes a matter of helping the child build the necessary bridges among the phonological, syntactic, and morphologic elements to create the integrated form of the language. In addition, if DVD is correctly viewed as a disorder in the organization of movement, transitions, and timing, treatment plans should include a variety of dynamic speech and language contexts for practice. As Ayres[4] has observed with reference to praxis disorders in general, if our treatments consist solely of drilling the child on particular constant sequences of movements, those sequences will become automatic. But we will not have addressed the underlying disorder, which is one of planning sequences that are not yet automatic. We must focus instead on either providing tasks that are new enough to be a challenge to the motor planning mechanism, yet familiar enough to be achievable, or focus on the application of learned speech skills to new contexts. For some children with DVD, simply repeating a well-learned word with their eyes closed, with a different intonation pattern, or within a new play routine is a monumental challenge.

Some of the traditional treatment approaches for DVD are helpful precisely because they incorporate components that facilitate the integration of language elements. Touch cues,[82] for example, provide supplemental cues to the child about positioning and movements of the articulators, which can facilitate oral motor planning for those children with reduced oral kinesthetic and proprioceptive awareness. Melodic intonation therapy[83] provides a suprasegmental frame for speaking, allowing the child to focus on verbal content. A pacing board serves a similar purpose, helping the child to sequence and transition from syllable to syllable or word to word with an external representation of structure (the board) and cross-modal (oral and manual) proprioceptive cues. These and other treatment approaches can be tailored to the age, sophistication, and motoric and linguistic strengths and weaknesses of the individual child to help him or her to analyze, organize, and successfully utilize speech and language structures.

Treatment with the Very Young Child

Treatment with the child under 3 years of age involves creating an environment to encourage increased exploration of the speech sound repertoire and to facilitate consistency in the use of meaningful syllable patterns.

Increasing variety in the speech sound repertoire is often a most difficult first step in the treatment process with the very young child and may be achieved more successfully when the child is focused on other movement activities. Depending on the child's overall motor status, this may best be done within the context of occupational or physical therapy sessions. Co-treatment is often a very effective approach at this beginning level for those children who demonstrate other types of apraxia and/or reduced muscle tone.[80] If co-treatment is either not appropriate or not feasible, the speech–language pathologist may wish to incorporate age-appropriate movement activities into therapy sessions.

Associating different pitches (high or low) or loudness levels with particular environmental sounds (eg, animals or vehicles) may be a first step in assisting the child to control some dynamic aspects of speech production. For the child with slightly more phonetic control, it is important to focus on the consistent use of specific phoneme sequences associated with meaning. Although the use of nonsense syllable drills has its place in an effective treatment program for the older child, decreasing frustration by increasing communicative effectiveness must be an immediate goal for very young children. Furthermore, nonsense drills are too abstract an activity to have any short-term or long-term success with the child under 3 years of age. Instead, use of meaningful syllable productions (eg, "go!", "pop!") to trigger an effect (eg, car going down a slide, clown popping up in a pop-up toy) in cause and effect play activities is highly motivating to the toddler.

In such activities the particular syllable chosen should be within the repertoire of the child, with the goal being consistent production of that syllable or string of syllables to produce the desired result. Associating different environmental sounds or syllable combinations (word approximations) with different actions and emotions increases the meaningful speech repertoire of the very young child in activities that are often engaging and repeated many times during the day with parents and other caregivers.

For the child between 18 and 36 months of age, it is also important to address the development of sequentially organized play themes as an aspect of the overall treatment plan. Such play should follow the course of development from context-bound schemes (eg, feeding a particular doll with a particular toy bottle) to individual repeated single schemes (eg, feeding a doll, feeding self, feeding mommy), unordered multischeme combinations (eg, feeding the doll then putting it to bed), and finally larger patterns of sequenced pretend play combinations (eg, pretending to pour tea into a cup, stirring it, having the doll drink it). The child should also be encouraged to develop flexibility with regard to referents (eg, feeding the doll with any toy bottle that happens to be available) and eventually to be able to use symbolic referents (eg, using a block as a baby bottle) and even imaginary referents (eg, shaping hand as if it held a baby bottle).

With some children, feeding skills and/or drooling will need to be addressed either within the speech–language therapy context or by other professionals, depending on the site and/or the training of the speech–language pathologist. Techniques may include providing oral stimulation and encouraging parents to do so at home through varied textures of foods and appropriate toys (eg, teething toys) and cueing the child tactually, auditorily, and/or visually to be aware of his or her drool and to swallow when needed.

Finally, the social skills and self-confidence of young children with DVD must also be considered in treatment planning. Many of these children are extremely shy as a result of their speech production difficulties; often they are reluctant to make eye contact, instead tilting their heads to the floor. This results not only in social isolation but also deprives the child of an important external source of information about articulatory performance: the faces of those who speak to him or her. For those who demonstrate this tendency, eye contact with the speaker should be encouraged when appropriate.[84] In some children with DVD, however, the additional performance load of making eye contact may be prohibitively "expensive."

Treatment with the Preschool and Early School-Age Child

A listing of the basic principles of a treatment program for the preschool and early school-age child is found in Table 5–2. Sometime between 3 and 4 years of age, a child begins to be able to accommodate a more structured and "metalinguistic" approach to treatment. At this point treatment objectives may be addressed through explicit speech production approaches and activities, and the use of nonsense words may be introduced for more direct speech production practice. This type of activity helps the child to master the purely motoric tasks of sequencing and transitioning speech sounds outside of the semantically loaded linguistic context, just as practicing scales and chords helps the piano student to

Table 5–2.   Basic Principles of a Speech Production Treatment
Program for Children with DVD

1. Main focus of treatment should be syllable structure control and organization within a variety of dynamic linguistic contexts.

2. A successful program is one that will facilitate correct production of varying syllable shapes and the organization of these shapes into longer and increasingly complex phonotatic patterns.

3. A sound-by-sound treatment plan that emphasizes phoneme production in isolation prior to moving to words and phrases does *not* address the hierarchical dynamic movement problem in DVD.

4. Auditory discrimination training does *not* address the problem.

5. Frequent, short sessions with breaks are most successful. Because DVD is a dynamic disorder, system fatigue is a problem.

6. Sessions should be divided into short parts:
   a. Warm-ups: Imitation of body and/or oral motor sequences.
   b. Practicing the scales: Syllable sequence drill activities. Establish consistent connected syllable productions from within the child's repertoire. Include sequences that vary articulatory positions, for example, from front to back ([bʌdʌgʌ] or "buttercup") or vice versa ([gʌdʌbʌ] or "go to bed").
   c. Learning the song: Meaningful single-word activities to include a core group of words that would increase overall intelligibility of speech.
   d. Changing the song: Short sentence activities starting with a key carrier phrase and changing one word, gradually increasing in length and complexity.

become more aware of finger positioning and to organize the fingers to transition from one note to another fluidly. Particularly for children with accompanying oral motor apraxia, this may facilitate the later integration of speech production skills into larger linguistic units.

As stated earlier, treatment plans should include a variety of dynamic speech contexts for practice with the goal of creating integrated linguistic wholes at higher levels. For this reason, principle 6 in Table 5–2 suggests the breakdown of a treatment session into parts with specific treatment methods to be employed in different portions of the session. However, some techniques may have more general usefulness. For example, the use of touch-cues[82] or other tactile systems[85] or a modified melodic intonation program[83] may be successfully incorporated during any portion of the session. We have found pacing boards to be a successful tool at both the word and sentence levels for providing visual and motor cues for the child attempting to smoothly merge phonetic parts into larger patterns.

Some related materials have also been useful for phonetic-level practice. A customized (ie, clinician-made) flip-book[Π] may be created by the clinician to accommodate the child's sound and syllable repertoire at any point in the treatment process. Individual sounds, syllables, or words may be written on each of four (or more) horizontal pages of small top-bound spiral notebooks.[¶] These pages

---

[Π]Many thanks to Suzanne Evans Morris who introduced the flipbook prototype to KS when they were working together at the Illinois State Pediatric Institute many years ago.

[¶]Alternatively, small slips of paper or small pictures (eg, 1-inch Mayer-Johnson[86] pictures) may be used in the spaces of a pacing board.

may be "flipped" individually to create different sound and syllable patterns for the child to repeat (eg, ba-bu-ba-bu), beginning with the consistent production of the same syllable repetitively (eg, ba-ba-ba-ba), which may be quite challenging for some young children or children with moderate-to-severe DVD. The goal of these (nonsense) syllable drills is to get the child to focus on movement patterns exclusive of word meanings. Variations of rate and stress may also be added to these drills to focus the child's practice on the dynamic organization of movement, transition, and timing. A similar commercially available product that focuses on the training of articulatory sound sequences by systematically varying movement patterns within words is *Moving Across Syllables*.[87]

"Key word" pictures (eg, a picture of a sheep paired with the syllable [ba], a ghost with [bu]) may be used in flip books with children who are not yet ready to associate sounds with letter symbols and/or by clinicians who feel uncomfortable with the use of nonsense syllables.[88] For children who cannot (or will not) produce nonsense or meaningful speech sequences under the explicit elicitation conditions of a flip book, practice in consistently producing the same phonetic target at a particular rate or with a particular intonation pattern may also be provided using counting books. Rather than counting the objects pictured, the clinician should point to and name each object as many times as it appears (eg, "Four dogs. Dog dog dog dog.") and encourage the child to do the same. The familiar book-reading context of this activity lowers the communication pressure on the child, who may therefore be better able to produce repetitive phonetic sequences.

At the level of short sentence activities, the use of predictable books (ie, books that repeat routinized verbal patterns) is an excellent source of motivating activities for children with emerging literacy skills. In addition to emphasizing repeated syntactic frames, these books provide movement (eg, Hop on Pop) and/or rhythm (eg, nursery rhymes) pattern practice and can be used as a framework for adapted melodic intonation therapy. For children without significant limb apraxia, the hand movements in finger plays (eg, Wheels on the Bus) sometimes provide a supportive nonlinguistic frame for the routinized linguistic content as well.

Introduction of new articulatory patterns has not been included as a treatment plan principle in Table 5–2 because it is not unique to a therapy program for DVD. Similar decision trees are followed for introducing new sounds, classes of sounds, or word shapes (eg, bisyllables) to children with DVD as for other types of developmental articulation problems, with the guiding principle being to maximize intelligibility. As indicated above ("Differential Diagnosis" section), however, certain classes of sounds or features (eg, vowels, voicing) are likely to require more emphasis than is required for children with "functional" phonological disorders. It is especially important to remember the additional difficulties that many children with DVD experience in producing vowels, especially those with a movement component (such as diphthongs and rhotic vowels), as errors in this class of phonemes often go unnoticed by speech–language pathologists.

The use of touch cues when introducing new placement positions is effective with many children in providing visual and tactile information to aid in distinguishing among various motor plans.[82] However, the articulatory focus implied by the use of touch cues does not imply that phonological principles are irrelevant to treatment. Because children with DVD have a strong tendency to have difficulty with entire classes of sounds or word shapes, therapy approaches that target phonological error patterns (eg, voicing, stopping, final consonant deletion, syllable reduction, etc) are quite appropriate if supplemented with placement information such as that provided by touch cues. Even more than with children with other phonological difficulties, goals should focus on successive approximations to correct production. For example, syllable closure (production of final consonants) may be achieved at the cost of accurate consonant production; the child may only be able to close syllables with one particular consonant at first (correctly saying, eg, [bʊk] for "book" but also [buk] for "boot" and [bok] for "boat"), or may only be able to produce CVC's in which both consonants are identical (eg, [gɔg] for "dog", [taet] for "cat" etc). Similarly, attempts at correct vowel productions may affect adjacent consonants; this should not influence the clinician to defer continuing focus on the vowel in favor of additional, perhaps unnecessary, emphasis on the surrounding consonants.[89]

Contrary to tradition, the nature of DVD as we now understand it implies that the training of particular sounds in isolation does not address the underlying problem. This has been our clinical experience, as well as that of many others.[15,83,84] In fact, new sounds should not be practiced in only one context; they should be inserted into a variety of movement contexts as soon as possible because the difficulty for children with DVD is not isolated sound production but production of phonemes within changing phonetic contexts (Table 5–2, principle 3). It is important to remember Ayres'[4] caution against drilling children with DVD on only particular constant sequences of movements. Sequences that are drilled will become automatic, and it is important for increasing intelligibility and decreasing frustration that the child establish a functional core vocabulary. But overlearning one set of words does not address the underlying disorder, which is one of planning sequences that are not yet automatic. We must focus on both providing tasks that are an achievable challenge for the motor planning mechanism and on the application of learned speech skills to new contexts. These two basic goals—establishing a functional vocabulary and addressing the fundamental motor planning component of the disorder—must be carefully balanced in the treatment of each individual child.

Finally, although it is necessary to deal with both phonetics and other aspects of language in treatment for DVD, the adage about old form-new content and vice versa certainly applies to planning intervention for these children. The emphasis in any one activity should be on either phonetic performance or on some other aspect of linguistic structure. New syntactic and morphological structures should be introduced using phonetic strings that are already within the child's phonetic repertoire. Conversely, more complex phonetic plans should be addressed in contexts of familiar sentence frames (or in nonsense words). In our experience, asking the child to divide attention between phonetic and other linguistic plans is counterproductive and slows the rate of progress in either area. This principle may require altering traditional protocols for grammatical intervention. For example, both of the authors have found it far more successful to introduce new morphological concepts (eg, plural) using phonetically easier morphological variants, despite the developmental order in which these forms are more typically acquired. The -es plural, for instance, can be approximated with a syllable (eg, [hauʔəʔ] for "houses"). The -s and -z plurals, which are developmentally earlier in typical children, are articulatorily more difficult in themselves and often require the production of a final consonant cluster as well. The same reasoning applies to other sibilant-final morphemes in English (possessive and third person singular) and to regular past tenses (-ed versus -t and -d variants). The introduction of a phonetically easier form allows the child to acquire a new grammatical meaning despite limited speech production capabilities.

Additional Treatment Considerations with Older Children

As the child matures, it becomes increasingly important for him or her to take responsibility for the design and success of his or her own treatment program. For the child with a long course of therapy, it may be appropriate to consider an occasional treatment break, even though further treatment may be needed later on. Not only may a break be important for the child psychologically, but therapeutically it allows a period of time for the child to stabilize and make newly learned abilities automatic before moving on to acquire additional new skills.

Many children with DVD are competent—albeit not gifted—users of English phonological structures by the middle-school years. Remaining speech production difficulties are likely to lie in the production of unfamiliar multisyllabic words, complex consonant clusters, certain particularly difficult phonemes (eg, [s]), and the like; these may be treated using adaptations of the techniques described above. Situations with higher levels of communication pressure, such as public speaking, may also continue to cause a breakdown in phonetic planning skills.

Depending on the child's educational level and the curriculum requirements, however, the primary focus of treatment may shift to address oral and written **language** issues in older children. For example, some children with DVD who do not have difficulty learning the decoding skills necessary for reading may nonetheless demonstrate problems with written language when words are integrated into longer more complex chunks of prose. In an ongoing longitudinal study, one of the authors (KS) is finding that children with a history of DVD demonstrate difficulty with text cohesion that becomes more apparent in the middle elementary grades as they engage in more extensive written language tasks. The use of "semantic organizer" approaches to writing instruction[90] as well as explicit discussion of literary cohesive devices are helpful treatment techniques.

Finally, it is increasingly important that older children with DVD be explicitly taught strategies for advocating for themselves with teachers and other school staff to maximize their academic potential. For example, the student may need to inform his or her teachers that he or she needs additional time to formulate an oral response, or that he or she will be able to speak more fluently if permitted to present oral reports one-on-one to the teacher, rather than in front of the entire class. As the child enters the middle elementary grades it becomes increasingly less appropriate for the parent to act as the primary advocate in day-to-day situations with teachers. Discussion of realistic speech expectations with the child often provides a motivating force for developing effective self-advocacy skills.

Use of Augmentative Communication Systems

The goal in the introduction of any augmentative system is to maximize speech intelligibility to facilitate independent communication. Many children with DVD develop a natural gesture and/or pantomime system on their own to increase successful communication. The use of natural augmentative gestures and facial expressions should be encouraged and indeed modeled, especially for children who are very young or severely affected.

With preschool and school-age children, the decision to introduce an augmentative communication system must be made on a case-by-case basis. Some families and children eagerly accept the idea of such a system because it reduces the frustration of communication attempts. For others it is not a feasible alternative. Often the level of frustration faced by the child and his family will be the determining factor in cases involving young children. If the motivation is only on the part of the speech–language pathologist, and the parents and child have minimal difficulty communicating, the probability of success is significantly lowered. In these cases, working on related skills and activities (eg, developing scanning skills and attention to visual input as a prerequisite to the possible future use of a communication board, encouraging use of creative gestures as a possible prerequisite to sign language) may be the best policy in case it becomes clear later to all concerned that oral communication will need to be supplemented in some way.

If the decision to introduce an augmentative system has been made, the issue of type of system must be addressed. One critical variable is the role that this system will play in the child's overall communication profile: is the augmentative system a supplement for a child who is often able to get his or her point across orally, or will it serve as his or her primary communication mode? For many children with severe DVD another critical variable in choosing such a system is the extent to which other motor abilities are impaired. Often the decision of whether to introduce sign as a system to augment speech at greater than the single-word level is dependent on this variable; if the child's ability to motor-plan a sequence of manual postures is as impaired as his or her ability to motor plan sequences of articulatory postures, manual language is usually not helpful. Many other factors, such as portability, ease of use for both communication partners, and communication needs must also be considered. A comprehensive augmentative communication assessment, such as that proposed by Shane and Bashir,[91] will assist in the resolution of many of these questions.

Future Directions

In 1984, Jaffe[92] suggested that, "Speech and language pathologists have an unprecedented opportunity to ask pertinent questions, to share their clinical experiences in evaluation and treatment, and to conduct research in this area." Unfortunately, although more basic research in DVD has continued, clinical research is still sorely lacking. Many treatment techniques have been proposed by the present authors and many others; the majority of these have not been subjected to objective efficacy studies.[81] Prognostic indicators for initial progress in therapy and for long-term success in speech, language, and academics are virtually unknown. Given the severity and potential longevity of the impairments in

DVD, it is vital that the most efficient and effective intervention strategies for different disorder profiles within the symptom complex be identified and verified as soon as possible.

Co-occurring characteristics also warrant further investigation. Specifically, there have been anecdotal reports by speech–language pathologists that some children with histories of motor planning problems for speech that may be largely resolved by the middle-school years also demonstrate difficulties with language comprehension stemming from central auditory processing disorders (CAPD). It is interesting to speculate why these problems may co-exist. Is there a common substrate that might account for deficits in both of these areas? Auditory processing is dependent on the rate, phonetic accuracy, and sequential order in which auditory information passes through the auditory system; praxis includes the analogous operations of timing, accurate coordination of movements, and sequential linking of individual segments. The pervasive transitions and coarticulatory effects that complicate computer recognition of speech may cause similar difficulties for linguistic input as well as output for some children with DVD. In this sense, DVD and CAPD may be flip sides of the same coin.

As we write this chapter, much about the classification, assessment, and treatment of DVD remains a puzzle. There is much work yet to be done. Many clarifying pieces of this puzzle will be found through careful longitudinal case studies on the part of all who value the art and science of clinical research.

References

1. Deputy PN: The need for description in the study of developmental verbal dyspraxia. *Australian Journal of Human Communication Disorders* 1984; 12(2):3–13.
2. Hall PK: At the center of controversy: Developmental apraxia. *American Journal of Speech-Language Pathology* 1992; 1(3):23–25.
3. Robin DA: Developmental apraxia of speech: Just another motor problem. *American Journal of Speech–Language Pathology* 1992; 1(3):19–22.
4. Ayres AJ: *Developmental Dyspraxia and Adult-Onset Apraxia*. Torrance CA, Sensory Integration International, 1985.
5. Strub RL, Black FW: *Organic Brain Syndromes: An Introduction to Neurobehavioral Disorders*. Philadelphia, F.A. Davis Co., 1981, p 232.
6. Kimura D, Archibald Y: Motor functions of the left hemisphere. *Brain* 1974; 97:337–350.
7. Darley FL, Aronson AE, Brown JR: *Motor Speech Disorders*. Philadelphia, W.B. Saunders Co., 1975.
8. Collins M, Rosenbek JC, Wertz RT: Spectrographic analysis of vowel and word duration in apraxia of speech. *Journal of Speech and Hearing Research* 1983; 26:217–224.
9. Martin AD: Some objections to the term apraxia of speech. *Journal of Speech and Hearing Disorders* 1974; 39:53–64.
10. Lebrun Y: Apraxia of Speech: The History of a Concept, in Square-Storer P (ed): *Acquired Apraxia of Speech in Aphasic Adults: Theoretical and Clinical Issues*. New York, Taylor and Francis, 1989, pp 3–19.
11. Rosenbek JC, Kent RD, LaPointe LL: Apraxia of Speech: An Overview and Some Perspectives, in Rosenbek JC, McNeil MR, Aronson AE (eds): *Apraxia of Speech: Physiology, Acoustics, Linguistics, Management*. San Diego, College-Hill Press, 1984, pp 1–72.
12. Betsworth MK, Hall PK: *The Presence of Variability in Developmental Apraxia of Speech*. Paper presented at the American Speech-Language-Hearing Association Annual Convention, St. Louis, November 1989.
13. Bridgeman E, Snowling M: The perception of phoneme sequence: A comparison of dyspraxic and normal children. *British Journal of Disorders of Communication* 1988; 23:245–252.
14. Pollock KE, Hall PK: An analysis of the vowel misarticulations of five children with developmental apraxia of speech. *Clinical Linguistics and Phonetics* 1991; 5(3):207–224.
15. Bashir AS, Strand KE: *Developmental Verbal Dyspraxia: Issues Related to Clinical Assessment and Management*. Workshop presented at Braintree Hospital Center for Communication Disorders, Braintree, MA, 1990.

16. Byrd K, Cooper EB: Apraxic speech characteristics in stuttering, developmentally apraxic, and normal speaking children. *Journal of Fluency Disorders* 1989; 14:215–229.
17. leNormand MT, Chevrie-Muller C: A follow-up case study of transitory development apraxia of speech: 'L'enfant a voyelles'. *Clinical Linguistics and Phonetics* 1991; 5(2):99–118.
18. Ekelman BL, Aram DM: Syntactic findings in developmental verbal apraxia. *Journal of Communication Disorders* 1983; 16:237–250.
19. Crary MA, Landess S, Towne R: Phonological error patterns in developmental verbal dyspraxia. *Journal of Clinical Neuropsychology* 1984; 6(2):157–170.
20. Snowling M, Stackhouse J: Spelling performance of children with developmental verbal dyspraxia. *Developmental Medicine and Child Neurology* 1983; 25:430–437.
21. Williams R, Ingham RJ, Rosenthal J: A further analysis for developmental apraxia of speech in children with defective articulation. *Journal of Speech and Hearing Research* 1981; 24:496–505.
22. Hall PK: The occurrence of developmental apraxia of speech in a mild articulation disorder: A case study. *Journal of Communication Disorders* 1989; 22:265–276.
23. Aplin DY.: Classification of dyspraxia in hearing-impaired children using the Q-technique of factor analysis. *Journal of Child Psychology and Psychiatry* 1987; 28(4):581–596.
24. Henry CE: The development of oral diadochokinesia and non-linguistic rhythm skills in normal and speech-disordered young children. *Clinical Linguistics & Phonetics* 1990; 4(2):121–137.
25. Shuster LI, Ruscello DM, Haines KB: *Acoustic patterns of developmental apraxia of speech.* Paper presented at the American Speech-Language-Hearing Association Annual Convention, St. Louis, November 1989.
26. Pebenito R, Fisch CB, Fisch ML: Developmental Gerstmann's syndrome. *Archives of Neurology* 1988; 45:977–982.
27. Cermak SA, Ward EA, Ward LM: The relationship between articulation disorders and motor coordination in children. *American Journal of Occupational Therapy* 1986; 40(8):546–550.
28. Ayres AJ, Mailloux ZK, Wendler CLW: Developmental dyspraxia: Is it a unitary function? *Occupational Therapy Journal of Research* 1987; 7(2):93–110.
29. Conrad KE, Cermak SA, Drake C: Differentiation of praxis among children. *American Journal of Occupational Therapy* 1983; 37(7):466–473.
30. Iloeje SO: Developmental apraxia among Nigerian children in Enugu, Nigeria. *Developmental Medicine and Child Neurology* 1987; 29:502–507.
31. Yoss K, Darley R: Developmental apraxia of speech in children with defective articulation. *Journal of Speech and Hearing Research* 1974; 17:399–416.
32. Guyette T, Diedrich W: A Critical Review of Developmental Apraxia of Speech, in Lass M (ed): *Speech and Language: Advances in Basic Research and Practice,* vol. 5. New York, Academic Press, 1981, pp 1–48.
33. Aram D: Assessment and treatment of developmental apraxia. *Seminars in Speech and Language* 1984; 5:2. Preface.
34. Rappaport L, Urion D, Strand K, Fulton AB: Concurrence of congenital ocular motor apraxia and other motor problems: An expanded syndrome. *Developmental Medicine and Child Neurology* 1987; 29:85–90.
35. Dewey D, Roy EA, Square-Storer PA, Hayden D: Limb and oral praxic abilities of children with verbal sequencing deficits. *Developmental Medicine and Child Neurology* 1988; 30:743–751.
36. Crary MA, Anderson P: *Speech and Motor Performance in Developmental Apraxia of Speech.* Paper presented at the American Speech-Language-Hearing Association Annual Convention, Atlanta, November 1991.
37. Blakely R: *Screening Test for Developmental Apraxia of Speech.* Tigard, OR, CC Publications, 1980.
38. Aram DM, Horwitz SJ: Sequential and non-speech praxic abilities in developmental verbal apraxia. *Developmental Medicine and Child Neurology* 1983; 25:197–206.
39. Velleman SL, Huntley R, Lasker J: *Is It DVD or Is It Phonological Disorder?* Paper presented at the American Speech-Language-Hearing Association Annual Convention, Atlanta, November 1991.
40. Hodson BW: *The Assessment of Phonological Processes* (revised). Austin, Pro-Ed., 1986.
41. Shriberg LD, Kwiatkowski J, Rasmussen C: *Prosodic Competence, Severity, and Intelligibility in Speech-Delayed Children.* Paper presented at the American Speech-Language-Hearing Association Annual Convention, St. Louis, November 1989.
42. Robin DA, Hall PK, Jordan LS, Gordan AJ: *Developmentally Apraxic Speakers' Stress Production: Perceptual and Acoustic Analyses.* Paper presented at the American Speech-Language-Hearing Association Annual Convention, Atlanta, November 1991.
43. Kent RD, Rosenbek JC: Acoustic patterns of apraxia of speech. *Journal of Speech and Hearing Research* 1983; 26:231–249.
44. Kent RD, Forner LL: Speech segment durations in sentence recitations by children and adults. *Journal of Phonetics* 1980; 8:157–168.
45. Smith BL: Temporal aspects of English speech production: A developmental perspective. *Journal of Phonetics* 1978; 6:37–67.

46. Walton JH, Pollock KE: Acoustic validation of vowel error patterns in developmental apraxia of speech. *Clinical Linguistics and Phonetics* 1993; 7(2):95–111.

47. Trost JE, Canter GJ: Apraxia of speech in patients with Broca's Aphasia: A study of phoneme production accuracy and error patterns. *Brain and Language* 1974; 1:63–79.

48. Odell K, McNeil MR, Rosenbek JC, Hunter L: Perceptual characteristics of consonant production by apraxic speakers. *Journal of Speech and Hearing Disorders* 1990; 55:345–359.

49. Macken M, Barton D: The acquisition of the voicing contrast in English: A study of voice onset time in word-initial stop consonants. *Journal of Child Language* 1979; 7:41–74.

50. Marion MJ, Sussman HM, Marquardt TP: The perception and production of rhyme in normal and developmentally apraxic children. *Journal of Communication Disorders,* 1993; 26:129–160.

51. Stackhouse J: An investigation of reading and spelling performance in speech disordered children. *British Journal of Disorders of Communication* 1982; 17:52–59.

52. Aten J: *The Denver Auditory Phoneme Sequencing Test.* Houston, College-Hill Press, 1979.

53. Stackhouse J: Segmentation, Speech, and Spelling Difficulties, in Snowling MJ (ed): *Children's Written Language Difficulties.* Philadelphia, NFER-Nelson, 1985, pp 96–115.

54. Kirk SA, McCarthy JJ, Kirk WD: *Illinois Test of Psycholinguistic Abilities,* rev. ed. Urbana, University of Illinois Press, 1969.

55. Goldsmith JA: *Autosegmental and Metrical Phonology.* Cambridge, MA, Basil Blackwell, Inc., 1990.

56. MacNeilage PF, Davis BL: Acquisition of Speech Production: Frames then Content, in Geannerod M (ed): *Attention and Performance XIII: Motor Representation and Control.* Hillsdale, NJ, Lawrence Erlbaum, 1990, pp 453–476.

57. Oller K: *Transcription and Categorization of Child Speech and Infant Sounds.* Short course presented at the annual meeting of the American Speech-Language-Hearing Association, Seattle, Washington, 1990.

58. Stoel-Gammon C: Phonological skills of 2-year-olds. *LSHSS* 1987; 18:323–329.

59. McCune L: First Words: A Dynamic Systems View, in Ferguson CA, Menn L, Stoel-Gammon C (eds): *Phonological Development: Models, Research, Implications.* Timonium, MD, York Press, 1992, pp 313–336.

60. Vihman MM, Velleman SL, McCune L: How Abstract is Child Phonology? Towards an Integration of Linguistic and Psychological Approaches, in Yavas M (ed): *First and Second Language Phonology.* San Diego, Singular Press, 1994, pp 9–44.

61. de Boysson-Bardies B, Sagart L, Durand C: Discernible differences in the babbling of infants according to target-language. *Journal of Child Language* 1984; 11:1–15.

62. Menn L: *Control and Contrast in Beginning Speech: A Case Study in the Development of Word Form and Word Function.* Unpublished doctoral dissertation, University of Illinois-Champaign-Urbana, University of Illinois, 1976.

63. Flax J, Lahey M, Harris K, Boothroyd A: Relations between prosodic variables and communicative functions. *Journal of Child Language* 1991; 18:3–19.

64. Shriberg LD, Kwiatkowski J, Rasmussen C: *Prosodic Competence, Severity, and Intelligibility in Speech-Delayed Children.* Presentation at the annual meeting of the American Speech-Language-Hearing Association, St. Louis, 1989.

65. Wetherby AM, Prizant BM: *Communication and Symbolic Behavior Scales.* USA, Riverside Publishing Co., 1990.

66. Lowe M, Costello A: *The Symbolic Play Test.* London, National Foundation of Educational Research, 1976.

67. Ekelman B, Aram D: Spoken syntax in children with developmental verbal apraxia. *Seminars in Speech and Language* 1984; 5(2):97–110.

68. Blakely R: *Test for Apraxia of Speech and Oral Apraxia—Children's Battery.* Rochester, MN, Mayo Clinic, 1977.

69. Stoel-Gammon C, Stone JR: Assessing phonology in young children. *Clinics in Communication Disorders* 1991; 1(2):25–39.

70. Ingram D: *Procedures for the Phonological Analysis of Children's Language.* Baltimore, University Park Press, 1981.

71. Grunwell P: *Phonological Assessment of Child Speech (PACS).* San Diego, College Hill Press, 1985.

72. Bernhardt B: Developmental implications of nonlinear phonological theory. *Clinical Linguistics and Phonetics* 1992; 6(4):259–282.

73. Bernhardt B: The application of nonlinear phonological theory to intervention with one phonologically disordered child. *Clinical Linguistics and Phonetics* 1992; 6(4):283–316.

74. Bankson NW, Bernthal JE: *Bankson-Bernthal Test of Phonology.* Chicago, Riverside Publishing Co., 1990.

75. Lowe R: *Assessment Link Between Phonology and Articulation (ALPHA).* East Moline, IL, LinguiSystems, Inc., 1986.

76. Khan L, Lewis N: Khan-Lewis *Phonological Analysis.* Circle Pines, MN, American Guidance Service, Inc., 1986.

77. Shriberg L, Kwiatkowski J: *Natural Process Analysis.* New York, John Wiley, 1980.
78. Oller DK: The Emergence of the Sounds of Speech in Infancy, in Yeni-Komshian G, Kavanaugh JF, Ferguson CA (eds): *Child Phonology: Production,* vol. 1. New York, Academic Press, 1980, pp 93–112.
79. Stark RE: Stages of Speech Development in the First Year, in Yeni-Komshian G, Kavanaugh JF, Ferguson CA (eds): *Child Phonology: Production,* vol. 1. New York, Academic Press, 1980, pp 73–92.
80. Jaroma M, Danner P, Koivuniemi E: Sensory integrative therapy and speech therapy for improving the perceptual motor skills and speech articulation of a dyspractic boy. *Folia Phoniatrica* 1984; 36:261–266.
81. Pannbacker M: Management strategies for developmental apraxia of speech: A review of literature. *Journal of Communication Disorders* 1988; 21:363–371.
82. Bashir A, Grahamjones F, Bostwick R: A touch-cue method of therapy for developmental verbal apraxia. *Seminars in Speech and Language* 1984; 5(2):127–137.
83. Helfrich-Miller K: Melodic intonation therapy with developmentally apraxic children. *Seminars in Speech and Language* 1984; 5(2):119–126.
84. Marquardt T: *Developmental Apraxia of Speech: Characteristics, Diagnosis and Treatment.* Presentation at South Carolina Speech-Language-Hearing Association Convention, North Myrtle Beach, SC, 1986.
85. Chumpelik D: The prompt system of therapy: Theoretical framework and applications for developmental apraxia of speech. *Seminars in Speech and Language* 1984; 5:139–153.
86. Johnson RM: *The Picture Communication Symbols Book.* Solana Beach, CA, Mayer-Johnson Co., 1985.
87. Kirkpatrick J, Stohr P, Kimbrough D: *Moving Across Syllables.* Tucson, Communication Skill Builders, 1990.
88. Jeffery KL, Phippen AS: *Initiation of Therapy: Remediation Exercises for the Severely Apraxic Child.* Presentation at the annual meeting of the American Speech-Language-Hearing Association, St. Louis, 1989.
89. Blakely RW: Treatment of Developmental Apraxia of Speech, in Perkins W (ed): *Dysarthria and Apraxia.* New York, Thieme-Stratton, Inc., 1983, pp 25–33.
90. Pehrsson RS, Robinson HA: *The Semantic Organizer Approach to Writing and Reading Instruction.* Rockville, MD, Aspen Publishers, Inc., 1985.
91. Shane H, Bashir A: Criteria for the adoption of an augmentative communication system: Preliminary considerations. *Journal of Speech and Hearing Disorders* 1980; 45:408–414.
92. Jaffe MB: Neurological Impairment of Speech Production: Assessment and Treatment, in Costello JM (ed): *Speech Disorders in Children.* San Diego, College-Hill Press, 1984, pp 157–186.

6

Phonological and Speech Production Characteristics of Children Following Traumatic Brain Injury: Principles Underlying Assessment and Treatment

THOMAS F. CAMPBELL, PH.D., AND CHRISTINE A. DOLLAGHAN, PH.D.

Introduction

Traumatic brain injury (TBI) is the most common acquired cause of disruption in the normal process of speech and language acquisition. Seatbelt laws and bicycle helmet campaigns notwithstanding, approximately one million children in the United States sustain head injuries each year. Approximately one sixth of these are severe enough to warrant hospitalization.[1]

Interest in understanding the effects of traumatic brain injury on communication skills has grown steadily over the past decade. As a prerequisite to establishing principles of evaluation and rehabilitation, recent studies have focused on characterizing the long-term syntactic,[2] semantic[3] and pragmatic[4] sequelae of TBI in children. To date, considerably less attention has been given to describing the phonological and speech production characteristics of these children.

TBI typically exerts devastating and shattering forces on the cranium and its contents. Predictably, it has important effects on the perceptual, motor, and cognitive-linguistic mechanisms that underlie phonological and speech production abilities. Unlike those children who display circumscribed unilateral lesions,[5] the diffuse cortic and subcortic damage often associated with TBI can result in complex speech production deficits that pervade all levels of the phonological and speech production system.

In this chapter we consider the issues associated with assessing and treating phonological and speech production deficits in children who have experienced TBI. To begin, we present a brief summary of the epidemiology and neuropathologic processes of brain injury. We then turn to what little is known about the speech production characteristics of this population and present a framework for assessment. We conclude by identifying principles underlying management of these children's speech production deficits.

Epidemiology and Etiology

Annegers[6] reported that the annual incidence of closed head injury (defined as concussion with loss of consciousness) in children under 15 years of age is approximately 220 per 100,000 children. These data are consistent with other incidence studies that have reported rates ranging from 117 to 295 per 100,000 children.[7,8] The lowest rates (117 to 150 per 100,000) are reported for children ages 0 to 4 years,[9–11] and the highest (250 to 500 per 100,000) for individuals 15 to 19 years of age.[6,8,12] Across all age levels, males are more prone to having head injuries than females,[13] with a reported ratio of approximately two males to every female.[1,11,12]

The major causes of head trauma in children appear to change with age.[1,8] Frankowski[9] reported that the majority of head injuries sustained by children 1 to 4 years of age result from falls (50%), followed by pedestrian accidents (20%) and motor vehicle accidents (17%). Recent studies also indicate that a significant number of head injuries in infants and young children are the result of parental neglect and abuse.[14,15] For children 5 to 9 years of age, the primary cause of injury is pedestrian accidents (39%), with motor vehicle accidents (26%), falls (19%), and bicycle accidents (9%) being significant contributors. In the teenage years, motor vehicle accidents are the cause of more than 50% of reported head injuries.

Neuropathology

Much has been written about the pathophysiological correlates of TBI. Pang,[16] Bigler,[17] and Richardson[18] provide comprehensive reviews of the physics of TBI and the mechanisms associated with brain injury. A brief discussion of the neuropathologic mechanisms that underlie TBI will provide the basis for understanding the wide range of speech production abilities found in these children.

Pang[16] defined primary head injuries as those that occur at the time of impact. Primary injuries result in permanent disruption of brain structures and are not believed to be affected by drug, medical, or behavioral treatments. Examples of primary head injuries include rotational shearing strains within the cortic and subcortic structures,[18] as well as contusions and lacerations resulting from the impact of the temporal and frontal lobes with the irregular antero-medial surfaces of the skull.[17] The dominant neurophysiological mechanism underlying severe primary head injury is diffuse axonal damage in the white matter;[18–20] these individuals are believed to have the poorest long-term outcome.[16]

Secondary brain injuries are superimposed on the primary damage and result from ischemia, brain edema, intracranial hematomas, subarachnoid hemorrhage, increased intracranial pressure, infections, and seizures.[18] Secondary injuries are more amenable to prevention and treatment than are primary injuries.[14,16]

One of the most important and distinguishing characteristics of TBI is the extent to which it tends to be diffuse, having effects on nearly all cortic and subcortic structures. The resulting behavioral deficits are correspondingly wide ranging and may vary tremendously from child to child, depending on such factors as injury type, injury severity, and age. For example, skull fractures and subdural hematomas appear to be more common in very young children than in older children. This fact has been attributed to the increased flexibility of the bones of the skull, as well as the presence of open skull sutures, which absorb impact, in this population.[21] Similarly, the neurological damage incurred in falls and blunt force trauma, common causes of injury in young children, may be quite different from the acceleration-related injuries associated with motor vehicle accidents in older children and adolescents. Such interactions make it exceedingly difficult to predict either the eventual outcome or the recovery course in survivors of pediatric head injury and make clear the need to consider each child an "N of 1" in planning assessment and intervention services.

General Deficits Following Childhood TBI

Prior to focusing on the phonological and speech production skills of children with TBI, it is worth noting that many such children exhibit impairments in their cognitive, motoric, linguistic, and communicative abilities that persist beyond the first year of recovery.[18] A number of authors have addressed specific findings in these areas.[2,22,23] Although significant individual variation exists, the available literature suggests that many TBI children exhibit ongoing deficits in their ability to learn new information,[24,25] to perform fine motor tasks at normal levels of speed and accuracy,[18] and to produce and comprehend linguistic forms rapidly and readily, especially in situations with high processing demands.[18,26] Acknowledgment of these general areas of deficit provides a backdrop for a specific examination of phonological and speech production characteristics of children following TBI—the issue to which we now turn.

Phonological and Speech Production Deficits Following Childhood TBI

Despite the interest in the sequelae of pediatric brain injury noted above, very little information exists concerning these children's speech production skills. In previous investigations, few children have received comprehensive speech evaluations, and information on these children's speech production abilities, if mentioned at all, has been reported in general and anecdotal form. In addition, there are few published accounts of the changes in speech abilities during the recovery process.

The anecdotal reports that have appeared in recent years do suggest the presence of speech production deficits following TBI. One of the most commonly mentioned deficits is decreased speech intelligibility, generally presumed to result from motor planning and motor speech problems, including dysarthria and apraxia of speech.[27-31] Prosodic and voice deficits also have been reported, with abnormalities in verbal fluency, speech rate, word and sentence stress, loudness, pitch, and resonance among those mentioned.[32,33]

Detailed descriptions of TBI children's phonological and articulation skills are particularly sparse. In one of the most comprehensive reviews to date, Thompson[31] described the articulation deficits associated with a variety of pediatric neuropathologies that can occur in the prenatal, perinatal, and postnatal periods. Thompson's review primarily focused on the speech production deficits related to developmental dysarthria and apraxia of speech, TBI being only one of many possible etiologies. For children with developmental dysarthria, all subsystems that support speech production may be impaired, including respiration, phonation, resonance, and articulation. According to Thompson, the articulation errors displayed by such children are quite varied but often include particular difficulties with the production of fricatives, affricates, and liquids in all word positions. Similarly, Thompson reported that the articulatory characteristics of children with apraxia of speech vary widely. The most commonly reported speech symptoms include vowel and consonant distortions, additions, cluster reduction, and articulatory groping. Although it has been hypothesized that dysarthria is more common than apraxia of speech following TBI in children,[29] data on the incidence of each of these motor speech disorders is unavailable. Whether there are differences in the nature and resolution of these speech disorders after TBI and other acquired neurodevelopmental disabilities is also unknown.

Jordan, Ozanne, and Murdoch[34] provide one of the few long-term outcome studies that mention articulatory proficiency specifically in TBI children. They reported that the articulation abilities of 20 8- to 16-year-old children who had sustained TBI at least 12 months previously were not significantly different from those of a group of age-matched uninjured subjects based on the articulation subtest of the Neurosensory Center Comprehensive Examination of Aphasia (NCCEA).[34,35] Data were not reported on the speech intelligibility of these children during conversation nor on longitudinal changes in articulation skills.

A Longitudinal Investigation of Phonological and Speech Production Deficits in Childhood TBI

Over the past 5 years we have examined the expressive language and speech skills of children and adolescents with TBI in a more comprehensive fashion than previous studies.[2,36,37] Using developmentally appropriate measures of speech and language functioning in reasonably naturalistic tasks, we obtained language samples from these survivors seven times during the 1-year period immediately following the injury. The first sampling session occurred after the children and adolescents were discharged to a rehabilitation hospital and showed some evidence of intentional communication. To create some yardstick for "typical" performance, each brain-injured subject was age-matched with a normally developing noninjured child whose speech and language were sampled on the same schedule and with the same procedures. Due to the lack of longitudinal descriptive studies concerning the speech production abilities of TBI children, it is instructive to summarize the results from the analyses performed on the language samples obtained from this select group of children, all of whom received less than 38 hours of speech and language treatment over the year following their injury.

Our work thus far has focused on nine children and adolescents ranging in age from 5:8 to 16:2 (years:months) at the time of injury. Four of the subjects were male and five were female. Each subject spoke English as a first language, and none had received speech, language, or psychological treatment prior to injury. In addition, all subjects had been functioning in normal classrooms prior to injury. Eight of the brain-injured subjects sustained closed head injuries from motor vehicle accidents, and the remaining child experienced an open head injury. All subjects were judged to be severely head-injured, meaning that they were unconscious for a minimum of 72 hours and received Glasgow Coma Scores of less than 11 (on a 15-point scale) for this time interval. For more extensive demographic, neurologic, cognitive, and linguistic data on these children, refer to Campbell and Dollaghan.[2]

In an initial investigation,[2] we reported data on seven global measures of expressive speech and language output (including total number of utterances, total number of words, mean length of utterance in morphemes, percentage of complex utterances, percentage of utterances with mazes, and percentage of consonants correct). Not surprisingly, significant differences were found between the head-injured and noninjured groups on every one of the seven indices at the first sampling session, which occurred approximately 1 month postinjury. However, by the final sampling session at approximately 13 months postinjury, the groups differed on only one of these measures, with the brain-injured children producing significantly fewer utterances than their matched controls.

How did these severely brain-injured subjects' speech production skills change over this 12-month period? The data presented in Figure 1 address this question with respect to changes in the Percentage of Consonants Correct (PCC)[38] for the brain-injured (BI) and normal (N) subjects during a 12-minute conversation. As originally reported, there was a significant difference in the mean PCC for the brain-injured (87%) and normal (98%) groups at the first sampling session. By the final session, there was no significant difference in the mean performance of BI (95%) and normal (98%) groups. As can be seen, the PCCs of the individual normal subjects (small open circles) were quite stable across the sampling sessions, with performance generally above 95% correct. For the individual brain-injured subjects (small filled circles), there were measurable increases in PCC across the sampling sessions, with six of the nine subjects producing at least 95% of their consonants correct at the final session. This result was somewhat surprising given the severity of these subjects' head injuries and suggests that their ability to correctly produce consonant phonemes in naturalistic conversation was reasonably close to that of their normal controls by 12 months following injury.

Did all brain-injured subjects actually reach the level of consonant articulation accuracy of their matched control subjects as the recovery period progressed? To further examine this question, a "normal performance quotient"[39] was calculated for each subject pair. The normal performance quotient was computed by dividing each brain-injured subject's PCC by the PCC of his or her matched control subject. A quotient of 1.0 indicates performance equal to that of the uninjured subject. As shown in Figure 2, six TBI subjects had performance quotients of 1.0 by the final session; all TBI subjects had performance quotients of at least 0.8 by sampling session 5, which occurred approximately 3 months post injury.

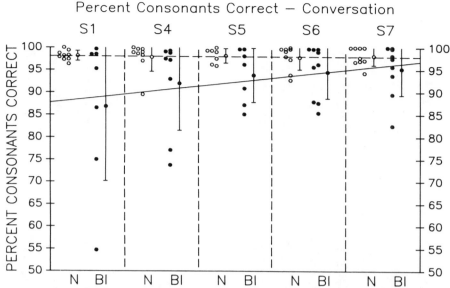

Figure 6–1. Percentage of Consonants Correct (PCC) for the normal (N) and brain-injured (BI) subjects at sampling sessions 1, 4, 5, 6, and 7. Small circles represent data from individual subjects; large circles represent group means. Filled circles represent data from brain-injured subjects; open circles represent data from normal subjects. Vertical lines represent one standard deviation above and below each group mean. Regression lines for the brain-injured (solid line) and normal (broken line) subjects are also shown.[2]

Based on these PCC results, it is tempting to conclude that the speech production deficits of most of these TBI children had resolved within 1 year after injury. However, PCC is a general index of consonant production and does not capture differences in articulatory precision or prosodic aspects of speech production. Clinical experience with these subjects suggested the need to examine articulation in more detail, as well as to consider other components of their speech production systems. To describe the segmental and nonsegmental characteristics of these children's speech in more detail, a series of analyses were performed on conversational language samples obtained from these children at the final session, approximately 13 months post injury.[40] These analyses included measures of phonemic and phonetic error types, ratings of prosodic and voice characteristics using the Prosody-Voice Screening Profile (PVSP),[41,42] and independent subjective listener ratings of speech clarity and speaking rate. The results of these analyses appear in Table 6–1 and can be summarized as follows:

1. Deletions of singleton consonants were the most common phonemic-level error; substitutions were noted in only two of the nine subjects.

2. Phonetic-level errors occurred in eight of the nine subjects. Inappropriate nasalization and lateralization of sibilants [s, z, ʃ] were common, and weak articulation and devoicing errors were also observed in approximately one-half of these subjects.

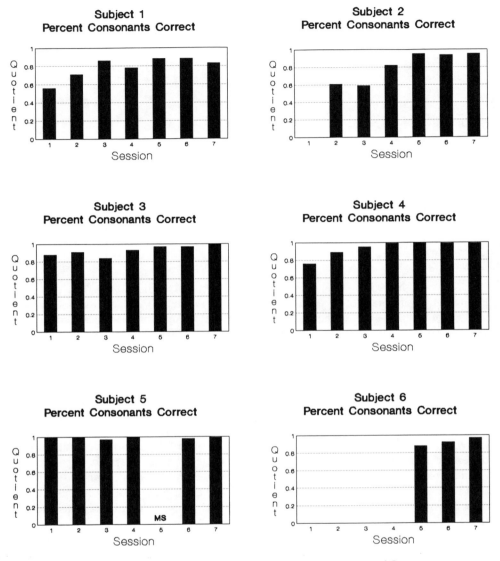

Figure 6–2. The "normal performance quotient" for the percentage of Consonants Correct for the nine subjects at each session. A quotient of 1.0 indicates that the brain-injured subject reached the level of performance of his or her control subject.[2]

3. Clinically significant deficits on the Prosody-Voice Screening Profile were found in all subjects but one at the final sampling session. Deficits in phrasing (word repetitions) were observed in seven of these subjects; six exhibited deficits in speaking rate and word/sentence stress. Four of the subjects displayed deficits in voice quality.

4. Naive listeners rated 108-second-long spontaneous samples obtained in a video narration condition[26] using direct magnitude estimation procedures

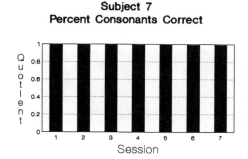

Subject 7
Percent Consonants Correct

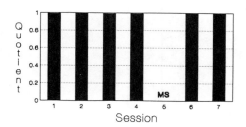

Subject 8
Percent Consonants Correct

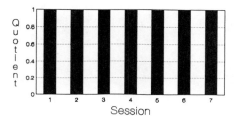

Subject 9
Percent Consonants Correct

Figure 6–2. *Continued.*

described in Campbell and Dollaghan.[36] Briefly, on two different occasions listeners judged a set of randomly ordered samples from brain-injured and control subjects with respect to speech clarity and speaking rate. The spontaneous speech of five of nine TBI subjects was rated significantly less clear than that of their normal control subjects; these same five TBI subjects were rated as having significantly slower speaking rates than their control subjects.

The results of these studies suggest that these subjects experienced a significant recovery of phonemic-level skills over a period of approximately 13 months. However, precision of articulation and suprasegmental aspects of speech production remained compromised in the majority of these subjects such that naive listeners judged their communication skills to be significantly poorer than those of matched controls.

Critical Issues Underlying Management of Speech Production Deficits

Appropriate management of speech production deficits in children who have sustained TBI requires close linkages between evaluation and treatment. As mentioned previously, the diffuse brain damage that often accompanies TBI can result in speech deficits that have their origins at one or more levels of the phonological and speech production system. Whether a child's speech problem is occurring at the perceptual, organizational, or motor-articulatory level

Table 6–1. Speech Production Characteristics of Nine Severely Brain-Injured Subjects, Approximately 13 Months Post Injury

Speech Production Component	Brain Injured Subjects								
	Subject 1	Subject 2	Subject 3	Subject 4	Subject 5	Subject 6	Subject 7	Subject 8	Subject 9
Percent Consonants Correct	82%	89%	100%	98%	95%	94%	100%	98%	100%
Phonemic Error Types	Deletion of final consonants [θ, ð, d, k, s, z, l, r]; Cluster reduction in word initial and final positions; Unstressed syllable deletion	Deletion of final consonants [z, tʃ, t, k]; Deletion of initial consonants [t, ð, k]	None	Deletion of [l] in word final position	Deletion of final consonants [l, l]; Deletion of initial consonants [ð, w]; Unstressed syllable deletion; Substitution of t/f	Deletion of [k] in final position; Cluster reduction in final position	None	None	None
Phonetic Error Types	Lateralization of [s]; Inconsistent nasalization of vowels; Weak articulation of stop consonants; Palatalization of [ð]	Lateralization of [s]; Inconsistent nasalization of vowels; Weak articulation of stop consonants; Devoicing of voiced stops; Trilled articulation of final stops	Inconsistent nasalization of vowels; Devoicing of voiced stops and fricatives	Lateralization of [s] and [z]	Lateralization of [s]; Weak articulation of stop consonants	Consistent nasalization of vowels and consonants; Weak articulation of all consonants	None	Substitution of ð/s; Lateralization of [s] and [z]; Inconsistent nasalization of vowels	Lateralization of [s]; Lateralization of [ʃ]
Prosody-Voice Characteristics	Deficits in phrasing, rate, and word/sentence stress	Deficits in rate, word/sentence stress, and pitch	Deficits in phrasing, rate, word/sentence stress, and nasal resonance	Deficits in phrasing, rate, word/sentence stress, and laryngeal quality	Deficits in phrasing	Deficits in phrasing, rate, word/sentence stress, loudness, pitch, and laryngeal quality	Deficits in phrasing	Deficits in phrasing, rate, words/sentence stress, and nasal resonance	Normal
Perceptual Ratings of Speech Clarity and Speaking Rate	Speech clarity significantly poorer than normal control subject	Speech clarity and speaking rate significantly poorer than normal control subject	Speech clarity and speaking rate significantly poorer than normal control subject	Speech clarity and speaking rate significantly poorer than normal control subject	Normal	Speech clarity and speaking rate significantly poorer than normal control subject	Normal	Speaking rate significantly poorer than normal control subject	Normal

could have clear implications for the selection of appropriate intervention goals.[43]

Our approach to evaluation and intervention of speech deficits in children with TBI draws heavily from methods used both with speech-delayed children and traumatically brain-injured adults. However, as would be expected there are some basic principles of management that differ from those used in the assessment and treatment of speech-delayed children and brain-injured adults. As a prelude to the discussion of specific principles of evaluation and intervention, we present a brief overview of five general issues that are critical to the clinical management of children with TBI.

A Broad-Based View of Phonological Disorders

Kamhi[44] and Fey[43] argue that the clinical management of children with speech delays requires a broad-based model of phonological disorders that includes articulatory, phonological, and cognitive components. Such a view is particularly relevant for children who have sustained traumatic brain injuries. Assessment and treatment procedures that focus solely on one specific aspect of the speech production system are far too restrictive to serve the needs of such a heterogeneous population of children with such widely varying speech production characteristics. In the evaluation and treatment of the speech production deficits of these children, it is constructive to conceptualize the term "phonological" in a similar fashion to that proposed by Shriberg and Kwiatkowski[45] (p.228). In their classification system, the term "phonological" is employed " . . . as a cover term to encompass the entire speech production process, from the underlying representations to phonological rules to the behaviors that produce the surface forms of speech." We believe that the term should also encompass speech perception and phonological memory components.[46,47] This broader definition of phonology emphasizes the need to consider potential disruptions at all of these levels, as well as the interactions among them, in assessing speech production deficits in children with TBI.

Developmental Impact

Seeking to understand how brain damage influences behavioral outcome is a problematic undertaking even in the case of adults who have finished the language acquisition process and who demonstrate circumscribed, focal lesions. The difficulties inherent in this endeavor are magnified in child survivors of TBI who are still acquiring language and whose diffuse lesions can reasonably be said to have left no anatomic structure or physiological function of the brain completely untouched.

Efforts to understand the effects of TBI on children's phonological skills are seriously complicated by the fact that such injuries disrupt the developmental course both of the neurological and the linguistic systems. The relationship between age at onset and the short-term and long-term effects of pediatric TBI is extremely poorly understood, but a growing body of evidence suggests that the traditional, plasticity-oriented view that "the earlier the onset, the greater the recovery" is at best a gross oversimplification.[48,49] For example, a growing body of evidence suggests that focal brain injury to very young children may have persistent effects on linguistic skills.[50-52] Whether such effects are permanent or similar in severity to those resulting from comparable lesions in adults remains unclear.[53] Even less is known about the impact of diffuse, traumatic injury on the developing brain and linguistic system. On the one hand, anatomic and physiological maturation of the central nervous system is ongoing during childhood, with nearly logarithmic increases in glial cells, synaptic connections, and dendritic arborization during the first few years of life, and myelinization that progresses through year 10.[21] These facts might suggest a greater opportunity for the operation of various hypothesized recovery mechanisms such as modifications of neural connections and vicarious functioning or "re-organization" of the brain, but empirical work on these possibilities is in its infancy. On the other hand, a number of investigators have suggested that behavioral skills that require new learning on the part of the child are particularly vulnerable to the effects of TBI.[20,24,33,54]

For all of these reasons, efforts to characterize and facilitate the phonological skills of children after TBI require consideration of the point along the developmental continuum at which the injury interrupted phonological abilities. The possibility that such skills may never become established to within normal levels of function must be seriously entertained given findings that TBI adults rarely attain preinjury levels of performance on rapid, precise motoric and information processing tasks.[18]

Premorbid Status

A related issue concerns the fact that all children are not equally at risk for TBI. Research has shown that children with attention deficits, intellectual impairments, behavioral difficulties, or those from families at risk are proportionally more likely to sustain TBI.[56] All of these premorbid factors have been related to the rate and success of speech and language development. The possibility that development prior to injury may not have been proceeding normally must be examined for every TBI child. In cases in which evidence exists to suggest a delay or disorder in speech or language production prior to the injury, expectations concerning rate or ultimate extent of recovery must be adjusted accordingly.

Heterogeneity of Deficit

The heterogeneity issue with respect to phonological deficits in TBI children is captured by Yorkston and Beukelman's[32] (p 252) comment concerning adults: "The picture emerging from clinical experience with TBI is one of wide variability in type, pattern, and severity of motor speech disorders. These disorders following TBI may be temporary or persistent, mild or severe, compatible with other deficits or disproportionately severe, and they may or may not be accompanied by other language and cognitive disorders."

Although communication disorders are rarely static phenomena, the child-specific physiological and developmental facts noted above suggest that changes may occur more rapidly and over a more protracted time period in TBI children than in either TBI adults or children with other etiologies.[18] Measuring such dynamic changes in such a heterogeneous population in a valid and reliable fashion is no small task. We have argued elsewhere[2,26,36] that monitoring changes in TBI children requires the use of measures that can be administered repeatedly in maximally naturalistic speaking situations without loss of reliability. Given the potential synergy among phonological, linguistic, motoric, and cognitive processes,[32] the unit of analysis may have to be determined individually for each child in accordance with his or her particular pattern of deficits.

Social Validation

A final issue concerns the need to consider the impact of the brain-injured child's phonological deficits in relation to the other sequelae of the injury. The effects of a traumatic insult on the neurological system are likely to be widespread. As a result, decisions about whether to select phonological skills from among the many potential intervention targets can only be made by considering the clinical significance of the phonological sequelae for the child's disability.[32] Social validation procedures[36] represent one obvious and straightforward way to estimate the clinical significance of a child's speech production deficits and thus their priority for intervention.

Assessment of Phonological and Speech Production Skills Following TBI

In what follows, we briefly note some of the distinguishing features of assessments aimed at specifying the speech production deficits of child survivors of TBI. There are a substantial number of children with TBI for whom augmentative and alternative modalities of communication will be necessary, but our comments are directed toward children who can use speech as their primary mode of communication.

Although many of the assessment procedures for this population will be familiar to speech–language pathologists, there are several considerations that are specific to children with TBI. Table 6–2 lists suggested basic areas to be included in a comprehensive evaluation of speech production. In this section, we highlight some of the issues specific to assessing these children.

A prerequisite to the assessment of speech production abilities in every TBI child is information on medical, neurologic, and neuropsychologic status. Such information will often change rapidly as the child emerges from coma and will suggest the point at which an initial assessment can be administered. These data will also aid in modifying assessment activities as necessary to allow the child to participate and aid in interpreting results.

While overall communicative assessment is an obvious priority from the earliest stages of recovery, we suggest that formal speech production assessment be postponed until the point at which the child makes some effort at intentional verbal communication. Of course, this does not preclude the use of activities designed to assist the child in reaching this point, such as re-establishing voluntary phonation.

Table 6–2.   Essential Components of the Phonological and
Speech Production Assessment

---

1.   Pre-Morbid Developmental Function
   Academic, cognitive, linguistic, and psychosocial function
   Special emphasis should be given to phonological and articulatory development
      (e.g., pre-injury phonemic and lexical inventories as well as speech intelligibility)

2.   Oral-Speech Motor Function
   Evaluation of the structure and function of all the speech subsystems including res-
      piratory, laryngeal, velopharyngeal, and articulatory (i.e., lips, mandible, tongue,
      teeth). Assessment of function should include speech and non-speech tasks.
   Diadochokinetic rates should be obtained to examine sequential ordering of conso-
      nants and vowels as well as difficulties with articulatory movement (e.g.,
      /pʌtʌkʌ/,/pætikek/)

3.   Collection of Speech Samples in a Variety of Contexts with Varying Processing
   Demands
      Conversation, on-line narration, single-word articulation tests, repetition of mono-
      syllabic and multisyllabic words

4.   Description of Segmental Speech Abilities
   Phonetic inventory
   Phonemic inventory
   Range of syllable shapes
   Phonological rules (normal and abnormal)
   Results should be compared across speaking contexts to determine if deficits vary
      with processing demands (e.g., conversation versus narration; single-word tasks
      versus multisyllabic word tasks)

5.   Description of Nonsegmental Speech Abilities
   Prosody (phrasing and fluency, speech rate, word and sentence level stress)
   Voice (loudness, pitch, laryngeal quality, nasal resonance)

6.   Social Validation Assessment
   Listeners' perceptual ratings of various aspects of speech production (e.g., speech
      intelligibility, speech naturalness, speaking rate, voice, etc.)
   These data may be used to determine the contribution of specific components of the
      speech production process to overall speech intelligibility. They can also be
      employed to determine the severity of speech production deficits relative to other
      cognitive and linguistic disorders.

One of the most important, though often neglected, areas for assessment is the child's level of premorbid developmental function, including information on cognitive, linguistic, academic, and especially phonological and articulatory abilities. Caregivers, teachers, and school records serve as primary sources of information concerning the child's preinjury phonemic inventory and speech intelligibility. The availability of video and audiorecording equipment in many homes may make it possible to obtain actual samples of preinjury speech production. This information may influence expectations about the extent and rate of recovery of speech skills after injury and guide decisions regarding treatment targets and procedures.

As shown in Table 6–2, evaluation of the entire motor speech system, including measures of respiratory, laryngeal, velopharyngeal, and articulatory function, is crucial in children who have suffered major bodily injuries in addition to central nervous system damage.[57] Yorkston and Beukelman[32] provide an excellent overview of methods for determining adequacy of respiratory support and laryngeal and velopharyngeal dysfunction, many of which can be adapted for use with children; see also Jaffe, Mastrilli, Molitor, and Valko.[29]

Another TBI-specific issue concerns the need for ongoing assessment. The recovery process is likely to vary substantially from child to child; only by systematic monitoring of speech production changes can the speech–language pathologist make principled decisions about the need for and timing of any intervention aimed at speech production skills. Spontaneous connected speech samples are the procedure of choice for this purpose; Shriberg[58] provides evidence that samples as short as 225 words in length yield valid and reliable data for analysis. The advantages of using spontaneous connected samples have been discussed elsewhere but are particularly obvious for children who will require multiple assessments over a protracted period of time. For this population, we also suggest that speech–language pathologists consider obtaining samples in more demanding (ie, fast-paced or complex) contexts, such as video narration or production of multisyllabic words. Comparing samples from less and more demanding contexts often reveals difficulties in TBI children's speech and language production when processing demands are high.[4,26,30,36] This information often aids in interpreting the variability observed by parents and teachers in the speech production skills of a child with TBI. Such information is also relevant in providing the child with practice in speech production tasks systematically graded in processing complexity. Such guided practice may facilitate the child's ability to maintain intelligibility in demanding speaking situations, such as those encountered in many academic contexts.

Another point specific to assessing the child with TBI is the need to include formal analyses of suprasegmental aspects of speech production in addition to the standard battery of segmental measures. Shriberg and Kwiatkowski's Prosody-Voice Screening Profile[41] is a major advance in standardizing such evaluations and is constructed such that it can be administered quickly and repeatedly. Depending on the results of this measure, specific aspects of prosody and voice may be targeted for assessment with more detailed, acoustic analyses (eg, speaking rate measured in syllables per second).

As with every child suspected of having a speech production deficit, it is important to have information concerning phonetic inventory, phonemic inventory, range of syllable shapes, and phonological rules. Although our data suggest a relative "sparing" of phoneme production skills, at least for children injured in the later stages of phonological development, the frequent occurrence of phonetic-level errors up to 13 months postinjury indicates the need to monitor these skills carefully. In addition, for the child injured in the early stages of phonological development, it is reasonable to expect significant effects on subsequent acquisition, particularly if perceptual and cognitive functions are impaired. The lack of information on these effects in young children represents one of many gaps in the current literature on this population.[59]

A final, critically important issue concerns the relative priority assigned to the child's speech production deficits in the context of his or her other cognitive, motoric, and linguistic impairments. Speech production deficits may be among the most noticeable or "describable" problems to the child's family and teachers, but efforts aimed at remediating less obvious deficits of cognition or language processing may have a more significant impact on the child's ultimate level of functioning. It is crucial that the speech–language pathologist work with other team members to set priorities for addressing the child's various impairments and to educate parents and others if speech production deficits are not among the top treatment priorities for the child.

Treatment of Speech Production Deficits Following TBI

The lack of information concerning speech production skills following TBI in childhood makes it difficult at present to determine the extent to which the deficits exhibited by children with TBI are similar to those of children with other etiologies. In addition, some spontaneous recovery of speech production skills is likely for many children with TBI, as are speech sound changes resulting from maturation in younger children with TBI. These facts make the evaluation of treatment efficacy imperative in this population. A number of investigators have described methods for achieving this end, using techniques as simple as repeated measurements on both "target" skills (specific treatment goals) and similar skills not being treated actively.[60–63]

For children with TBI, overt speech production deficits may result from impairments in one, some, or all components of the communication system, from "higher" cognitive processes involved in utterance formulation to lexical representation and access, phonological and phonetic coding, and motor output. In addition, among the most common sequelae in these children are deficits in memory and fine motor skills[18,22] that are obviously fundamental to speech production as well. Planning intervention for children with such a wide range of possible contributing factors requires tailoring treatment ends and means to the individual pattern of deficits exhibited by each child.

The specific focus and methods of treatment will largely depend on a child's assessment profile across the areas summarized in Table 6–2. As noted previously, there is little descriptive information concerning the speech production deficits of children following TBI; even less has been written concerning how best to intervene to remediate these deficits. Thus, at present, planning intervention for such children requires that the clinician draw on the existing literature concerning children with developmental phonological and speech-motor deficits, as well as on the literature concerning adults with TBI. Thompson[31] pointed out that many treatment objectives and techniques for children with acquired apraxia of speech are derived from and in many cases identical to those employed with speech-delayed children. Similarly, there appears to be no alternative to using principles derived from treatment designed for adult dysarthric speakers in planning intervention for children whose speech is dysarthric following TBI.

We suggest that there are four distinct orientations to intervention that may be appropriate in organizing intervention programs for speech production deficits following TBI in children; these are summarized in Table 6–3. Any one of these or some combination of them may be appropriate to consider in designing

Table 6–3.   Examples of Intervention Approaches for the Treatment of Speech
Production Deficits in Traumatic Brain-Injured Children

Phonological

   Procedures to expand inventories of phones, phonemes and syllable shapes, and to
   establish phonological contrasts; emphasis is placed on improving speech intelligibility (Weiner, 1981;[70] Shriberg & Kwiatkowski, 1982b;[71] Fey, 1992;[43] Stoel-Gamon, 1985;[72]
   Elbert & Gierut, 1986;[64] Bernthal & Bankson, 1988;[73] Gierut, 1989;[74] Hodson & Paden,
   1991[75]).

Motor-Articulatory

   Procedures to facilitate articulatory placement and motoric aspects of sound production
   (McDonald, 1964;[65] Winitz, 1969;[76] Shelton & McReynolds, 1979;[77] Vaughn & Clark,
   1979;[78] Bernthal & Bankson, 1981;[79] Hardy, 1983;[80] Passy, 1985;[81] Pannbacker, 1988;[82]
   Thompson, 1988;[31] Murdoch, Ozanne & Cross, 1990;[83] Yorkston & Beukelman, 1991;[32]
   Jaffe, Mastrilli, Molitor & Valko, 1985[29]).

   Procedures for developing oral-motor strength and articulatory postures (Netsell &
   Cleeland, 1973;[84] Blakeley, 1983;[85] Haynes, 1985;[86] Ylvisaker, 1985;[87] Thompson, 1988;[31]
   Yorkston & Beukelman, 1991;[32] Love, 1992[88]).

Prosody-Voice

   Procedures to modify prosodic abnormalities including speaking rate, word/sentence
   stress and phrasing (Yorkston & Beukelman, 1977;[67] Helm, 1979;[89] Ylvisaker, 1985;[87]
   Yorkston, Beukelman & Bell, 1986;[90] Thompson, 1988;[31] Beukelman, Yorkston & Tice,
   1988;[91] Murdoch, Ozanne & Cross, 1990;[83] Shriberg, Kwiatkowski & Rasmussen,
   1990;[41] Yorkston & Beukelman, 1991[32]).

   Procedures for promoting respiratory, laryngeal and velopharyngeal function (Hardy,
   1983;[80] Prator & Swift, 1984;[92] Ylvisaker, 1985;[87] Thompson, 1988;[31] Yorkston &
   Beukelman, 1991;[32] Love, 1992[88]).

Compensatory

   Compensatory articulation strategies for individuals with severe motor impairments to
   maximize speech potential (Yorkston, Beukelman & Bell, 1986;[90] Pannbacker, 1988;[82]
   Collins, Rosenbek & Donahue, 1982;[93] Murdoch, Ozanne & Cross, 1990;[83] Yorkston &
   Beukelman, 1991;[32] Love, 1992[88]).

   Procedures to provide the child with specific strategies for repairing communication
   breakdowns when they occur, making the child a "self-responsible communicator"
   (Dollaghan & Kaston, 1986;[68] Dollaghan, 1987[69]).

---

intervention for a child with TBI, depending on his or her pattern of speech production deficits.

For example, if assessment reveals an incomplete phonemic or phonetic inventory, the focus of treatment is likely to be phonological, with the emphasis on
establishing contrasts among speech sounds and increasing intelligibility.[64] The
objectives and procedures described by the authors listed in Table 6–3 will provide a starting point in designing a program for children whose problems seem
to include developing the categories and contrasts necessary for an adequate
phonological system. For the child whose phonemic system appears relatively
intact but who exhibits difficulty with precision of articulation, motor-articulatory approaches to intervention may be most appropriate.[65] As shown in the second column of Table 6–3, these approaches emphasize motor learning activities
aimed at improving articulatory precision and may encompass techniques to

develop oral-motor strength for those children with obvious deficits in muscle strength and tone.[32]

Our data suggest that deficits in prosody and voice, including slow speaking rate and stress assignment errors, are likely to persist for at least 1 year following pediatric TBI. For children whose deficits include prosody and voice variables, it may be appropriate to employ the types of procedures discussed by authors listed in the third column of Table 6–3. For example, cues and acoustic or visual feedback concerning the optimal speaking rate for a particular child may be employed. Structured practice procedures, such as contrastive stress drills, may contribute to increased automaticity of correct production at the syllabic or lexical levels.[41]

A compensatory orientation toward intervention may be needed when a reasonable period of appropriate treatment has resulted in a lack of clinically significant change in speech production skills.[63] In such cases, treatment may best be oriented toward providing the child and his or her listeners with augmentative and compensatory techniques to increase intelligibility in the face of persistent speech production deficits. Examples include the use of external cues for the child and his or her listeners, such as the alphabetic supplementation method described by Beukelman and Yorkston.[32,67] Treatment aimed at providing the child with strategies for recognizing and repairing the communication breakdowns that result from persistent speech production deficits may also be useful.[25,68,69]

Of course, the speech profile alone is not sufficient when planning intervention in the child who is recovering from TBI. Cognitive sequelae such as deficits in attention, working memory, and judgment[25] may preclude the use of treatment methods requiring sustained, controlled effort or "focus"[66] on the part of the child, making direct remediation of speech production deficits a very difficult task. In such cases, the clinician may need to explore the extent to which the child's cognitive deficits can be addressed prior to focusing on speech production skills. Unfortunately, virtually no empirical evidence exists concerning the extent to which such cognitive deficits can be remediated, although Ylvisaker and Szekeres[94] provide examples of treatment activities aimed at improving metacognitive and executive functioning in adolescents following TBI. In addition, Sohlberg and Mateer's[95] description of cognitive rehabilitation strategies for adults provides a more specific framework and set of treatment procedures that clinicians may find helpful as they attempt to address these deficits in children.

Conclusions

In this chapter we have attempted to present the contradictory reality of phonological and speech production deficits of children with TBI who are both similar to and different from other children exhibiting phonological and speech production impairments. Speech–language pathologists will need to rely on their knowledge of the entire array of phonological and speech production deficits, assessment methods, and treatment techniques in approaching these children, with their generally diffuse and catastrophic physical and neurological damage. We would summarize the major themes of this chapter as follows:

1. The diffuse brain damage that is associated with TBI can result in speech production deficits at one or all levels of the speech production system. Consequently, appropriate assessment and treatment of children with TBI require a broad-based model of phonological disorders that considers disruptions at all levels as well as the interactions among them.

2. The relationship between age at injury and subsequent development of speech production abilities is poorly understood. Nevertheless, consideration must be given to premorbid phonological status and the point along the speech development continuum at which the injury occurred when interpreting assessment results, planning intervention goals, and predicting outcome.

3. The phonological and speech production abilities of TBI children can change dramatically over time. Therefore, reliable and valid procedures for monitoring longitudinal change must be employed to determine the need for and timing of intervention.

4. In determining intervention goals, phonological and speech production deficits must be prioritized relative to other cognitive, motor, and linguistic deficits. Social validation procedures can be important adjuncts to more traditional methods for determining the clinical significance of a TBI child's speech production impairments.

5. Available information on the nature and resolution of phonological deficits in these children is extremely limited. This necessitates the use of assessment and treatment objectives and methods developed for other populations as starting points for clinical management.

Suggested Readings

Beukelman, D.R. and Yorkston, K.M.: *Communication Disorders Following Traumatic Brain-Injury: Management of Cognitive, Language, and Motor Impairments,* Austin, Texas: Pro-ed, 1991.

Bigler, E.D.: *Traumatic Brain Injury: Mechanisms of Damage, Assessment, Intervention and Outcome,* Austin, Texas: Pro-ed, 1990.

Campbell, T.F. and Dollaghan, C.A.: Expressive language recovery in severely brain-injured children. *Journal of Speech and Hearing Disorders* 1990; 55: 567–581.

Richardson, J.T.F.: *Clinical and Neuropsychologic Aspects of Closed Head Injury,* London: Taylor and Francis, 1990.

Ylvisaker, M.: *Head Injury Rehabilitation: Children and Adolescents,* San Diego, California: College-Hill Press, 1985.

References

1. Goldstein FC, Levin H: Epidemiology of Traumatic Brain Injury: Incidence, clinical characteristics, and risk factors. In Bigler RD (ed): *Traumatic Brain Injury: Mechanisms of Damage, Assessment, Intervention and Outcome.* Austin, TX: Pro-ed, 1990, pp 51–64.
2. Campbell TF, Dollaghan CA: Expressive language recovery in severely brain-injured children. *JSHD* 1990; 55:567–581.
3. Jordan FM, Murdoch BE, Buttsworth DL: Closed-head-injured children's performance on narrative tasks. *Journal of Speech and Hearing Research* 1991; 34:572–582.
4. Dennis M, Barnes MA: Knowing the meaning, getting the point, bridging the gap, and carrying the message: Aspects of discourse following closed head injury in childhood and adolescence. *Brain and Language* 1990; 39:428–446.
5. Shriberg LD, Aram DM: Speech production characteristics of children with unilateral brain lesions. In process.
6. Annegers, JF: The epidemiology of head trauma in children. In Shapiro K (ed): *Pediatric Head*

Trauma. Mount Kisco, NY: Futura, 1983, pp 1–10.

7. Klauber MR, Barrett-Connor E, Marshall LF, Bowers SA: The epidemiology of head injury: A prospective study of an entire community—San Diego County, CA, 1978. *American Journal of Epidemiology* 1981; 113:500–509.

8. Annegers JF, Grabow JD, Kurland LT, Laws ER: The incidence, causes, and secular trends of head trauma in Olmstead County, Minnesota, 1935–1974. *Neurology 1980;* 30:912–919.

9. Frankowski, RF: Head injury mortality in urban populations and its relation to the injured child. In Brooks BF (ed): *The Injured Child.* Austin, TX: University of TX Press, 1985, pp 20–29.

10. Frankowski RF, Annegers JF, Whiteman, S: The descriptive epidemiology of head injury in the United States. In Becker DP, Povlishock JD (eds): *Central Nervous System Trauma Research Status Report—1985.* Bethesda, MD: National Institutes of Neurological and Communicative Disorders and Stroke, National Institutes of Health, 1985, pp 33–43.

11. Klauber MR, Barrett-Connor E, Hofstetter CR, Micik, SH: A population-based study of nonfatal childhood injuries. *Preventative Medicine* 1986; 15:139–149.

12. Kraus JF, Black MA, Hessol N, Ley P, Rokaw W, Sullivan C, Bowers S, Knowlton S, Marhsall, L: The incidence of acute brain injury and serious impairment in a defined population. *American Journal of Epidemiology* 1984; 119:186–201.

13. Cooper, PR: Epidemiology of head injury. In Cooper PR (ed): *Head Injury.* Baltimore, MD: Williams and Wilkins, 1982, pp 1–14.

14. Bagnato SJ, Feldman H: Closed head injury in infants and preschool children: Research and practice issues. *Infants and Young Children* 1989; 2:1–13.

15. Billmire ME, Myers PA: Serious head injury in infants: Accident or abuse? *Pediatrics* 1985; 75:340–342.

16. Pang, D: Pathophysiologic correlates of neurobehavioral syndrome following closed head injury. In Ylvisaker M (ed): *Head Injury Rehabilitation: Children and Adolescents.* San Diego, CA: College Hill Press, 1985, pp 3–70.

17. Bigler ED: Neuropathology of traumatic brain injury. In Bigler ED (ed), *Traumatic Brain Injury: Mechanisms of Damage, Assessment, Intervention and Outcome.* Austin, TX: Pro-Ed, 1990, pp 13–49.

18. Richardson JTE: *Clinical and Neuropsychological Aspects of Closed Head Injury.* London: Taylor and Francis, 1990.

19. Adams JH, Mitchell DE, Graham DI, Doyle D: Diffuse brain damage of the immediate impact type. *Brain.* 1977; 100:489–502.

20. Jordan FM: Speech and language disorders following childhood closed head injury. In Murdoch BE (ed): *Acquired Neurological Speech/Language Disorders in Childhood.* New York: Taylor and Francis, 1990, pp 124–147.

21. Raimondi AJ, Hirschauer J: Clinical criteria: children's coma score and outcome scale for decision making in managing head-injured infants and toddlers. In Raimondi AJ, Choux M, DiRocco C (eds): *Head Injuries in the Newborn and Infant.* New York: Springer Verlag, 1986, pp 141–150.

22. Levin H, Benton AL, Grossman RG: *Neurobehavioral Consequences of Closed Head Injury.* New York, NY, Oxford University Press, 1982. 23. Cooper JA, Flowers CR: Children with a history of acquired aphasia: Residual Language and Academic Impairments. *JSHD* 1987; 52:251–262.

24. Rutter M: Psychological sequelae of brain damage in children. *American Journal of Psychiatry* 1981; 138:1533–1544.

25. Ylvisaker M, Szekeres SF: Metacognitive and executive impairments in head-injured children. *Topics in Language Disorders* 1989; 9:34–49.

26. Dollaghan CA, Campbell TF, Tomlin R: Video narration as a language sampling context. *JSHD* 1990; 55:582–590.

27. Brink JD, Garrett AL, Hale WR, Woo-Sam J, Nickel VL: Recovery of motor and intellectual function in children sustaining severe head injuries. *Developmental Medicine and Child Neurology.* 1970; 12:565–571.

28. Stark RE: Dysarthria in children. In Darby JK (ed): *Speech and Language Evaluation in Neurology: Childhood Disorders.* New York: Grune and Stratton, 1985, pp 185–218.

29. Jaffe MB, Mastrilli JP, Molitor CB, Valko A: Intervention for motor disorders. In Ylvisaker M (ed), *Head Injury Rehabilitation: Children and Adolescents.* San Diego, CA: College-Hill Press, pp 167–194.

30. Ylvisaker M: Language and communication disorders following pediatric head injury. *The Journal of Head Trauma Rehabilitation* 1986; 1:48–56.

31. Thompson CK: Articulation Disorders in the Child with Neurogenic Pathology. In Lass LJ, McReynolds LV, Northern JL, Yoder DE (eds): *Handbook of Speech-Language Pathology.* Philadelphia, PA: DC Becker, 1988, pp 548–591.

32. Yorkston KM, Beukelman DR: Motor speech disorders. In Beukelman DR, Yorkston KM (eds): *Communication Disorders Following Traumatic Brain Injury: Management of Cognitive, Language and Motor Impairments.* Austin, TX: Pro-Ed, 1991, pp 251–315.

33. Ylvisaker M: Communication outcome in children and adolescents with traumatic brain injury. *Journal of Neuropsychologic Rehabilitation* 1993; 3(4):367–387.
34. Jordan FM, Ozanne AE, Murdoch BE: Long-term speech and language disorders subsequent to closed head injury in children. *Brain Injury* 1988; 2:179–185.
35. Spreen O, Benton AL: *Neurosensory Center Comprehensive Examination of Aphasia.* University of Victoria, Victoria, Australia: 1969.
36. Campbell TF, Dollaghan CA: A method for obtaining listener judgments of spontaneously produced language: Social validation through direct magnitude estimation. *Topics in Language Disorders* 1992; 12:42–55.
37. Dollaghan CA, Campbell TF: A procedure for classifying disruptions in spontaneous language samples. *Topics in Language Disorders* 1992; 12:56–68.
38. Shriberg LD, Kwiatkowski J: Phonological disorders III: A procedure for assessing severity of involvement. *JSHD* 1982c; 47:256–270.
39. Bagnato SJ, Mayes DD: Patterns of developmental and behavioral progress for young brain-injured children during interdisciplinary intervention. *Developmental Neuropsychology* 1986; 2:213–240.
40. Campbell TF, Dollaghan CA: Segmental and nonsegmental speech characteristics of children and adolescents following traumatic brain injury. In progress.
41. Shriberg LD, Kwiatkowski J, Rasmussen C: Prosody-Voice Screening Profile [PVSP]: *Scoring Forms and Training Materials.* Tucson, AZ: Communication Skill Builders, 1990.
42. Shriberg LD, Kwiatkowski J, Rasmussen C, Lof GL, Miller JF: *The Prosody-Voice Screening Profile (PVSP): Psychometric Data and Reference Information for Children.* Technical Report No. 1. Tucson, AZ: Communication Skill Builders, 1990, pp 1–54.
43. Fey, ME: Articulation and phonology: Inextricable constructs in speech pathology. *LSHSS* 1992; 23:225–232.
44. Kamhi AG: The need for a broad-based view of phonological disorders. *LSHSS* 1992; 23:261–268.
45. Shriberg LD, Kwiatkowski J: Phonological disorders I: A diagnostic classification system. *JSHD* 1982a; 47:226–242.
46. Baddeley AD: *Working Memory.* Oxford, England: Oxford University Press. 1986.
47. Gathercole SE, Baddeley AD: Phonological memory deficits in language disordered children: Is there a causal connection? *Journal of Memory and Language* 1990; 29:336–360.
48. Woods BT, Grey S: Language deficits after apparent clinical recovery from childhood aphasia. *Annals of Neurology* 1978; 6:405–409.
49. Levin H, Eisenberg HM, Wigg NR, Kobayashi K: Memory and intellectual ability after head injury in children and adolescents. *Neurosurgery* 1982; 11:668–673.
50. Aram DM, Ekelman BL, Rose DF, Whitaker HA: Verbal and cognitive sequelae following unilateral lesions acquired in early childhood. *Journal of Clinical and Experimental Neuropsychology* 1985; 7:55–78.
51. Aram D, Ekelman B, Whitaker H: Spoken syntax in children with acquired unilateral hemisphere lesions. *Brain and Language* 1986; 27:75–100.
52. Thal DJ, Marchman V, Stiles J, Aram D, Trauner D, Nass R, Bates E: Early lexical development in children with focal brain injury. *Brain and Language* 1991; 40:491–527.
53. Feldman HM, Holland AL, Kemp S, Janosky JE: Language development after unilateral brain injury. *Brain and Language* 1992; 42:89–102.
54. Ewing-Cobbs L, Fletcher JM, Levin HS: Neuropsychological sequelae following pediatric head injury. In Ylvisaker M (ed): *Head Injury Rehabilitation: Children and Adolescents.* San Diego, CA: College Hill Press, 1985, pp 71–90.
55. Szekeres S, Ylvisaker M, Holland A: Cognitive rehabilitation therapy: A framework for intervention, in Ylvisaker M (ed): *Head Injury Rehabilitation: Children and Adolescents.* San Diego, CA, College-Hill Press, 1985, pp 219–246.
56. Rutter M, Chadwick O, Shaffer D: Head injury. In Rutter M (ed): *Developmental Neuropsychiatry.* New York: Guilford Press, 1983, pp 83–111.
57. Horn LJ, Garland DE: Medical and orthopedic complications associated with traumatic brain injury. In Rosenthal M, Griffith ER, Bond MR, Miller JD (eds): *Rehabilitation of the Adult and Child with Traumatic Brain Injury.* Philadelphia, PA, FA Davis, 1990, pp 107–126.
58. Shriberg LD: *User's Manual: Programs to Examine Phonetic and Phonological Evaluation Records (PEP-PER).* Madison, WI: University of Wisconsin, Software Development and Distribution Center, 1986.
59. Marchman VA, Miller R, Bates EA: Babble and first words in children with focal brain injury. *Applied Psycholinguistics* 1991; 12:1–22.
60. Fey M: *Language Intervention with Young Children.* San Diego, CA: College-Hill Press, 1986.
61. McReynolds LV, Thompson, CK: Flexibility of single-subject designs. Part I: Review of the basics of single-subject designs. *JSHD* 1986; 51:194–203.

62. Kearns KP: Flexibility of single-subject experimental designs. Part II: Design selection and arrangement of experimental phases. *JSHD* 1986; 51:204–213.
63. Bain BA, Dollaghan CA: The notion of clinically significant change. *LSHSS* 1991; 22:264–270.
64. Elbert M, Gierut J: *Handbook of Clinical Phonology*. Austin, TX: Pro-ed, 1986.
65. McDonald ET: *Articulation Testing and Treatment: A Sensory-Motor Approach*. Pittsburgh, PA:Stanwix House, 1964.
66. Shriberg LD, Kwiatkowski J, Gruber FA: *Speech-Sound Normalization in Developmental Phonological Disorders*. Miniseminar presented at the annual meeting of the American Speech-Language-Hearing Association. San Antonio, TX, 1992.
67. Beukelman DR, Yorkston KM: A communication system for the severely dysarthric speaker with an intact language system. *JSHD* 1977; 42:265–270.
68. Dollaghan C, Kaston N: A comprehension monitoring program for language-impaired children. *JSHD* 1986; 51:264–271.
69. Dollaghan C: Comprehension monitoring in normal and language-impaired children. *Topics in Language Disorders* 1987; 7:45–60.
70. Weiner F: Treatment of phonological disability using the method of meaningful minimal contrast: Two case studies. *JSHD* 1981; 46:97–103.
71. Shriberg L, Kwiatkowski J: Phonological disorders II: A conceptual framework for management. *JSHD* 1982b; 47:242–256.
72. Stoel-Gammon C, Dunn C: *Normal and Disordered Phonology in Children*. Austin, TX: Pro-ed, 1985.
73. Bernthal J, Bankson N: *Articulation and Phonological Disorders* 2nd ed. Englewood Cliffs, NJ: Prentice-Hall, 1988.
74. Gierut J: Maximal opposition approach to phonological treatment. *JSHD* 1989; 54:9–19.
75. Hodson BW, Paden EP: *Targeting Intelligible Speech. A Phonological Approach to Remediation—1991* 2nd ed. Austin, TX: Pro-ed, 1991.
76. Winitz H: *Articulatory Acquisition and Behavior*. Englewood Cliffs, NJ: Prentice-Hall, 1969.
77. Shelton R, McReynolds L: Functional articulation disorders: Preliminaries to treatment. In Lass N (ed): *Speech and Language Advances in Basic Research and Practice*. New York: Academic Press, 1979, pp 1–111.
78. Vaughn GR, Clark RM: *Speech Facilitation: Extraoral and Intraoral Stimulation Technique for Improvement of Articulation Skills*. Springfield, IL: Charles C Thomas, 1979.
79. Bernthal J, Bankson N: *Articulation Disorders* Englewood Cliffs, NJ: Prentice-Hall, 1981.
80. Hardy JC: *Cerebral Palsy*. Englewood Cliffs, NJ: Prentice Hall, 1983.
81. Passey J: *Cued Articulation*. Victoria, Australia: J Passey, 1985.
82. Pannbacker M: Management strategies for developmental apraxia of speech: A review of the literature. *Journal of Communication Disorders* 1988; 21:367–371.
83. Murdoch BE, Ozanne AE, Cross JA: Acquired childhood speech disorders: Dysarthia and Apraxia. In Murdoch BE (ed): *Acquired Neurologic Speech-Language Disorders in Childhood*. New York: Taylor and Francis, 1990.
84. Netsell R, Cleeland C: Modification of lip hypotonia in dysarthria using EMG feedback. *JSHD* 1973; 40:170–178.
85. Blakeley RW: Treatment of developmental apraxia of speech. In Perkins WH (ed): *Dysarthria and Apraxia*. New York: Thieme-Stratton, 1983.
86. Haynes S: Developmental apraxia of speech: Symptoms and treatment. In Johns DF (ed): *Clinical Management of Neurogenic Communication Disorders* 2nd edition. Boston, MA: Little Brown, 1985 pp 259–266.
87. Ylvisaker M: *Head Injury Rehabilitation: Children and Adolescents* San Diego, CA: College-Hill Press,1985.
88. Love RJ: *Childhood Motor Speech Disability*. New York: Macmillan Publishing Company, 1992.
89. Helm NA: Management of palilalia with a pacing board. *JSHD* 1979; 44:350–353.
90. Yorkston KM, Beukelman DR, Bell KR: *Clinical Management of Dysarthric Speakers*. Boston, MA: Little Brown, 1986.
91. Beukelman D, Yorkston K, Tice R: *Pacer/Tally*. Tuscon, AZ: Communication Skill Builders, 1988.
92. Prator RJ, Swift RW: *Manual of Voice Therapy*. Boston, MA: Little Brown, 1984.
93. Collins M, Rosenbek J, Donahue E: The effects of posture on speech in ataxic dysarthria. *ASHA* 1982; 24:767.
94. Ylvisaker M, Szekeres S: Metacognitive and executive impairments in head-injured children and adults 1989; *Topics in Language Disorders* 9:34–49.
95. Sohlerg M, Mateer C: *Introduction to Cognitive Rehabilitation*. New York: Guilford, 1989.

Part III
Sensory Factors

7

Hearing Impairment in Infants and Toddlers: Identification, Vocal Development, and Intervention

CAROL STOEL-GAMMON, PH.D., AND MARGARET M. KEHOE, M.SC.

Speech communication involves, among other things, a complex interaction of physical, physiologic, and linguistic processing on the part of the speaker as well as the listener. To communicate verbally, the speaker must (1) formulate an idea, (2) encode it into words by retrieving the appropriate items from a "mental dictionary," (3) generate a set of neural commands for the production of the words selected, and (4) execute the motor movements needed to generate the appropriate speech sounds. Reception of a spoken message by the listener also involves the following series of steps, which begin with auditory sensation and end with the perception of the message: (1) The sound wave transmitted by the speaker activates the auditory system; (2) nerve impulses are transmitted to the brain; (3) the string of sounds is analyzed perceptually and parsed into linguistically meaningful chunks by comparing the input with the stored forms of words and phrases; and (4) the listener recognizes the intended message.

The stream of sounds used to convey a message is heard not only by the intended recipient of the message, the listener, but also by the producer of that message, the speaker. Speakers listen to their own output and compare their productions with an internal representation (ie, a stored version in the mental dictionary) of the words or phrases they intend to say. If there is a mismatch between the output and the intended form, the production is modified so that it better matches the intended form. Although this comparison of one's own output with an internal representation (auditory feedback) is considered secondary in the speaker–listener loop, distortion or delay in this type of feedback has been shown to cause difficulties with production patterns—speech becomes slurred or distorted.[1]

One of the essential elements underlying the production and comprehension of speech is an intact peripheral and central auditory system. The system must be sensitive to sounds in the frequency range of 500 to 4000 Hz (the frequency range of the majority of speech sounds) and must be able to detect small differences in frequency and durational characteristics of phonemes. Individuals with a substantial hearing loss have difficulty engaging in the types of speaker–listener interactions described above. Such individuals have difficulty decoding a message because the incoming sound wave produced by the speaker does not activate the hearing mechanism in the same way that it would in an individual with normal hearing. Thus, the basic auditory and perceptual processes that underlie the recognition and interpretation of words are impaired. Hearing loss also affects the speaker in the speech chain. Even those individuals who display normal speech patterns prior to hearing loss often develop atypical patterns after the loss, with the change attributed largely to an inability to monitor their own productions due to distortions in auditory feedback.

Although the speaker–listener chain is based on interactions between adults, children can successfully engage in these interactions provided the messages conveyed are relatively simple. In the event of a hearing loss in early childhood, particularly one that occurs prior to the onset of speech, multiple aspects of the speech chain are affected. In the most severe cases, the child is not capable of perceiving spoken language at all; in such a case, the child could observe facial movements associated with speech, but would hear nothing (much like a hearing person watching television with the sound turned off). In cases of less severe hearing impairment, the auditory system might be activated by some portions of the sound wave, but the signal would be lacking sufficient information to discriminate the complete range of speech sounds. Even minor distortion in the speech signal can affect discrimination of phonetically similar words such as *Pete* versus *beat* or *sun* versus *fun*. Thus, hearing loss would affect all aspects of the speech chain for the "listener," from sensitivity to speech sounds to recognition of the intended message.

When hearing loss occurs in infancy or early childhood, before the individual has acquired language, speech production patterns are severely affected in several ways. If a child's hearing level is not adequate to support accurate perception, the production representations stored in the mental dictionary would be based on a degraded input signal and thus would be markedly different from those of hearing peers. Moreover, the auditory feedback loop would be markedly impaired, preventing online comparisons of output with the stored representation. However, some aspects of early speech–language development are left intact. For example, infants with hearing impairment begin to vocalize shortly after birth just like their normal peers. This age-appropriate onset of prelinguistic vocal productions is presumably due to normal development of the vocal-motor system underlying speech. Thus, the motor ability to produce sounds is unimpaired even though the auditory ability to perceive those productions is affected.

The purpose of this chapter is to examine the effects of hearing impairment on early vocal and verbal development of infants and toddlers. The chapter is divided into three sections that deal with three different aspects of hearing loss in infancy. We begin with a discussion of early identification of hearing loss. This topic is important for two reasons: First, we cannot determine the effects of hearing impairment on speech development unless we can identify babies who have such an impairment; second, appropriate intervention programs depend on early identification and implementation. The second section summarizes research on vocal and verbal development of infants and toddlers with and without hearing impairment. In the final section, we discuss intervention programs for the hearing impaired. Intervention in this population involves a two-pronged approach, one aimed at enhancing the *reception* of the speech and the other at improving *production*. Our discussion centers around sensory aids for the perception of speech (which, in turn, should help speech production). A discussion of intervention programs that focus on speech production is presented in Chapter 9. A set of suggested readings is provided at the end of this chapter.

Identification of Hearing Loss

Incidence

Any discussion of *identification* of hearing loss must be linked to figures regarding the *incidence* of this condition; a statement of the incidence must, in turn, take into consideration whether the baby is born into a well-baby nursery (WBN), is a graduate of a neonatal intensive care unit (NICU), or manifests "high-risk" criteria. High-risk and NICU infants have a higher incidence of transient and permanent hearing loss than the general population of newborns. Incidence figures for educationally significant hearing loss in infant and toddler populations vary, but the most frequently cited results are 1 in 1000 in a WBN[2] and 1 in 50 for children born "at-risk" or in a NICU.[3] Other reports suggest that the incidence of significant audiological problems in NICU babies may be slightly higher and range up to 4 and 5%.[4,5] Prevalence figures for hearing-impaired school age children are higher than for infants and toddlers due to the inclusion of milder degrees of hearing loss, unilateral hearing loss, and nonpermanent hearing loss due to conductive pathology.

Lundeen[6] reported hearing impairment prevalence rates in the United States using data collected by the National Speech and Hearing Survey (NSHS) Team during the 1968/1969 school year. This data base included the audiometric results of 38,000 school children in grades 1 through 12. The percentage of children with pure tone averages greater than 25 decibels (dB) was 2.63%. The NSHS sample reveals considerably lower prevalence rates than the other frequently cited prevalence study in which 5% of children showed a significant hearing loss in at least one ear.[7] Because the NSHS study is based on a larger sample of children and uses more modern audiometric standards, Lundeen considers it the most accurate prevalence statistic for school age children.

Identification

Early identification of hearing impairment is the first goal of any audiological program. The second goal is to provide appropriate intervention to maximize the chance for optimal speech, language, cognitive, and psychosocial development. The earlier intervention is initiated, the greater the opportunity to reduce the impact of hearing impairment.[8] In recent years, significant technological advances in hearing testing have led to attempts to lower the age of identification.

In particular, advances in noninvasive electrophysiological techniques that do not require behavioral responses, such as Auditory Brainstem Response (ABR) and Otoacoustic Emissions (OAEs), and refinements in behavioral procedures have enhanced early identification efforts. The ABR test measures neuroelectric activity generated by the auditory nerve and brainstem in response to auditory stimuli and has become established as a valid and reliable measure for screening hearing loss in newborns.[9] It approximates behavioral audiometric thresholds in the mid- to high-frequency region and is unaffected by sleep states or sedation.[10] Although ABR has the disadvantage of yielding a high false-positive rate, it is still considered the most efficient tool for the neonatal population.

OAEs also offer potential for clinical application in the pediatric setting.[11,12] OAEs are low-level acoustic signals from the cochlea that can be measured in the ear canal using an inserted microphone. Although the mechanism by which they are produced is not completely understood, they are believed to reflect processes associated with the outer hair cells.[11] There are two types of emissions: spontaneous (SOAEs) and elicited (EOAEs). The latter type can be measured in the majority of children and adults with normal hearing and hence has the greatest clinical potential.[13,14] The magnitude of the OAEs corresponds closely with hearing loss up to 40 dB in young children; they are typically absent for loss greater than 40 to 50 dB.[11] Because the goal of most neonatal screening programs is to identify infants at risk for loss greater than 30 dB, OAEs serve as an excellent screening tool. Comparative studies employing ABR and OAEs in neonate and infant screening suggest that OAEs may be equivalent to ABR in terms of sensitivity and specificity,[15] although further investigation of OAEs is needed.

Visual Reinforcement Audiometry (VRA) is the most commonly used test procedure for the screening and assessment of hearing loss in infants and toddlers 6 months to 2 years of age. In VRA, a head turn response to auditory stimuli is reinforced with an attractive visual event such as the activation of an automated toy. Since its original conception by Suzuki and Ogiba in 1960,[16] investigators have refined the technique by exploring which stimulus parameters, visual reinforcers, and assessment strategies are most effective with young children.[17] In general, most normal-hearing infants condition easily to the task and respond at levels of 20 dB or better.[18] However, VRA does have limitations. Around 2 years of age, toddlers tend to lose interest in the task and display more rapid habituation of responses.[19] Strategies for increasing the rate of responses at this age range, through the use of novel reinforcers and session breaks, have been shown to be effective.[18] VRA continues to be a vital tool in the identification of hearing loss in infants and young children.

A strong commitment to early identification of hearing impairment in the United States is reflected in a position statement prepared by the Joint Committee on Infant Hearing in 1990.[20] The committee is composed of representatives from the American Speech–Language Hearing Association (ASHA), American Academy of Otolaryngology-Head-Neck Surgery, the American Academy of Pediatrics, the Council on Education of the Deaf, and directors of speech and hearing programs in state health and welfare agencies. The committee's statement expands pre-existing risk criteria for neonates and infants and makes separate recommendations for audiological screening. Neonates at risk for hearing impairment should be screened for hearing loss prior to discharge from the hospital or no later than 3 months of age. Infants should be screened within 3 months after being identified as at risk. Initial screening of neonates and infants less than 6 months of age should include ABR. Evaluation after 6 months should include behavioral testing and/or ABR.

Despite the strong commitment and the increased efforts to identify hearing loss as early as possible, the average age of identification remains disappointingly high. Reports range between 12 months and 2 years. Elssman, Matkin, and Sabo[21] indicate an average age of identification of 19 months regardless of whether the infant was high risk. Mace, Wallace, Whan, and Stelmachowicz[22] report a mean age of identification of 2.1 years, with factors such as greater degree of hearing loss and additional handicapping conditions contributing to earlier identification.

Delay in identification of hearing loss and in appropriate intervention results from a number of factors. First, up to 50% of children with hearing loss are not detected by the high risk register.[21] Without a comprehensive neonatal screening program, these children's chances for early identification are minimized. Second, the failure of professionals to support parents' early suspicions of hearing loss is also a factor.[23,24] Finally, once a hearing loss has been identified the child should receive appropriate amplification as soon as possible. All too often, however, delays of as much as 6 months may occur between identification and fitting of amplification. For example, Stein et al[25] reported that the median age of enrollment in a habilitation program was around 20 months for both NICU and WBN graduates regardless of the earlier diagnosis for infants in the NICU group. Amplification may be delayed due to medical management of a middle ear condition, concern about a fluctuating hearing loss, or a conservative approach to hearing aid fitting.

The difficulties of identifying hearing-impaired infants in the United States has led to the proposal of a new model for early identification. In March 1993, the National Institutes of Health conducted a Consensus Development Conference on the Early Identification of Hearing Impairment in Infants and Young Children.[26] The outcome of the conference was the recommendation of universal screening for all infants under the age of 3 months. The advantage of universal screening is that ideally all infants with hearing loss will be identified prior to the development of speech and language. A disadvantage of universal screening is the increased cost of screening all newborns. However, it was the committee's opinion that the additional expense could be offset by the use of new test techniques such as OAEs that are rapid and easy to administer. Implementation of these recommendations will expand our data base of hearing-impaired infants, thus increasing our understanding of the effects of hearing loss on vocal development.

For many years the prime means of identifying hearing loss in infancy and early childhood was not through an assessment of hearing, but rather through the recognition of atypical patterns of speech and language development. The following sections summarize the similarities and differences in the patterns of prelinguistic and early linguistic development in infants and toddlers with normal hearing and hearing impairment.

Prelinguistic Vocal Development

Infants with Normal Hearing

Infants produce a variety of vocalizations during the first year of life, beginning with simple birth cries and progressing through an ordered sequence of stages to complex babbling with identifiable syllables and adult-like intonation patterns. The productions can be divided into two general categories: (1) *reflexive* vocalizations such as cries, coughs, and involuntary grunts reflecting the physical state of the infant; and (2) *nonreflexive* vocalizations like "cooing" or "jargon babbling" that are nonautomatic productions that contain many phonetic features found in adult languages. Regardless of the linguistic community in which they are being raised, all infants seem to pass through the same stages of vocal development. In this section, we will describe these stages and the approximate ages associated with each using the frameworks of Oller[27] and Stark.[28] Although commonly referred to as "stages," the periods described here are not discrete, and vocalization types typically overlap from one stage to another. A new stage is marked by the appearance of vocal behaviors not observed in the preceding period.

STAGE 1: REFLEXIVE VOCALIZATIONS (BIRTH TO 2 MONTHS)

This stage is characterized by a majority of reflexive vocalizations such as crying, fussing, and vegetative sounds like coughing, burping, and sneezing. In addition, some vowel-like sounds may occur. The vocalizations of this period are partially determined by the infant's anatomic structure. In newborn babies, the vocal tract resembles that of a nonhuman primate in which the oral cavity is small and almost totally filled by the tongue, and the larynx is high in the neck with little separation of the oral and nasal cavities.[29] This configuration limits the range of sound types that can be produced. Rapid growth of the head and neck area in the stages that follow allows production of a greater variety of sounds.

STAGE 2: COOING AND LAUGHTER (2 TO 4 MONTHS)

During this stage, infants begin to make some comfort-state vocalizations often referred to as "cooing" or "gooing" sounds. These vocalizations contain consonant-like and vowel-like productions formed in the back of the mouth. Crying typically becomes less frequent and much to parents' delight sustained laughter and infant chuckles appear.

STAGE 3: VOCAL PLAY (4 TO 6 MONTHS)

In this period, it seems as though babies are testing their vocal apparatus to determine the range of vocal qualities they can produce. The period is characterized by the appearance of a wide variety of phonation types, including yells, whispers, squeals, and growls. Rudimentary syllables of consonants and vowels occasionally occur, and some babies produce long series of raspberries (bilabial trills) and sustained vowels.

STAGE 4: CANONICAL BABBLING (6 MONTHS AND OLDER)

The prime feature of this period is the appearance of sequences of consonant-vowel syllables with adult-like timing. For the first time, babies sound as though they are actually trying to produce words, and a sequence such as [mama] or [dada] may lead parents to report that their baby has begun to call them by name. Although the baby is indeed producing something like "mama" or "daddy," in most cases there is no evidence that the productions are semantically linked to an identifiable referent. Multisyllabic utterances in this period are typically categorized as *reduplicated* babbles (ie, strings of identical syllables like [bababa]) or *variegated* babbles (syllable strings with varying consonants and vowels). While both types of utterances occur in the canonical stage, reduplicated babbles predominate initially, and at about 12 to 13 months variegated babbles emerge as the more frequent type.

STAGE 5: JARGON BABBLE (9 MONTHS AND OLDER)

This stage overlaps both with the canonical stage and with the early period of meaningful speech. It is characterized by the appearance of long strings of syllables uttered with a variety of stress and intonational patterns. To many adults, it seems as though children are speaking in whole sentences—making statements, asking questions—but are using their "own" language rather than the standard language spoken by older children and adults around them.

The Link between Babble and Speech

Studies focusing on the relationship between babble and speech show strong links between the phonological patterns of late babbling and early meaningful speech. Regardless of the language being acquired, productions in this period contain a high proportion of CV syllables in which the consonantal elements are stops, nasals, or glides.[30,31] Individual differences have been noted and those patterns that appear in a particular child's nonmeaningful vocalizations also occur in his earliest words.[32] Other links between babble and speech include: (1) the age of onset of canonical babble and age of onset of meaningful speech; (2) frequency of canonical syllables and acquisition of a 50-word vocabulary; (3) use of consonants in canonical babble and level of phonological development at 3 years of age (see Stoel-Gammon[33] for a summary of these studies). The late onset of canonical babble and/or reduced use of consonants in the prelinguistic period appears to be linked to delays in the acquisition of speech and language.[34–36]

To summarize, the research on prelinguistic vocal development shows that infants pass through a predictable sequence of stages from cries and vegetative noises in the first month to jargon babble at the end of the first year. The form of productions in the later stages of prelinguistic development shares many features with children's early words; in both, stops, nasals, and glides occur with greatest frequency, and CV is the most common syllable shape. Longitudinal studies spanning the prelinguistic and linguistic periods suggest that performance on particular aspects of babbling in the first year is linked to subsequent linguistic performance.

Infants with Hearing Loss

Comparisons of the productions of normal-hearing (NH) and hearing-impaired (HI) infants and toddlers allow us to examine the effects of hearing impairment on early language development. Investigations of young subjects with hearing impairment have tended to center around the following set of questions:

1. Do babies with HI vocalize in the first year of life?
2. Do HI babies vocalize as frequently as their NH peers?
3. Is the form of vocalization (ie, sound types and stages) produced by babies with HI the same as that of their NH peers?
4. Is degree of hearing loss associated with differences in patterns of prelinguistic vocalizations among subjects with HI?

Although we have some information regarding these questions, our knowledge is limited by the size and nature of the database on HI subjects. As noted in the previous section, detection of hearing impairment in infancy was relatively rare prior to the 1980s and, in spite of the recent advances in assessment procedures, is not a routine occurrence today. Much of the work currently available comes from data collected before the use of electrophysiological techniques for identifying loss in infancy was common and is consequently limited to single cases or small groups of subjects. Methodological differences in data collection and data analysis also make it difficult to make valid comparisons of research on HI subjects and to determine similarities and differences between vocal development of HI and NH groups. The following sections provide an overview of the research to date.

DO BABIES WITH HEARING LOSS VOCALIZE?

There is general agreement that the answer to this is affirmative. Just like their hearing peers, babies with HI begin to vocalize shortly after birth and continue to do so in the months that follow.

DOES HEARING LOSS AFFECT THE FREQUENCY OF VOCAL PRODUCTIONS?

There is a lack of consensus regarding the answer to this question. A number of investigators reported that frequency of vocalization tends to increase with age for hearing subjects but to decrease with age for subjects with HI.[37-41] In contrast, Stark's[42] careful examination of frequency of vocalizations (measured by number of utterances per minute) of 11 HI subjects, aged 15 to 24 months, led to the conclusion that the frequency of vocalization of the HI subjects was similar to that of younger hearing subjects at the same stage of vocal development. She also noted that rate of vocal output increased for subjects in both groups as they passed to higher stages of development.

Stark's finding that HI and NH babies have the same rate of vocalization if they are matched for stage, rather than age, is not supported by two case studies that show that babies with HI vocalize as frequently as their *age-matched* peers. Oller, Eilers, Bull, and Carney[43] followed the vocal development of a girl with profound sensorineural bilateral hearing loss from 8 to 13 months, and Kent, Osberger, Netsell, and Hustedde[44] compared the vocal development of twin boys from 8 to 15 months: one boy was NH, and the other had a profound sensorineural bilateral loss. In these longitudinal case studies, the HI subjects vocalized as frequently as hearing subjects in the same age range.

Thus, there are conflicting findings regarding the answer to this question. The different outcomes may be due to individual variation across subjects, to differences in degree of hearing loss of the HI subjects, or to early (and presumably better) amplification in the longitudinal studies. Further research on larger groups of subjects is needed to provide a clear answer to this question.

HOW DOES HEARING LOSS AFFECT THE STAGES AND PATTERNS OF
VOCAL DEVELOPMENT?

Relatively little early research addressed this question prior to the 1980s. The few available studies before that time suggested that early vocal development of HI infants was indistinguishable from their NH peers. Mavilya[39,40] followed the vocal development of four subjects from 3 to 6 months: three subjects had severe-to-profound hearing loss; the other had normal hearing. She reported that prior to 5 to 6 months all four subjects produced similar types of vowels and consonants, including some consonant-vowel combinations. At around 6 months, the frequency of vocalizations of the HI babies decreased substantially, while the rate for the NH subject increased. Her findings provide support for the presence of similarities between HI and NH vocal development during the first 6 months.

Lenneberg's widely cited research[45,46] showed no differences in the developmental patterns of babies with and without HI during the first year after birth. (No information regarding the degree of hearing loss was provided.) According to Lenneberg, the HI infants began cooing at 2 to 3 months and started "babbling" (producing canonical syllables) at 6 to 7 months, similar to their NH peers. Group differences emerged only after 12 months of age when the HI subjects failed to begin producing words. Although Lenneberg's findings are intriguing, his conclusions regarding group differences are weakened by the fact that they appear to be based on data from only two HI subjects (see discussion by Gilbert[47]).

In spite of the small numbers of subjects and possible methodological inadequacies of data collection and analysis, the work of Mavilya and Lenneberg led many researchers to conclude that hearing loss had little effect on vocal development in the first year of life. Thus, texts on language development cite Lenneberg's research and make statements such as: "Children babble even if they themselves are deaf and cannot hear their own sounds . . . The onset of babbling occurs at about the same age in deaf as in hearing children, and it is similar in form. ."[48] Research carried out since 1980, however, has raised serious doubts about this view. The more recent studies show differences between subjects with HI and NH in at least two domains: (1) age at onset of canonical babbling; and (2) size and composition of the consonantal inventory.

Oller and colleagues[43,49] have suggested that apparent similarities in vocal output of HI and NH subjects may be a consequence of inadequate description and categorization of infant vocalizations. According to Oller, transcriptions of infant vocalizations should always be made in conjunction with a "metaphonological" categorization scheme based on the stages of vocal development.[50] Using this stage framework, Oller and Eilers[49] demonstrated differences between NH and HI subjects in the onset of the canonical babbling stage: the 21 infants with NH began producing canonical syllables between 6 and 10 months, while the age of onset for the 9 subjects in the HI group ranged from 11 to 25 months. Moreover, after entering the canonical babbling stage, the infants with HI produced fewer canonical syllables per utterance than did the NH subjects.

In addition to a late onset of canonical babbling, infants with hearing loss evidence different patterns of speech sound production. In their investigation of nonmeaningful productions of 11 NH and 11 HI subjects, Stoel-Gammon and Otomo[51] found that subjects in the NH group evidenced an increase in the size of the consonantal inventory with age, whereas the consonantal repertoires of subjects in the HI group either decreased in size or remained constant over time. Even subjects with a moderate conductive loss due to atresia adhered to this pattern. The study also reported that the HI subjects produced fewer utterances with canonical syllables (supporting Oller and Eiler's[49] findings) and more utterances with glottal sequences (eg, [ʔʌʔʌʔʌ]). In addition, the range of vowel productions in the output of subjects with HI is also restricted.[42,44]

Of particular interest is one of the HI subjects in Stoel-Gammon and Otomo's sample[51] who experienced normal vocal development until she was stricken with a severe case of meningitis at 8 months of age that caused a profound hearing loss. Samples gathered at 11 and 19 months showed a substantial decrease in her consonantal repertoire during this period in spite of normal hearing and age-appropriate onset of canonical babbling prior to her illness.

Stoel-Gammon[52,53] compared the composition of the consonantal inventories (analyzing both types and tokens) for subjects in the Stoel-Gammon and Otomo study[51] and reported several differences. Compared with NH infants, subjects in the HI group produced more labial consonants and fewer alveolar consonants; more nasal consonants and fewer oral stop consonants; more syllabic consonants (including syllabic fricatives); and more glottal consonants. The findings on composition of phonetic inventories among HI subjects in this study are supported by the reports of Lach, Ling, Ling, and Ship[54], Stark[42], and Yoshinaga-Itano, Stredler-Brown, and Jancosek[55].

Another difference between HI and NH subjects was the nature of change in phonetic inventory.[53] Among the NH subjects, change in the place and manner features of consonantal classes was unidirectional; for the HI subjects, it was typically U shaped. For example, analysis of 44 samples from NH subjects showed that the mean proportion of stops increased from 18% for subjects 5 to 7 months of age, to 40% at the 8- to 13-month range, to 43% at 14 to 18 months; the mean proportion of labials showed a decreasing trend over the three age periods from 59 to 37 and 32%. In contrast, for the 28 HI samples, the mean occurrence of stops at three age periods was 21% (at 5 to 12 months); it fell to 7% (at 15 to 21 months) and then rose to 18% (at 22 to 39 months); for labials, the comparable figures show a rise in mean proportion followed by a fall: 37, 91, and 75%. (One obvious difficulty in comparing the vocal development of NH and HI subjects is evident in the foregoing comparisons: the NH subjects cease babbling around 18 to 21 months, but most HI subjects continue to produce nonmeaningful utterances in the second and third year of life; once the NH subjects stop babbling, age-related comparisons of nonmeaningful productions are not possible.)

HOW DOES DEGREE OF HEARING LOSS AFFECT PRELINGUISTIC VOCALIZATIONS?

Only a few studies have directly examined the relationship between degree of hearing loss and prelinguistic vocal development. Stoel-Gammon and Otomo[51] noted that the vocalizations of *all* subjects in the HI group differed from those of the NH subjects, but that the nature and magnitude of difference was less for those subjects with a moderate loss. The consonantal inventory of one subject who had a moderate conductive loss (associated with atresia) was reduced compared with the NH subjects, but distribution of the inventory in terms of sound classes nearly matched that of the NH subjects. In her study of 11 subjects, aged 15 to 24 months, Stark[43] stated that degree of loss did not appear to be closely related to stage of vocal development; she did note, however, that none of the subjects with profound loss had entered the stage of canonical babble.

The largest data set that addresses the issue of degree of hearing loss comes from Yoshinaga et al,[55] who studied the vocal development of 91 infants and toddlers with sensorineural loss from birth to 3 years of age. Infants with Pure Tone Averages (PTA) of 70 dB or less were classified as "hard of hearing"; those with PTAs greater than 70 dB were classified as "deaf." Group comparisons of the productions of consonants and vowels showed only a few statistically significant differences: subjects in the deaf group produced significantly fewer tokens of the consonants [t, d, l, s] and the vowels [e] and its diphthongized counterpart [eɪ]. Interestingly, the consonants most affected by degree of loss were the alveolars, a sound class produced infrequently by the HI subjects in Stoel-Gammon's comparison[52,53] of phonetic inventories of HI and NH subjects.

To summarize, the available data suggest that hearing loss, even in the moderate range, has a detrimental affect on vocal development. Based on Yoshinaga-Itano's study,[55] we can conclude that differences in degree of hearing loss are associated with relatively minor changes in segmental inventories during the prelinguistic period. In contrast, the relationship between degree of loss and speech production skills during the period of meaningful speech is directly correlated: the greater the loss, the greater the difficulty in learning to produce intelligible speech.[8]

Explanations and Implications

Several recurrent themes emerge from this comparison of vocal development in HI and NH subjects. First, HI infants vocalize in the first months of life in much the same way as their NH peers but fail to enter the canonical babbling stage within the appropriate time frame (by 9 to 10 months). Second, the vocalizations of HI subjects differ from the NH subjects in syllabic structure and in characteristics of the consonant and vowel sounds that occur. Third, vocal characteristics of HI subjects show only slight variations that can be attributed to differences in degree of hearing loss. The goal of this section is to present some possible explanations for the patterns of vocal development among HI babies and to discuss implications of hearing loss for prelinguistic and early linguistic development.

LATE ONSET OF CANONICAL BABBLE

The reasons for the late onset of canonical babble remain unclear. We know that it cannot be attributed to anatomic or structural differences among the HI population or to difficulties with motor movement (although lack of practice in production may be associated with a lack of motor control). A major difficulty in pinpointing the causes for failure to produce canonical babble is the fact that we do not exactly know why most hearing babies enter the stage at around 6 to 7 months. Presumably, anatomic and muscular changes occurring in the first 6 months play an important role. As noted earlier, the infant's vocal tract resembles that of a nonhuman primate in the early months, but with growth in the head and neck area in the third and fourth months, the larynx lowers, and the tongue fills a smaller portion of the oral cavity.[29] Prior to these changes, it would not be possible to produce the consonant and vowel-like sounds that occur in the canonical stage.

The onset of the canonical period may also be related to an emergent motor pattern that appears around 6 months. Babies begin to produce repetitive body movements such as waving their arms, kicking, and opening and closing their hands.[56,57] The temporal synchrony in onset of these "rhythmic stereotypies" of the limbs and the appearance of repeated CV syllables has led some researchers to suggest that canonical babbling represents a vocal analogue (opening and closing of the jaw) of other repetitive body movements.[58] According to this line of reasoning, it would follow that a delay in the onset of canonical babble would be linked to a general delay in motor development and not to a loss in hearing acuity.

The finding that hearing loss is associated with significant delays in the onset of canonical babbling suggests that while both age-appropriate anatomic and structural growth and normal motor development may be necessary for the appearance of CV syllables, they are *not* sufficient. In addition to these factors, the onset of canonical babble is dependent on the ability to perceive speech—presumably the speech of others, although it is possible that hearing one's own vocalizations might be sufficient. The best way to determine whether the critical cue is external input or self-vocalizations is to locate hearing infants whose exposure to speech is limited to their own productions. In an attempt to do just this, Lenneberg[45] examined productions of one or two hearing babies (the number of subjects is unclear) born to deaf parents. He reported that even though these babies were exposed to limited amounts of adult speech, their babbling was indistinguishable from that of hearing babies raised by hearing parents, suggesting that exposure to one's own vocalizations is sufficient to trigger the onset. Given that these findings are based on one or two subjects, they should be replicated with larger samples before any firm conclusions can be drawn.

If we conclude that the late onset of canonical babble in HI subjects is due primarily to their inability to hear speech input, an important question still remains: Why do HI babies begin to produce canonical syllables at 12, or 14, even 24 months? One possible explanation is that the age of onset in these subjects is linked to amplification. Evidence to support a link between age at amplification and age of appearance of canonical syllables is lacking at present. Longitudinal studies must be carried out before this relationship can be fully understood.

INVENTORY DIFFERENCES

Most researchers have noted unusually high proportions of labial consonants in the productions of HI subjects. The probable cause for the high incidence of this sound class is relatively straightforward—consonants articulated with lip movements have a visual component that is lacking in consonants produced at other places of articulation. Because auditory cues are greatly reduced, HI subjects presumably pay attention to the visual cues and reproduce the oral gestures associated with labial and labiodental productions. Research by Kuhl and Meltzoff[59] has shown that NH infants 3 to 4 months of age pay attention to the visual cues associated with speech sound production and can link specific oral movements with specific sound types. Stoel-Gammon[52] noted that the younger subjects in her study (4 to 20 months) produced fewer labials than the older subjects (18 to 39 months) and hypothesized that the influence of visual cues may increase with age.

Possible explanations for the findings that HI subjects produce fewer alveolars and fewer stop consonants are more speculative. In discussing the relatively high proportion of nasals and fricatives and the low proportion of stops in the HI samples she analyzed, Stoel-Gammon[52] suggested a link between amount of tactile and kinesthetic feedback and frequency of occurrence of consonantal types. Nasals and fricatives can be prolonged and thus would provide a good deal of tactile and kinesthetic feedback. In contrast, stops are of short duration, giving less feedback, and thus might be produced less frequently.

The paucity of alveolar consonants in productions of HI subjects is puzzling. Locke[30] noted that the alveolar stop [d] is among the most frequent consonantal types in the nonmeaningful productions of NH infants. Interestingly, Yoshinaga's study[55] showed that production of alveolars appears to be the *only* sound class that is sensitive to the degree of hearing loss–the greater the loss, the fewer alveolars (see discussion above). Just why this is the case remains unclear.

IMPLICATIONS OF A LACK OF PRACTICE AND OF AUDITORY FEEDBACK

Speech has a skill component, and, as with any skilled activity, practice increases the control and precision with which a movement is performed. The more a baby produces the movements that shape the vocal tract to produce particular sounds and sound sequences, the more automatic those movements become, and the easier it is to execute them in producing meaningful speech. In a recent study of the transition from babble to speech in NH infants, Vihman[60] noted that the syllables a particular child used in forming early words tended to be the same syllables that occurred frequently in that subject's babbling samples. One ramification of this observation is that babies who have many different CV syllables in babbling would be at an advantage in early word acquisition because they would have a larger repertoire of forms to which meaning can be attached. Because HI subjects produce relatively few CV syllables in the prelinguistic period, they would have relatively few forms to which they could attach meaning.

Practice in the production of speech-like vocalizations is also important in feedback. As noted in the introduction, speakers are themselves listeners; thus, even in the prelinguistic period, infants are exposed to two types of vocal input; the speech of others and their own productions. The importance of the feedback loop for prelinguistic vocal development was emphasized by Fry[61] (p 189), who stated: "As sound-producing movements are repeated and repeated, a strong link is forged between tactual and kinesthetic impressions and auditory sensations that the child receives from his own utterances." Awareness of the links between one's own oral-motor movements and the acoustic signal that results is a prerequisite to auditory-vocal matching that underlies word production. The more a child babbles, the greater the opportunity to establish the feedback loops necessary for producing and monitoring his own speech. Infants who vocalize infrequently, as do some babies with HI, would have fewer opportunities to establish this loop.

Practice and feedback are not independent aspects of early vocal development. Practice involves the repeated production of sounds; feedback involves hearing and monitoring these productions. It is possible to have practice without auditory feedback, but feedback cannot occur in the absence of practice. Although babies with HI have a normally developing vocal apparatus that would allow them to practice the movements associated with the production of CV syllables, they would only receive tactile and kinesthetic feedback from oral movements. Their hearing loss would severely limit the auditory feedback they would receive.

Lack of practice also affects the timetable of speech and language development. Locke and Pearson[62] examined the linguistic development of a young, cognitively normal girl who was tracheotomized and "generally aphonic" from 5 to 20 months. Although she was exposed to speech from the adults around her, she vocalized infrequently and consequently had little opportunity to form auditory or tactile feedback loops based on her own output. Following decannulation (ie, removal of the tube that prevented normal respiration) just prior to 21 months, there was a marked increase in the frequency of vocal output; interestingly, only six of the 909 utterances recorded by the researchers met the criteria for canonical syllables. In addition to the lack of well-formed syllables, the speech output was characterized by a limited repertoire of consonantal types. Locke and Pearson noted that her speech was similar to that of HI subjects studied by Stoel-Gammon and Otomo[51] and Oller and Eilers.[49] These findings, though limited to a case study of a single child, serve to highlight the importance of practice and auditory feedback in the normal vocal development.

EFFECTS OF HEARING LOSS ON SPEECH AND LANGUAGE DEVELOPMENT

The prelinguistic period is a time during which the building blocks used in perception and production are formed. Given the link between babble and speech–language development in NH children, hearing loss during the prelinguistic period takes on increased importance. Research suggests that even if, by some miracle, a prelinguistically deaf baby were to have her hearing fully restored at 12 months, her speech patterns would remain atypical for some time. On the perceptual side, she would have to learn the associations between spoken forms and objects and actions in the world around her. On the production side, she would need to go through the "practice and feedback" exercises that NH infants engage in prior to beginning to talk; these exercises would give the phonetic forms she could use in the production of words and create the feedback loops that would allow her to monitor her own productions (see Chapter 9).

In light of the importance of prelinguistic vocalization to later speech development, early detection and habilitation of hearing loss take on increased importance. Fitting the child with appropriate amplification represents a first step.

Recent advances in hearing aids and sensory devices, such as cochlear implants and tactile aids, hold the promise of providing improved habilitation programs for the young child. These are described in the section that follows.

Sensory Aids and Speech Production

An important area of research in the habilitation of hearing impaired children is the evaluation of newly developed sensory aids such as cochlear implants and tactile aids. Because the fitting of such sensory devices to the infant population is relatively recent, there are no studies that deal only with this group. The investigations that have been conducted report results on subjects ranging in age from 2 to 18 years. Although speech production abilities have been less extensively studied than speech perception skills, they are still considered to be an important benefit of any sensory aid for the deaf.[63] A series of studies during the last 10 years have focused on assessing and comparing the benefits of different devices.[64-67] One of the key issues in measuring change is the use of appropriate assessment tools.

Studies have incorporated both traditional measures of speech production and more experimental analysis procedures. Two frequently used "traditional" tests employed in the evaluation of sensory aids are Ling's[68] Phonetic Level Speech Evaluation (PLE) and Phonological Level Speech Evaluation (Phonological). The PLE evaluates imitated production of suprasegmental speech patterns, vowels and diphthongs, singleton consonants, and consonant clusters. The phonological speech evaluation examines the consistency of suprasegmental patterns and phoneme production in spontaneous speech. Both tests, but the PLE in particular, rely on a complex coding system that is strongly dependent on listener judgments. A number of methods have been used to quantify performance on the PLE so that comparisons can be made between sensory devices and test setting.[64,66] Kirk and Hill-Brown[64] used these measures with children who had received the House Ear Institute (HEI) single channel implant to evaluate benefits of implant experience. They found a significant increase in imitation of segmental and suprasegmental aspects of speech and in spontaneous speech production at 6 months postimplant and a maintenance of these skills at 1 year postimplant.

The PLE has also been used in the speech production protocol of pediatric recipients of the Cochlear Corporation Nucleus multichannel implant.[66,69] Significantly higher scores were obtained in segmental and suprasegmental subtests of the PLE and in the phonological evaluation at postimplant testing. Tobey and Hasenstab[69] noted that suprasegmental skills appeared to plateau after 1 year of implant use, whereas imitative and spontaneous segmental skills appeared to improve progressively with greater implant experience. A recent study by Tye-Murray and Kirk[70] showed an increase in the number and variety of vowels and diphthongs produced by children wearing the Nucleus device. Comparison of performance on the vowel and diphthong subtests of the PLE with production of vowels and diphthongs in spontaneous speech yielded only weak correlations between the two, suggesting that results on the PLE do not necessarily reflect spontaneous speech performance. In a similar vein, Shaw and

Coggins[71] reported unacceptably low levels of inter-observer reliability with the PLE, posing a strong challenge to the frequent use of this instrument in device evaluation.

Many times, candidates for sensory aids may have such poor speech production and linguistic skills that traditional assessment procedures may not be suitable. With this in mind, Osberger et al[65] developed a new analysis scheme to be utilized with young deaf children who have very limited speech-production ability. Vocalizations from an elicited 6-minute speech sample are judged to be "speech," "speech-like," "nonspeech," or "other," and the number of vocalizations in each category are tallied. This type of analysis has been used to evaluate the effectiveness of different devices in promoting development of speech skills.[63] Another way of monitoring device performance is to examine changes in speech production when the speech processor is turned on and off. Tobey et al[66] conducted acoustic analyses of the vowel /ɛ/ when the implant was in use and when it was not and found significantly lower second formant values in the "off" condition. This suggests a more centralized vowel production when auditory feedback is absent.

Information on speech production benefits from tactile aid use has been less well documented than with cochlear implants. Many reports are of an anecdotal nature but still suggest that use of a tactile aid will lead to increased frequency of vocalization, maintenance of voicing, and more appropriate voice quality.[72] Oller, Eilers, Vergara, and LaVoie[73] found that young deaf children's productions of consonants and vowels greatly improved when a tactual vocoder was introduced into their school training program. Weisenberger and Kozma-Spytek[67] reported that the Tacticon, a multichannel electrotactile device, had facilitative effects on the speech production skills of a group of profoundly HI children. Higher scores were obtained on listener rating scores recorded during connected discourse tracking with the device turned on versus off.

The results of these studies and numerous others seem to indicate that the sensory information delivered via a cochlear implant or tactile device has beneficial consequences for speech production. Taken together, these studies show improvement in the imitative and spontaneous production of suprasegmental and segmental aspects of speech. In general, greater changes have been observed in the imitative productions of vowels and simple consonants than in spontaneous speech.[67,70] However, the results are somewhat less dramatic than originally anticipated. In addition, the impact of these results is lessened by methodological issues common to studies of this nature. These issues include small sample sizes, unequal cell numbers, absence of control groups, and paucity of normative data regarding test procedures. Determining the efficacy of new advances in sensory aids remains a challenging research issue.

Cochlear implants and tactile devices have received enormous research attention in recent years due to their experimental nature. Yet we must not forget that the majority of HI children are not fitted with implants or tactile aids but with personal hearing aids. Improvements in hearing aid technology, such as use of directional microphones, noise suppression, and digital circuitry, should lead to enhanced speech perception abilities and ultimately superior speech production skills. In addition, the widespread use of FM systems and other listening devices in the classroom designed to combat the negative effects of noise and distance, should facilitate speech perception and production skills. Gains in speech production should also be evaluated in light of these new developments in amplification.

Acknowledgments

Preparation of this chapter was supported in part by a grant from NIDCD (DC0052) and by the Virginia Merrill Bloedel Hearing Research Center at the University of Washington.

Suggested Readings

Folsom R: Identification of hearing loss in infants using auditory brainstem response: Strategies and program choice. *Sem Hear* 1990; 11:333–341.

Kirk K, Hill-Brown C: Speech and language results in children with a cochlear implant. *Ear Hear* 1985; 6 (suppl):36S–47S.

National Institutes of Health: *Consensus Development Conference on Early Identification of Hearing Impairment in Infants and Young Children*, 1993.

Norton S: Application of transient evoked otoacoustic emissions to pediatric populations. *Ear Hear* 1993; 14:64–73.

Oller DK, Eilers RE: The role of audition in babbling. *Child Dev* 1988; 59:441–449.

Stoel-Gammon C, Otomo K: Babbling development of hearing-impaired and normally hearing subjects. *J Speech Hear Disorders* 1986; 51:33–41.

Stoel-Gammon C: Prelinguistic vocalizations of hearing-impaired and normally hearing subjects: A comparison of consonantal inventories. *J Speech Hear Disorders* 1988; 53:302–315.

Tobey E, Hasenstab MS: Effects of a nucleus multichannel cochlear implant upon speech production in children. *Ear Hear* 1991; 12(suppl):48S–54S.

Yoshinaga-Itano C, Stredler-Brown A, Jancosek B: From phone to phoneme: What we can understand from babble. *Volta Rev* 1992, 94:283–314.

References

1. Denes PB, Pinson EN: *The Speech Chain: The Physics and Biology of Spoken Language.* Baltimore: Waverly Press, Inc., 1963.

2. Feinmesser M, Tell L: Neonatal screening for detection of deafness. *Arch Otolaryngol* 1976; 102:297–299.

3. Schulman-Galambos C, Galambos R: Brainstem evoked response audiometry in newborn hearing screening. *Arch Otolaryngol* 1979; 105:86–90.

4. Sanders R, Durieux-Smith A, Hyde M, Jacobson J, Kileny P, Murnane O: Incidence of hearing loss in high risk and intensive care nursery infants. *J Otolaryngol* 1985; 14(suppl):28–33.

5. Stein L, Ozdamar O, Kraus N, Paton J: Follow-up of infants screened by auditory brainstem response in the neonatal intensive care unit. *J Pediatr* 1983; 103:447–453.

6. Lundeen C: Prevalence of hearing impairment among school children. *LSHSS* 1991; 22:269–271.

7. Eagles E, Wishik S, Doerfler L, Melnick W, Levine H: Hearing sensitivity and related factors in children. *Laryngoscope* (monogr suppl) 1963.

8. Hirsh I: Teaching the deaf child to speak. In Smith F, Miller GA (eds): *The Genesis of Language.* Cambridge, MA: MIT Press, 1966, pp 207–216.

9. Hyde ML, Malizia K, Riko K, Alberti PW: Audiometric estimation error with ABR in high risk infants. *Acta Otolaryngol* 1991; 111:212–219.

10. Folsom R: Identification of hearing loss in infants using auditory brainstem response: Strategies and program choice. *Sem Hear* 1990; 11:333–341.

11. Norton S: Application of transient evoked otoacoustic emissions to pediatric populations. *Ear Hear* 1993; 14:64–73.

12. Prieve B: Otoacoustic emissions in infants and children: Basic characteristics and clinical application. *Sem Hear* 1992; 13:37–52.

13. Bonfils P, Uziel A, Pujol R: Evoked oto-acoustic emissions from adults and infants: Clinical applications. *Acta Otolaryngol* 1988; 105:445–449.

14. Norton S, Widen J: Evoked otoacoustic emissions in normal-hearing infants and children: Emerging data and issues. *Ear Hear* 1990; 11:121–127.
15. Stevens J, Webb H, Hutchinson J, Connell J, Smith M, Buffin J: Click evoked otoacoustic emissions compared with brainstem electric response. *Arch Dis Childhood* 1989; 64:1105–1111.
16. Suzuki T, Ogiba Y: A technique of pure-tone audiometry for children under three years of age: Conditioned orientation reflex (COR) audiometry. *Rev Laryngol Otol Rhinol* 1960; 81:33–45.
17. Thompson G, Wilson W: Clinical application of visual reinforcement audiometry. *Sem Hear* 1984; 5:85–99.
18. Thompson G, Thompson M, McCall A: Strategies for increasing response behavior of 1- and 2-year old children during visual reinforcement audiometry (VRA). *Ear Hear* 1992; 13:236–240.
19. Primus M, Thompson G: Response strength of young children in operant audiometry. *J Speech Hear Res* 1985; 28:539–547.
20. Joint Committee on Infant Hearing 1990 Position Statement. *ASHA* 1991; 33(suppl 5):3–6.
21. Elssmann S, Matkin N, Sabo M: Early identification of congenital sensorineural hearing impairment. *Hear J* 1987; 40:13–17.
22. Mace A, Wallace K, Whan M, Stelmachowicz P: Relevant factors in the identification of hearing loss. *Ear Hear* 1991; 12:287–293.
23. Mahon W: Hearing care for infants and children: Issues in identification of hearing loss. *Ear Hear* 1987; 40:7–11.
24. Thompson M, Thompson G: Early identification of hearing loss: Listen to parents. *Clin Pediatr* 1991; 30:77–80.
25. Stein L, Jabaley T, Spitz R, Stoakley D, McGee T: The hearing-impaired infant: Patterns of identification and habilitation revisited. *Ear Hear* 1990; 11:201–205.
26. National Institutes of Health: Consensus Development Conference on Early Identification of Hearing Impairment in Infants and Young Children. Bethesda, MD: NIH, 1993.
27. Oller DK: The emergence of sounds of speech in infancy. In Yeni-Komshian GH, Kavanagh JF, Ferguson CA (eds): *Child Phonology, vol 1.* New York: Academic Press, 1980, pp 93–112.
28. Stark RE: Stages of speech development in the first year of life. In Yeni-Komshian GH, Kavanagh JF, Ferguson CA (eds): *Child Phonology,* vol 1. New York: Academic Press, 1980, pp 73–92.
29. Lieberman P, Crelin ES, Klatt DH: Phonetic ability and related anatomy of the newborn adult human Neanderthal man and the chimpanzee. *Am Anthropol* 1972; 74:287–307.
30. Locke JL: *Phonological Acquisition and Change.* New York: Academic Press, 1983.
31. Stoel-Gammon C: Phonetic inventories 15–24 months: A longitudinal study. *J Speech Hear Res* 1985; 28:505–512.
32. Vihman MM, Ferguson CA, Elbert M: Phonological development from babbling to speech: Common tendencies and individual differences. *Appl Psycholinguist* 1987; 7:3–40.
33. Stoel-Gammon C: Prelinguistic vocal development: Measurement and predictions. In Ferguson CA, Menn L, Stoel-Gammon C (eds): *Phonological Development: Models, Research, Implications.* Timonium, MD: York Press, 1992, pp 439–456.
34. Jensen TS, Boggild-Andersen B, Schmidt J, Ankerhus J, Hansen E: Perinatal risk factors and first year vocalizations: Influence on preschool language and motor performance. *Dev Med Child Neurol* 1988; 30:153–161.
35. Stoel-Gammon C: Prespeech and early speech development of two late talkers. *First Lang* 1989; 9:207–224.
36. Whitehurst GJ, Smith M, Fischel JE, Arnold DS, Lonigan CJ: The continuity of babble and speech in children with specific expressive language delay. *J Speech Hear Res* 1991; 34:1121–1129.
37. Anderson VA, Newby H: *Improving the Child's Speech,* 2nd ed. London, Oxford: University Press, 1973.
38. Maskarinec AS, Cairns GF, Butterfield EC, Weamer DK: Longitudinal observations of individual infant's vocalizations. *J Speech Hear Disorders* 1981; 46:267–273.
39. Mavilya MP: *Spontaneous Vocalization and Babbling in Hearing-Impaired Infants.* Unpublished doctoral dissertation, Teachers College, Columbia University, New York, 1969.
40. Mavilya MP: Spontaneous vocalization and babbling in hearing impaired infants. In Fant G (ed): *International Symposium on Speech Communication Abilities and Profound Deafness.* Washington, DC: Alexander Graham Bell Association for the Deaf, 1972, pp 163–171.
41. Meers HJ: *Helping Our Children to Talk.* London: Lonigan, 1968.
42. Stark RE: Phonatory development in young normally hearing and hearing-impaired children. In Hochberg I, Levitt H, Osberger M (eds): *Speech of the Hearing Impaired: Research, Training, and Personnel Preparation.* Baltimore: University Park Press, 1983, pp 251–266.
43. Oller DK, Eilers RE, Bull DH, Carney AE: Prespeech vocalizations of a deaf infant: A comparison with normal metaphonological development. *J Speech Hear Res* 1985; 26:47–63.
44. Kent RD, Osberger MJ, Netsell R, Hustedde CG: Phonetic development in identical twins differing in auditory function. *J Speech Hear Disorders* 1987; 52:64–75.

45. Lenneberg EH, Rebelsky GF, Nichols IA; The vocalizations of infants born to deaf and hearing parents. *Human Dev* 1965; 8:23–37.
46. Lenneberg EH: *Biological Foundations of Language.* New York: John Wiley & Sons, 1967.
47. Gilbert JHV: Babbling and the deaf child: A commentary on Lenneberg et al (1965) and Lenneberg (1967). *J Child Lang* 1982; 9:511–515.
48. deVilliers J, deVilliers P: Language Acquisition. Cambridge, MA, Harvard University Press, 1978.
49. Oller DK, Eilers RE: The role of audition in babbling. *Child Dev* 1988; 59:441–449.
50. Oller DK: Metaphonology and infant vocalization. In Lindblom B, Zetterstrom R (eds): *Precursors of Early Speech.* New York: Stockton Press, 1986, pp 21–35.
51. Stoel-Gammon C, Otomo K: Babbling development of hearing-impaired and normally hearing subjects. *J Speech Hear Disorders* 1986; 51:33–41.
52. Stoel-Gammon C: Prelinguistic vocalizations of hearing-impaired and normally hearing subjects: A comparison of consonantal inventories. *J Speech Hear Disorders* 1988; 53:302–315.
53. Stoel-Gammon C: *Prelinguistic Vocalizations of Hearing-Impaired and Normally Hearing Subjects.* Proceedings of the XIIth Congress of Phonetic Sciences. Aix-en-Provence France, Universite de Provence, 1991, pp 154–157.
54. Lach R, Ling D, Ling AH, Ship N: Early speech development in deaf infants. *Am Ann Deaf* 1970; 115:522–526.
55. Yoshinaga-Itano C, Stredler-Brown A, Jancosek B: From phone to phoneme: What we can understand from babble. *Volta Rev* 1992; 94:283–314.
56. Kent RD, Hodge M: The biogenesis of speech: Continuity and process in early speech and language development. In Miller J (ed): *Research on Child Language Disorders: A Decade of Progress.* Austin, TX: Pro-Ed, 1991, pp 25–53.
57. Thelen E: Rhythmical behavior in infancy: An ethological perspective. *Dev Psychol* 1981; 17:237–257.
58. MacNeilage PF, Davis BL: Acquisition of speech production: The achievement of segmental independence. In Hardcastle WJ, Marchal A (eds): *Speech Production and Speech Modeling.* Dordrecht: Kluwer, 1990, pp 55–68.
59. Kuhl PK, Melzoff AN: The bimodal perception of speech in infancy. *Science* 1982; 218:1138–1141.
60. Vihman MM: Early syllables and the construction of phonology. In Ferguson CA, Menn L, Stoel-Gammon C (eds): *Phonological Development: Models, Research, Implications.* Timonium, MD: York Press, 1992, pp 393–422.
61. Fry DB: The development of the phonological system. In Smith F, Miller GA (eds): *The Genesis of Language.* Cambridge, MA: MIT Press, 1966, pp 187–206.
62. Locke JL, Pearson DM: Linguistic significance of babbling: Evidence from a tracheostomized infant. *J Child Lang* 1990; 17:1–16.
63. Osberger M, Robbins A, Berry S, Todd S, Hesketh L, Sedey A: Analysis of the spontaneous speech samples of children with cochlear implants or tactile aids. *Am J Otol* 1991; 12(suppl):151–164.
64. Kirk K, Hill-Brown C: Speech and language results in children with a cochlear implant. *Ear Hear* 1985; 6(suppl):36S–47S.
65. Osberger M, Miyamoto R, McConkey Robbins A, Renshaw J, Berry S, Myres W, Kessler K, Pope M: Performance of deaf children with cochlear implants and vibrotactile aids. *J Am Acad Audiol* 1990; 1:7–10.
66. Tobey E, Angelette S, Murchison C, Nicosia J, Sprague S, Staller S, Brimacombe J, Beiter A: Speech production performance in children with multichannel cochlear implants. *Am J Otol* 1991; 12(suppl):165–173.
67. Weisenberger J, Kozma-Spytek L: Evaluating tactile aids for speech perception and production by hearing-impaired adults and children. *Am J Otol* 1991; 12(suppl):188–200.
68. Ling D: *Speech and the Hearing-Impaired: Theory and Practice.* Washington, DC: The Alexander Graham Bell Association for the Deaf, 1976.
69. Tobey E, Hasenstab MS: Effects of a nucleus multichannel cochlear implant upon speech production in children. *Ear Hear* 1991; 12(suppl):48S–54S.
70. Tye-Murray N, Kirk K: Vowel and diphthong production by young users of cochlear implants and the relationship between the phonetic level evaluation and spontaneous speech. *J Speech Hear Res* 1993; 36:488–502.
71. Shaw S, Coggins T: Interobserver reliability using the Phonetic Level Evaluation with severely and profoundly hearing-impaired children. *J Speech Hear Res* 1991; 34:989–999.
72. Weisenberger J: Tactile aids for speech perception and production by hearing impaired people. *Volta Rev* 1989; 91:79–100.
73. Oller DK, Eilers R, Vegara K, LaVoie E: Tactual vocoders in a multisensory program training speech production and perception. *Volta Rev* 1986; 88:21–36.

8

Otitis Media

JOANNE E. ROBERTS, PH.D., AND
SUSAN CLARKE-KLEIN, PH.D.

Introduction

Otitis media, next to the common cold, is the most common illness of early child-hood.[1,2] When a child has fluid in his or her middle ear, it is called *otitis media with effusion* (OME). Typically associated with an episode of OME is a mild con-ductive hearing loss that, because of the fluid, can persist for several months. It has been postulated for the young child in the formative stages of speech and language development, persistent and recurrent episodes of OME with associat-ed hearing loss may result in later difficulties in the development of speech and language and in academic problems.[3,4] Other researchers have questioned whether such a relationship exists between early OME and later development and have suggested no consistent relationship is present.[5-7] The purpose of this chapter is to review the epidemiology of OME, the possible linkage between OME and later speech–language development, and the literature examining this linkage. Implications for the phonological and articulation assessment and man-agement of young children experiencing OME are also described.

History and Pathophysiology

Definition and Epidemiology of Otitis Media

Otitis media means inflammation of the middle ear. Acute otitis media is differ-entiated from otitis media with effusion. When there is an infection in the middle ear, the condition is called acute otitis media (AOM). Symptoms such as fever, irritability, or an ear ache may occur. When there is fluid in the middle ear that is not infected, the condition is called otitis media with effusion (OME) or serous otitis media. Many children go back and forth between AOM and OME, and some show no symptoms even when they have AOM.

Otitis media is highly prevalent in early childhood, and is the most frequently recorded diagnosis in young children seen for illness-related office visits.[8] By age

3 years, approximately 71% of children have had at least one episode of otitis media, and 33% of children have had three or more episodes.[2] Howie, Ploussard, and Sloyer[9] reported that nearly all children have had at least one episode of otitis media by 6 years of age and approximately three fourths have their first episode before 2 years of age. Otitis media is highly prevalent in children between 6 and 12 months, although the incidence remains high throughout the preschool years, especially among children whose first episode of otitis media occurred during early infancy.[2,8] OME can continue for several weeks or even months after the onset of an AOM. Teele et al[2] found that after an episode of AOM, fluid persisted in 70% of children at 2 weeks, 40% at 1 month, 20% at 2 months, and 10% at 3 months.

Hispanic youngsters have the highest incidence of otitis media, followed by Caucasian, and then African-American children.[1] Other groups with a high incidence of otitis media are American Indians, Alaskan and Canadian Eskimos, children with family histories of otitis media, children from families of low socioeconomic status, and children from larger families.[8] Children from special populations including children with Down Syndrome, Apert Syndrome, Fragile X Syndrome, William's Syndrome, cleft lip, and/or cleft palate are also at increased risk for otitis media. The incidence of otitis media is also higher in children who attend childcare programs, are exposed to cigarette smoke, and were bottle fed rather than breast fed during the first few months of life.[8,10]

Hearing Loss Associated with OME

OME generally results in some hearing impairment, which continues as long as the effusion is present. The hearing loss is typically conductive and mild to moderate in degree, although no hearing loss may occur. When a child has OME, hearing levels from 15 to 40 dBL and averaging about 25 dBL. Permanent (sensorineural) loss is rare, occurring when an infection spreads through the round window membrane. Altered hearing sensitivity is no longer present once the effusion has resolved, although there is some electrophysiological evidence of auditory deficits in young children with histories of OME.[11,12]

Linkage of OME and Hearing to Speech Development

OME occurs most frequently during the developmental period, when children are achieving major milestones in speech perception and production. By way of review, recall that infants have the capacity to perceive phonetic contrasts that are not necessarily contrasts of their native language within the first few weeks of birth. Normally developing infants as young as 3 months are able to detect and discriminate acoustic cues that signal place and articulation (phonetic) contrasts. Infants typically begin to babble using consonant–vowel combinations at 6 months and start using sound patterns of their native language between 6 and 10 months. At or near the age of 10 months, infants also begin to comprehend meaningful speech and recognize prosodic features and speech sounds specific to their language environment. At this point, infants communicate through vocalizations and/or gestures using word-like sounds consistently. Children go on to produce their first recognizable words at about 1 year of age, and between 1.5 and 2 years there is onset of two-word utterances, rapid growth in vocabulary, accelerated phonological development (moving beyond the dominance of stops, nasals, and glide /w/), and perceptual differentiation of most of the phonemes of their native language. Over the next 2 years, vocabulary increases dramatically, as does the use of complex syllabic structures and expansion of the consonant inventory. By 4 years of age, phonemic and perceptual development are well established, although continued refinements take place over the next few years.

A young child acquires speech and language through listening and interacting with people in the environment. From the continuous flow of surrounding speech, the child learns to detect and organize speech into units, phonemically categorize these units, and then abstract the rules for his phonological system. Conversational speech, however, is not always a consistent and clear corpus of information. Speech occurs very rapidly such that words are often glossed over. Articulation varies greatly among speakers and even within the same speaker. For example, adjacent speech sounds, stress patterns, a speaker's state, and the environmental context all affect a speaker's articulation and the ability of a listener to comprehend a message. The comprehension of speech is also greatly influenced by background noise, which typically is only 10 to 15 dBL less than the intensity level of the speech signal.

The hearing loss associated with OME may place an additional burden on the young child learning to speak who does not have the same ability as older children and adults to use contextual cues or previous experience to decipher a message that often is unclear. Thus, segmenting communication, categorizing speech sounds, and acquiring phonological rules may be difficult for a child with OME.

Persistent or recurrent OME during the formative years of speech acquisition may affect the perception and development of speech in several ways. First, if fluctuating hearing loss is present, the child may receive a partial or inconsistent auditory signal and subsequently encode information incompletely and inaccurately into the database from which speech develops. Second, persistent (prolonged) or frequent (and varied) disruptions in auditory input may impede discrimination and development of speech.[13] Phonemes, particularly low energy speech sounds (eg, voiceless stops, stridents, and fricatives,) would be particularly affected. Morphologic markers (eg, "s" to mark plurality or possessive), short words ("to," "the") that are spoken rapidly, and inflections or markers that carry subtle nuances of language (eg, questions) may also be difficult to perceive and produce. (In a computer simulation of the hearing losses equivalent to those typically experienced during OME, Dobie and Berlin[14] found such patterns evident.) Thus, if the early ability to discriminate speech is a precursor to later phonological development, then even mild hearing losses associated with OME may place infants at a distinct disadvantage for recognizing, comprehending, and then producing language during the developmental years. Third, prolonged or frequent OME may also lead to problems in attending to auditory communication. Children may experience frequent changes in the intensity of signals, learn to tune out, and therefore develop attention difficulties. Fourth, the illness associated with OME (ie, the stuffy congested feeling and general malaise) may significantly restrict or alter the child's interactions with people and objects in the environment.[15] As a result, the child may have fewer opportunities to establish a knowledge base from which speech develops.

Differentiating Features and Characteristics of Children with OME

Overview of Studies

During the past decade numerous investigators have reported a relationship between early persistent OME and later speech processing and speech production. Children with a history of OME compared with children with few episodes of OME in early childhood have been reported to score lower on measures of speech processing[16–18] and speech production.[19,20] Although a growing number of studies have shown a significant relationship between OME and later measures of child development, other studies have not supported this conclusion.

The conflicting findings about the relationship of OME to later speech outcomes may in part be explained by methodological problems.[6,7] Specifically, the timing of the data collection (retrospective, prospective, or ambispective) and the research design (case-control, cross-sectional, or cohort) are critical to consider.

In regard to timing, several of the investigators examining the OME speech relationship relied on OME data collected retrospectively rather than prospectively. In a retrospective study, the OME and speech outcomes have occurred before the study began. Retrospective collection of OME data has typically been done through parent's recall of past events or review of medical records and thus has been more likely to contain measurement errors and/or lack of consistent measures. For example, some parents would be less accurate than others in recalling their children's medical histories, and some records are more complete than others. In contrast, data collected prospectively records the natural course of children's OME experiences and speech outcomes on a longitudinal basis from early infancy or at specified sampling intervals. Neither was observed before the beginning of the study. Such a procedure is likely to have greater objectivity and accuracy over time. Other studies have employed an ambispective data collection procedure in which the OME data were collected retrospectively and the developmental outcome data collected prospectively.

The research design employed in several studies has also limited the interpretation of the results. In case control studies subjects are chosen on the basis of whether they have speech–language problems. Children who exhibit speech/learning problems are compared with children who are developing normally and the history of OME is retrieved through parents' reports or a review of medical records. Case-control studies are especially susceptible to biases related to case and control selection. For example, the parents of children with speech disorders may be more likely to recall incidents of OME or to seek medical assistance than are the parents of children with normal speech and language development. In cross-sectional studies, OME and speech outcomes are measured at a given point in time (eg, at 5 years of age). These studies may not be useful in studying the developmental relationship between early childhood OME and speech–language development because measurements are made at only one time and the child's history of OME is not considered. Cohort studies, on the other hand, constitute a more rigorous methodology for assessing the relationship between speech development and OME. In cohort studies, children with different potential risk factors for speech delays (eg, children in childcare who do or do not experience OME) are compared with children not exposed to those risk factors and then followed to ascertain their developmental outcomes. Cohort studies avoid the biases of case and control selection because children are not selected to participate who already have the outcome (speech/language/learning difficulties) of interest. For more details of methodological procedures used in OME studies, see Roberts and Roush[21] and Roberts et al.[22]

Speech Perception and OME

RETROSPECTIVE STUDIES

Early studies reported a relationship of OME in childhood to auditory processing skills and collected the OME data retrospectively and the speech measures prospectively. Holm and Kunze[23] reported that children with a history of OME treated in ear, nose, and throat clinics scored poorer on tests of auditory association and auditory sequencing but not in auditory reception than children from other hospital clinics without a history of OME. Lewis[24] reported deficits of auditory sequential memory, auditory discrimination, and integration of phonemic elements for Australian Aboriginal children with chronic OME. Sak and Ruben[25] found that the auditory reception skills of 8- to 11-year olds with a history of OME differed from the skills of their siblings who did not have a history of OME, although auditory memory, association, or closure did not differ.

Hoffman-Lawless, Keith, and Cotton[26] investigated whether the auditory processing abilities of school-age children who had received surgical intervention for early middle ear infections that had persisted for 9 months or longer differed from the abilities of disease-free children. They reported differences between the groups at age 7 years on one of five auditory processing tasks administered (filtered speech), but no significant differences were found at age 9 years.

More recently, Thielke and Shriberg[27] assessed the relationship of OME and auditory processing abilities of Native American children (ages 3.8 to 5.8 years) with histories of OME before 2 years of age. They reported lower scores for these children in auditory memory, speech perception, and sound recognition. Zargi and Boltezar[28] examined the auditory processing abilities of 62 8- to 10-year olds from Slovenia with and without histories of OME before 2 years of age. Difficulties with auditory perception were evident in 88% of the children with histories of OME.

Other studies have reported a relationship between OME and specific aspects of speech processing. Clarkson, et al[29] reported that 5-year-old children with language delays and histories of OME had more difficulty phonemically categorizing stimuli and discriminating voice-onset-time than children with normal language abilities and no histories of OME. However, discrimination and categorization skills did not differ for children with and without a history of OME who had normal language. Jerger and colleagues[16] found that 2- to 5-year-old children with a history of OME as compared with children without a history of OME scored poorer in their recognition of monosyllabic words when background noise was present, although no differences were found for discrimination in quiet.

Two more recent studies found binaural masking level differences (BMLD) for tones related to children's previous OME experiences. BMLD measure the ability of the auditory system to detect subtle interaural difference cues of time and amplitude in noisy environments. Moore et al[18] found that the mean BMLD was reduced in 5- to 16-year-old children with a history of OME. Pillsbury et al[12] found the BMLD were reduced significantly before and after otologic surgery in children with a history of OME and hearing loss, especially for children with asymmetrical losses of hearing.

PROSPECTIVE STUDIES

One study examined the relationship between OME and later speech discrimination using both OME and speech data collected prospectively. Gravel and Wallace[17] examined listening abilities of 14 4-year-olds who were at high risk for OME due to low birthweight or asphyxia and 9 normal-birth babies who were followed since birth. They found that children who had experienced recurrent OME during infancy required a higher signal-to-noise ratio to perform as well as otitis-negative children. No differences were found between groups for discrimination in quiet.

Articulation Phonology and OME

Table 8–1 provides a description of the studies that have examined the relationship between children's OME experiences and their speech production skills. Each study is described by the number of subjects, timing of the data collection (retrospective, prospective, ambispective), study design (cohort, case-control, and cross-sectional), population, method of OME documentation, ages at which speech outcomes were assessed, and the significant and nonsignificant findings in speech production. Several of these studies are discussed below in more detail.

RETROSPECTIVE STUDIES

Early studies reported a relationship of OME to children's articulation[23,30] in which the OME data were collected retrospectively and the outcome data prospectively. Holm and Kunze[23] evaluated the speech and language skills of 16 children (ages 5 to 9 years) with chronic otitis media and documented fluctuating hearing losses. When the skills of the OME group were compared with otologically normal children, the OME children exhibited more articulation errors on a standardized test. Similarly, Needleman[30] explored the association of recurrent OME and speech errors and found that children between 3 and 8 years who had histories of OME with onset prior to 18 months misarticulated more consonants than subjects without a history of OME, although both groups made errors on the same sounds.

More recent studies have reported differences in the use of phonological processes in children with speech disorders with and without a history of OME.[20,31-33] Churchill et al[31] assessed the phonology of two groups of speech disordered 3- to 6-year-olds. One group had evidenced histories of OME during the first 2 years of life and the other had not. They reported that children with speech disorders and OME during the first 2 years of life evidenced significantly more stridency deletion (in both consonant singleton and cluster environments) than

Table 8–1. Studies of Articulation/Phonological Outcomes in Children with OME

Reference	n (control)	Timing	Design	Population	OME Documentation	Age Outcomes Assessed (years:months)	Articulation/Phonological Outcomes Significant	Nonsignificant
Holm and Kuntze, 1969[23]	16 (16)	A	Co	With and without OME; ENT & other clinics; low SES	Parent report; medical records	5:6–9:0	Consonant errors in words; TDTA	
Needleman, 1977[30]	20 (20)	A	Co	With and without OME; low–middle SES	Medical records	3:0–8:0	Consonant errors in words & continuous speech; TDTA	
Silva et al, 1982[61]	47 (355)	NC	Cr	Residents of New Zealand enrolled in health study; with and without OME	Parent report; typanometry; microscopic OME evidence	5:0	DASC	
Shriberg and Smith, 1983[34]	11 (11)	R	Ca	Referral to SLP speech delays; with and without OME	Clinic records	4:6–5:3	Consonant errors in continuous speech: I. Initial consonant change; II. Nasal consonant change	
Teele et al, 1984[19]	205	P	Co	With and without OME; low to high SES	Typanometry; otoscopy	3:0		GFTA
Schlieper et al, 1985[62]	13 (13)	A	Co	With and without OME; middle to high SES	Medical records	4:3	Consonant errors in continuous speech	
Hubbard et al, 1985[32]	24 (24)	A	Co	Cleft palate; early/late tubes	Medical records	5:0–11:0	Consonant errors in words; TDTA	
Bishop and Edmundson, 1986[36]	69 (48)	A	Ca/Co	Residents of England; with and without language disorders; with and without OME	Parent report	4:0–4:6		Percentage of phonological processes; NSA
Paden et al, 1987[20]	40	A	Co	With OME; tubes to be inserted	Medical records	1:6–3:6	Velar deviation/omissions; liquid deviations/omissions	

Study	N			Subjects	Data collection	Age	Outcome measures
van der Vyver et al, 1988[33]	10 (10)	A	Ca	Cerebral palsy; with and without OME	Review of records	7:0–11:0	postvocalic obstruent omission; elevated threshold at 500 Hz; early onset/late remission OME
Churchill et al, 1988[31]	15 (15)	R	Ca	Speech delays; with and without OME	Parent report	3:6	Consonant errors; final consonant deletion in singletons and clusters; ATAA
Roberts et al, 1988[38]	55	A	Co	Low SES	Tympanometry; otoscopy	2:6–8:0	Stridency deletions (singletons and consonant clusters); APP; Consonant errors; individual phonological processes; GFTA
Paden et al, 1989[35]	36	A	Co	With OME; with and without speech delays	Medical records tympanometry; otoscopy	1:6–3:6	Total phonological processes; GFTA
Teele et al, 1990[39]	194	P	Co	With and without OME; low–high SES	Tympanometry; otoscopy	7:0	Velar deviations; consonant cluster reduction; retest adequacy; time between onset and treatment of OME
Lous, 1990[37]	384	A	Co/Cr	Residents of Denmark; with and without OME	Tympanometry; otoscopy; parent report	6:0–8:8	Consonant errors in words; GFTA; Consonant errors in sentence repetition task; associations between phonology and type B (indicative of fluid) tympanogram

R, retrospective; P, prospective; A, ambispective; NC, not coded for cross-sectional because OME and outcome data were collected simultaneously at one point in time; Co, cohort; Ca, case control; Cr, cross-sectional; SES, socioeconomic status; TDTA, Templin-Darley Tests of Articulation; DASC, Dunedin Articulation Screening Scale; GFTA, Goldman-Fristoe Test of Articulation; NSA, Newcastle Speech Assessment; APP, Assessment of Phonological Processes; ATAA, Afrikaans Test of Articulation Abilities.

the children without histories of OME. Both groups exhibited deviations of /r/ targets. Shriberg and Smith[34] examined the speech of children with documented phonological "delays" and found that speech-disordered children with histories of early OME as compared to otologically normal children differed in two atypical phonological patterns: initial consonant deletions/substitutions and nasal sound substitutions.

The influence of OME on the phonological development of other special populations has also been studied. Hubbard et al[32] compared the phoneme productions of two groups of 24 children with repaired cleft palates who differed in their treatment for OME. Tube placement had been performed on one group initially at a mean age of 3.0 months. The children then received regular monitoring and replacements of middle ear tubes as necessary. The other group had the tube placement at 30.8 months or no tube placement. The investigators gathered information related to ear examination and/or myringotomy history by reviewing clinical and hospital records. The duration of active middle ear disease throughout the first 3 years of life was estimated based on the assumptions that OME had probably been present prior to and until myringotomy, and that myringotomy and tube placement had resolved the OME. Greater numbers of articulation errors were evident in the group with later tube placement. van der Vyver et al[33] examined the influence of OME on 7- and 11-year-olds with cerebral palsy, 10 of whom had an OME history and 10 without. Although both groups had articulation errors, the OME-positive children exhibited significantly more articulation errors than the control group, particularly on consonant singletons and final consonant clusters.

Paden, Novak, and Beiter[20] studied the phonological development of 40 children ranging in age between 18 and 35 months beginning 1 week prior to typanostomy tube placement. Phonological status was reassessed every 3 to 4 months until children had mastered target phonological patterns or reached 3 years of age. They found that children who did not catch up to their peers in phonological development by age 3 years evidenced deviations of velars, liquids, consonant clusters, and postvocalic singleton obstruents in combination with an elevated threshold at 500 Hz and history of early onset and late remission of OME. In a follow-up study, Paden, Matthies, and Novak[35] reported that at 4 years of age the children who continued to demonstrate phonological delays differed from children who had progressed phonologically in that they continued to evidence postvocalic singleton obstruent omissions, velar deviations, and stridency deletions. In addition, their phonological disorders were more severe than the other children when first assessed, and more time had elapsed between their initial diagnosis of OME and remission. Paden and colleagues devised a formula for predicting whether a child with OME would eventually require phonological intervention. Discriminant analysis was used to classify children as those who would require phonological intervention and those who would go on to evidence normal phonological abilities by age 4 years. Predictor variables included initial adequacy score, elapsed time from OME diagnosis to remission, and retest adequacy. The formula appeared to provide a means for predicting the need for phonological intervention with a high degree of accuracy.

Two other studies failed to find a significant relationship between OME and later phonological development.[36,37] Bishop and Edmundson[36] found that phonological process usage among language-disordered 4 year olds with and without histories of recurrent OME and a control group (without language disorders or otitis media history) did not differ. Lous[37] investigated the relationship of previous OME history, the presence of secretory otitis media, and phonological performance in Danish 7 year olds. He administered a phonological sentence repetition test (SITO) to 384 children and found no relationship between OME history and phonological performance. However, concurrent measures of phonology and tympanogram type (in the better ear) at age 7 years (cross-sectional design) indicated that children with bilateral type B curves (indicative of the presence of fluid) had lower phonological scores. The type of tympanogram explained 2 to 3% of the variance in phonological outcomes when compared with background variables (eg, gender, age, mother's socioeconomic status).

PROSPECTIVE STUDIES

Three studies examined the relationship between early OME and later phonological development using OME and speech data collected prospectively,[19,38,39] and the findings have been inconsistent. Roberts et al[38] studied 55 socioeconomically disadvantaged children attending a childcare program and whose medical history was followed prospectively during well and illness periods from birth. They found a significant relationship between the number of days of OME during the first 3 years of life and the total number of phonological processes used by children between the ages of 4.5 and 8 years. No significant relationship was reported for OME and individual phonological process usage or consonant errors.

Teele and colleagues[19,39] documented the OME history of 219 children in five health centers from birth through 7 years of age. Children's ears were examined using pneumatic otoscopy and tympanometry during routine and illness-related visits across this entire time span. These researchers found that OME during the first 3 years of life was not significantly associated at 3 years of age with lower scores on standardized measures of speech.[19] However, at age 7 years OME during the first 3 years of life was found to be associated with number of articulation errors on the Goldman Fristoe Test of Articulation.[39] Children with a history of OME had more articulation errors.

Summary

A large number of retrospective studies have found an association between OME and later speech processing and production; however, methodological issues as described earlier make these results somewhat questionable. The prospective studies examining the relationship of OME to later speech development have avoided many of the problems associated with past studies. These studies, however, are also limited in several ways. First, the findings are inconsistent, some reporting significant findings and others not. Second, when findings are statistically significant, the size of the effect is generally small and of uncertain clinical relevance. Third, the studies did not measure hearing status during OME episodes, even though the hearing loss associated with OME is believed to be the primary factor influencing speech development. Finally, the studies generally did not account for related factors that may have influenced children's speech skills, such as the quality of the child's language environment.

Further studies need to examine the relationship between a history of OME in early childhood and later phonological processing and development. Prospective cohort studies are needed to monitor subjects from early infancy, with repeated documentation of OME experience, hearing sensitivity, and phonological outcomes. Reliable and valid OME documentation procedures and measures of speech processing and production must be used, and these measures should be extended into the middle elementary school years. Hearing sensitivity should be documented during episodes of OME and routinely when children are well. Studies must also consider the multiple risk factors influencing a child's speech development, including factors that relate to both the child (eg, perceptual, language, motoric and cognitive abilities) and caregivers (quality of the home and daycare child-rearing environment). For example, a child with a nonresponsive caregiving environment may be more adversely affected by persistent OME than a child with a stimulating, responsive environment. A combination of variables should identify which children are most vulnerable to adverse OME consequences and must be considered in any study of the relationship between OME and later phonological development.

Evaluation/Assessment

Clearly, OME is highly prevalent in early childhood, and it's effect on later development is controversial. There is some indication in the literature that some children experiencing recurrent and persistent OME during the first few years of life may be at greater risk for later developmental difficulties. Until the nature of this relationship has been determined, practitioners need guidelines on the management of OME. The American Academy of Pediatrics[40] and more recently the American Academy of Audiology[41] and the American Speech-Language Hearing Association[42] reported their position on management of OME and stressed the importance of early identification and assessment of children with OME and associated hearing loss. The American Academies of Pediatrics, Family Physicians, and Otolaryngology-Head and Neck Surgery with the support of the Agency for Health Care Policy and Research of the United States Department of Health and Human Services are currently in the process of developing guidelines for the management of OME in young children.

The strategies discussed in the next two sections relate to the implications of OME based on a concern for articulation/phonological status and development. See Bluestone and Kleins[43] for a discussion of medical issues related to assessment and identification, Roberts and Schuele[44] for language and academic issues, and the American Public Health Association and American Academy of Pediatrics[45] and Roberts, Wallace, and Zeisel[46] for early childhood and health issues. Assessment recommendations based on a particular concern for phonological/articulation development in children with a history of OME are: (1) Screen for OME and associated hearing loss; (2) assess caregiver's concerns; and (3) assess articulation and phonological development.

Screen for OME and Associated Hearing Loss

Hearing and middle ear status should be screened in children who are at risk for

OME and subsequent developmental delays. Children at risk include those from the special groups described in an earlier section (definition and epidemiology of OME) as having a higher incidence of OME (eg, children with Down Syndrome, cleft lip or palate, children in childcare). For children experiencing more than 3 months of OME with continued medical management, hearing should be screened. Procedures for middle ear screening should follow the American Speech-Language-Hearing Association Guidelines for Screening for Hearing Impairment and Middle Ear Disease Disorders[47] and Joint Committee on Infant Hearing[48] and should include acoustic immittance measures (tympanometry) and pure tone audiometry or specialized behavioral and electrophysiological measures. For children failing the screening, appropriate audiological assessment and follow-up should be conducted.

Assess for Evidence of Articulation/Phonological (Phonetic/Phonemic) Deviations

The nature of the speech difficulties reported in the OME speech studies may suggest some direction for the assessment. First, some studies have shown that particular phonological processes have been associated with histories of OME (eg, postvocalic singleton obstruent omission, stridency deletion, consonant cluster reduction, velar and liquid deviations). Therefore, the assessment should provide several opportunities for each of these phonological patterns to occur. Second, if a child demonstrates speech deviations due to a history of OME, it is more likely to reflect deficiencies at the phonemic level (internal modifications, such as simplification processes, of the underlying phonological system) than at the phonetic level (misarticulations, related to poor maintenance of speed, mobility, or precision during sound production). Some children with a history of OME may evidence highly unintelligible speech, which can indicate a restricted phonemic repertoire.

The assessment of children with a history of OME should incorporate the same assessment procedures used for any child at risk for phonological difficulties. Fey[49] suggests the phonological evaluation should assess the child's: (1) phonetic inventory in isolated words and/or connected speech; (2) structure of syllables or words; (3) phonemic inventory or phonological contrasts; (4) source of the problems, that is, whether it is emanating from a perceptual, articulatory, or linguistic level; and (5) phonological rules, processes, or deviations that might reflect difficulty with the phonological system. If there is some indication that the nature of the disorder may be in part phonetic, probing for stimulability of speech targets would be useful.

Monitor for Early Evidence of Developmental Delays

The development of communication skills in any child with OME persisting for longer than 3 months should be monitored. Caregiver's concerns about the child's speech, language, hearing, and overall development may also be useful in identifying developmental problems. When a problem is observed in speech or language, the diagnostic evaluation of a speech–language pathologist should define the nature of the delay. Referral to an appropriate specialist is necessary for children at risk for other developmental difficulties.

Implications for Treatment

In developing intervention plans for the child with OME, the position statements from the professional organizations described in the last section (Academy of Pediatrics,[40] American Academy of Audiology,[41] and American Speech-Language-Hearing Association[42]) will be useful, as are the references on medical management,[43] language/academic interventions,[44] and early childhood practices.[45,46] Specific phonological/articulation treatment strategies for children with OME include: (1) Provide an optimal listening and language learning environment; (2) inform families and other caregivers about OME; (3) select speech intervention procedures; and (4) use amplification systems, when appropriate.

Provide an Optimal Listening and Language-Learning Environment

For a child with an OME-related speech difficulty, an optimal language-learning environment is essential. Although no studies have identified the best way to optimize the environment for children experiencing persistent OME, the same procedures used for children with hearing loss or speech–language delays should be appropriate. Gaining the child's attention and facing the child when speaking should increase his understanding of language. Some children may need verbal redirection to keep their attention focused on the speaker. For children in a preschool or childcare setting, preferential seating at the front of the class or near the teacher will help the child in listening to the teacher. In addition, having the child work in small groups and reducing background noise by installing washable draperies and shutting the door may help the child focus on the auditory signal. To encourage an optimal environment in which to learn speech, caregivers should respond to children's communicative attempts, provide frequent opportunities to participate in conversations, elaborate on conversational topics, and read to children frequently. These accommodations should benefit all young children but can be especially important for children experiencing hearing loss related to OME.

Inform Families and Other Caregivers Regarding OME and Their Child

Caregiver's concerns about the development of a child experiencing recurrent or persistent OME should be discussed. Sharing information with parents and other caregivers about topics they desire information about is essential. Possible topics are: the signs of hearing loss (eg, decreased attentiveness), nature of conductive hearing loss (eg, sounds and noise the child can and cannot hear), role of hearing in learning speech and language, factors increasing the incidence of OME (eg, "propping" baby bottles and cigarette smoke), signs or symptoms of OME (eg, congestion, pulling on ear), and management of OME (eg, completion of antibiotics). Information can be disseminated in workshops, presentations, and brochures.

For infants and toddlers with developmental difficulties, Public Law 99-457 requires that family concerns be addressed in a multidisciplinary team assessment. When indicated, an "Individualized Family Service Plan" (IFSP) must be developed in collaboration with family members to specify the needs of the child and family and the family's role in meeting the goals specified.[50] Similar intervention procedures are specified in an "Individualized Education Plan" (IEP) for children 3 years of age and older.

Select Speech Intervention Procedures

For a child who needs speech intervention, the type of deviation (ie, phonetic, phonemic, versus phonetic/phonemic) will dictate the type and focus of treatment procedures. Although the literature suggests some phonological characteristics may be more likely in a child with OME, each child's intervention plan should be based on his profile. Traditional phoneme-centered treatment is appropriate when speech-sound difficulties appear to be motor based. However, for other children whose difficulty is phonemic in nature, a phonological approach will be more appropriate.

A phonologically based assessment/treatment approach must provide information and intervention strategies that address deficiencies of (1) perception, (2) language organization, and (3) speech production.[51] Approaches that heighten the child's discrimination abilities may provide an effective intervention for some young children with OME. For example, Hodson and Paden[52] incorporate a listening component into therapy in which the child listens to amplified words containing the phonological targets. Kamhi[51] recommends sorting tasks based on the target phonological unit (eg, phoneme, feature, pattern) to enhance children's awareness. The minimal-contrast approach[53] may also be useful for a child experiencing OME.

Use of Amplification Systems

Low-gain hearing aids and FM sound field systems may be useful in therapy or in a classroom setting for some children experiencing mild-to-moderate hearing losses associated with OME, although there is limited empirical support for these aids. Ross, Brackett, and Maxon[54] describe how FM sound field amplification improves both the audibility of speech around the child and the signal-to-noise ratio without the need for wearable hearing aids. Benefits of mild amplification have been demonstrated in conjunction with intervention programs for children with articulation and phonological disorders.[55,56] Hodson and Paden[52] report that children with severely unintelligible speech can benefit from listening at a low level of amplification to words or stories that contain their target phonological pattern. Elliot, Longinotti, Clifton, and Meyer[57] reported that 6 and 10 year olds with normal hearing derived significant benefit from mild amplification in a consonant–vowel identification task. Although not widely used, sound field amplification has been successfully applied in classrooms of children with mild hearing losses and academic deficits (Monitored Amplification Resource Room Study)[58] and in regular classrooms.[59] Despite the benefits of low-gain hearing aids and FM sound field systems for children with OME, there are few studies of these aids and their use. For further discussion of the use of low-power FM and sound field amplification systems, see "Amplification as a Remediation Technique for Children with Normal Peripheral Hearing"[60] from the American Speech-Language-Hearing Association's Committee on Amplification for the Hearing Impaired.

Conclusion

OME is highly prevalent among young children, although the effects of recurrent and persistent OME on children's phonological development remain unclear. The results from prospective studies are inconsistent and suggest that a relationship between a history of OME and phonological development may occur for some but not all children. Continued research is needed to determine if there is such a relationship and the factors that, when combined with a history of OME, might influence children's perceptual processing and phonological development. In the interim, OME should be viewed as one possible risk factor for later speech difficulties. The phonological abilities of children who have experienced episodes of OME should be evaluated and, when necessary, treated using state-of-the-art procedures with the goal of minimizing any possible adverse developmental consequences of OME.

Acknowledgments

This chapter was supported by a grant from the Maternal and Child Health Program (MCJ-370599, Title V, Social Security Act), Health Resources and Services Administration, Department of Health and Human Services, and the United States Department of Education (H029K20342).

References

1. Teele DW, Klein JO, Rosner BA: Epidemiology of otitis media in children. *Ann Otol Rhinol Laryngol* 1980; 89(suppl 68):5–6.
2. Teele DW, Klein JO, Rosner BA: Epidemiology of otitis media during the first seven years of life in children in greater Boston: A prospective cohort study. *J Infect Dis* 1989; 160:83–94.
3. Downs M: The expanding imperatives of early identification. In Bess F (ed): *Childhood Deafness: Causation, Assessment, and Management.* New York: Grune and Stratton, 1977, pp 95–106.
4. Feldman H, Gelman R: Otitis media and cognitive development: Theoretical perspectives. In Kavanagh JF (ed): *Otitis Media Child Development.* Parkton, MD: York Press, 1986, pp 27–41.
5. Paradise JL, Rogers KD: On otitis media, child development, and tympanostomy tubes: New answers or old questions? *Pediatrics* 1986; 77:88–92.
6. Ruben JR, Bagger-Sjoback D, Downs MP, Gravel JS, Karakashian M, Klein JO, Morizono T, Pararella MM: Complications and sequelae. *Ann Otol Rhinol Laryngol* 1989; 98(suppl 139): 46–55.
7. Ventry I: Research design issues in studies of effects of middle ear effusion: Workshop on the effects of otitis media on the child. *Pediatrics* 1983; 71:644–645.
8. Bluestone CD, Klein JO: Otitis media, atelectasis tube dysfunction. In Bluestone CD, Stool SE, Scheetz MD (eds): *Pediatric Otolaryngology.* Philadelphia: W.B. Saunders Company, 1990, pp 320–486.
9. Howie V, Ploussard JH, Sloyer J: The "otitis prone" condition. *Am J Dis Child* 1975; 129:676.
10. Henderson FW, Giebink GS: Otitis media among children in day care: Epidemiology and pathogenesis. *Rev Infect Dis* 1986; 8:533–538.
11. Folsom R, Weber B, Thompson G: Auditory brainstem responses in children with early recurrent middle ear disease. *Ann Otol Rhinol Laryngol* 1983; 92:249–253.
12. Pillsbury HC, Grose JH, Hall JW: Otitis media with effusion in children. Binaural hearing before and after corrective surgery. *Arch Otol Head Neck Surg* 1991; 117:718–723.
13. Northern JL, Downs MP: *Hearing in Children,* 4th ed. Baltimore: Williams and Wilkins, 1991.
14. Dobie RA, Berlin CI: Influence of otitis media on hearing and development. *Ann Otol Rhinol Laryngol* 1979; 88(suppl 60):48–53.
15. Menyuk P: Development in children with chronic otitis media design factors in the assessment of language. *Ann Otol Rhinol Laryngol* 1979; 42:328–334.
16. Jerger S, Jerger J, Alford B, Abrams S: Development of speech intelligibility in children with recurrent otitis media. *Ear Hear* 1983; 4:138–145.

17. Gravel JS, Wallace IF: Listening and language at 4 years of age: Effects of early otitis media. *JSHR* 1992; 35:588–595.
18. Moore DR, Hutchings ME, Meyer SE: Binaural masking level differences in children with a history of otitis media. *Audiology* 1991; 30:91–101.
19. Teele DW, Klein JO, Rosner BA, The greater Boston otitis media study group: Otitis media with effusion during the first three years of life and development of speech and language. *Pediatrics* 1984; 74:282–287.
20. Paden EP, Novak MA, Beiter AL: Predictors of phonological inadequacy in young children prone to otitis media. *JSHD* 1987; 52:232–242.
21. Roberts JE, Roush J: Otitis media. In Levine MD, Carey WB, Crocker AC, Gross RT (eds): *Development–Behavioral Pediatrics*. Philadelphia: W.B. Saunders Co., 1992, pp 309–316.
22. Roberts JE, Burchinal MR, Davis BP, Collier AM, Henderson FW: Otitis media in early childhood and later language. *JSHR* 1991; 34:1158–1168.
23. Holm VA, Kunze HK: Effect of chronic otitis media on language and speech development. *Pediatrics* 1969; 43:833–839.
24. Lewis N: Otitis media and linguistic incompetence. *Arch Otol Head Neck Surg* 1976; 102:387–390.
25. Sak RJ, Ruben RJ: Effects of recurrent middle ear effusion in preschool years on language and learning. *Dev Behav Pediatr* 1982; 3:7–11.
26. Hoffman-Lawless K, Keith R, Cotton R: Auditory processing abilities in children with previous middle ear effusion. *Ann Otol* 1981; 90:543–545.
27. Thielke HM, Shriberg LD: Effects of recurrent otitis media on language, speech, and educational achievement in Memominee Indian children. *J Am Ind Educ* 1990; 30:25–33.
28. Zargi M, Boltezar IH: Effects of recurrent otitis media on auditory perception and speech. *Am J Otol* 1992; 13:366–372.
29. Clarkson RL, Eimas PD, Marean GC: Speech perception in children with histories of recurrent otitis media. *J Acoust Soc Am* 1989; 85:926–933.
30. Needleman H: Effects of hearing loss from early recurrent otitis media on speech and language development. In Jaffee BF (ed): *Hearing Loss in Children*. Baltimore: University Park Press, 1977; pp 640–649.
31. Churchill JD, Hodson JD, Jones BW, Novak RE: Phonological systems of speech-disordered clients with positive/negative histories of otitis media. *LSHSS* 1988; 19:100–106.
32. Hubbard TW, Paradise JL, McWilliams BJ, Elster BA, Taylor FH: Consequences of unremitting middle-ear disease in early life. *N Engl J Med* 1985; 321:1529–1534.
33. van der Vyver M, van der Merwe A, Tesner HEC: The effect of otitis media on articulation in children with cerebral palsy. *Brief Res Rep Int J Rehab* 1988; 11:386–389.
34. Shriberg LD, Smith AJ: Phonological correlates of middle-ear involvement in speech-delayed children: A methodological note. *Am Speech-Lang-Hear Assoc* 1983; 26:293–297.
35. Paden EP, Matthies ML, Novak MA: Recovery from OME-related phonologic delay following tube placement. *J Speech Hear Disord* 1989; 54:94–100.
36. Bishop DVM, Edmundson A: Is otitis media a major cause of specific developmental language disorders? *J Disord Commun* 1986; 21:321–338.
37. Lous J: Secretory otitis media and phonology when starting school. *Scand Audiol* 1990; 19:215–222.
38. Roberts JE, Burchinal MR, Koch MA, Footo MM, Henderson FW: Otitis media in early childhood and its relationship to later phonological development. *JSHD* 1988; 53:416–424.
39. Teele DW, Klein JO, Chase C, Menyuk P, Rosner BA: The greater Boston otitis media study group: Otitis media in infancy and intellectual ability, school achievement, speech, and language at age 7 years. *J Infect Dis* 1990; 162:685–694.
40. American Academy of Pediatrics: *Middle Ear Disease and Language Development: Policy Statement*. Elk Grove Village, IL: The Academy, 1984.
41. American Academy of Audiology: Public meeting on clinical practice guidelines for the diagnosis and treatment of otitis media in children. *Audiol Today* 1992; 4:23–24.
42. American Speech-Language-Hearing Association: *Statement on Diagnosis and Treatment of Otitis Media in Children*. Presentation to Agency for Health Care Policy and Research, Washington, DC, May 1992.
43. Bluestone CD, Klein JO: Intratemporal complications and sequelae of otitis media. In Bluestone CD, Stool SE, Scheetz MD (eds): *Pediatric Otology*. Philadelphia: W.B. Saunders Company, 1990, pp 487–545.
44. Roberts JE, Schuele CM: Otitis media and later academic performance: The linkage and implications for intervention. *Top Lang Disord* 1990; 11:43–62.
45. American Public Health Association and American Academy of Pediatrics: *Caring for Our Children: National Health and Safety Performance Standards: Guidelines for Out-of-Home Child Care Programs*. Washington, DC: APHA/AAP, 1992.

46. Roberts JE, Wallace IF, Zeisel SA: Otitis media: Implications for early intervention. *Zero Three* 1993; 13:24–28.
47. American Speech-Language-Hearing Association: Guidelines for screening for hearing impairments and middle ear disorders. *ASHA* 1990; 32(suppl 2):17–24.
48. Joint Committee on Infant Hearing: 1990 position statement. *ASHA* 1991; 33:3–6.
49. Fey ME: Clinical forum: Phonological assessment and treatment. Articulation and phonology: An addendum. *LSHSS* 1992; 23:277–282.
50. Congressional Record House: Education of the Handicapped Act Amendments of 1986. Washington, DC: September 1986.
51. Kamhi AG: Clinical forum: Phonological assessment and treatment. The need for a broad-based model of phonological disorders. *LSHSS* 1992; 23:261–268.
52. Hodson B, Paden E: *Targeting Intelligible Speech: A Phonological Approach to Remediation,* 2nd ed. Austin, TX: Pro-Ed, 1991.
53. Elbert M, Gierut JA: *Handbook of Clinical Phonology: Approaches to Assessment and Treatment.* San Diego: College Hill Press, 1986.
54. Ross M, Brackett D, Maxon AB: *Assessment and Management of Mainstreamed Hearing-Impaired Children: Principles and Practices.* Austin, TX: Pro-Ed, 1991.
55. Clifton L, Elliot L: CV identification thresholds for speech-language-learning disordered listeners. *J Acoust Soc Am* 1982; 71:857.
56. Gordon-Brannan M, Hodson BW, Wynne MK: Remediating unintelligible utterances of a child with a mild hearing loss. *Am J Speech-Lang Pathol* 1992; 1:28–38.
57. Elliot L, Longinotti C, Clifton L, Meyer D: Detection and identification thresholds for consonant-vowel syllables. *Percep Psychophy* 1981; 30:411–416.
58. Sarff LS, Ray H, Bragwell C: Why not amplification in the classroom? *Hear Aid J* 1981; 11:44–50.
59. Flexer C: Turn on sound: An odyssey of sound field amplification. *Educ Audiol Assoc Newsl* 1989; 5:6–7.
60. American Speech-Language-Hearing Association: Amplification as a remediation technique for children with normal peripheral hearing. *ASHA* 1991; 33(suppl 3):22–24.
61. Silva PA, Kirkland D, Simpson A, Stewart IQ, Williams SM: Some developmental and behavioral problems associated with bilateral otitis media with effusion. *J Learn Disabil* 1982; 15:417–421.
62. Schlieper A, Kisilevsky H, Mattingly S, Yorke L: Mild conductive hearing loss and language development: A one year follow-up study. *Dev Behav Pediatr* 1985; 6:65–68.

9

Articulation and Phonological Disorders in Hearing-Impaired School-Aged Children with Severe and Profound Sensorineural Losses

MARIETTA M. PATERSON, ED.D.

Introduction

It is generally accepted that the presence from birth or early childhood of organic hearing loss interferes with a child's development of speech and spoken language.[1,2–8] The study of early vocalization behavior and phonological development of hearing-impaired infants and young children is described by Stoel-Gammon and Kehoe in Chapter 7. Most information on phonological disorders of school-aged hearing-impaired students is derived from prelingually and early postlingually deafened children with permanent sensorineural hearing losses in the severe and profound range.[3,5,8,9] For children with permanent sensorineural hearing losses in the mild-to-moderate range, the auditory sensory deficit can often be managed with hearing aids and special learning support. Phonological development for these children might be expected to closely follow normal speech development, although some professionals are concerned that this population gets "lost in the cracks."[1,9] Children who suffer permanent sensorineural losses in the severe and profound range in early childhood have the greatest need for speech treatment during school age and will be the focus of the information presented in this chapter.

Professionals involved in the provision of direct services to school-aged hearing-impaired children often face an enormous variety of speech and spoken language learning needs in their students. These needs are related to the impact of hearing loss on speech and spoken language development and the results of highly varied early childhood learning experiences in a highly heterogenous hearing-impaired population. Many young hearing-impaired children benefit from early detection and early auditory–oral intervention and arrive at school with a phonological system well in place.[10–14] Other children arrive at school with little speech or speech patterns that require intense remediation.

The hearing-impaired child's spoken communication abilities also reflect the influence of differing educational philosophies, approaches, and methods.[15–18] There are a number of interrelated factors that account for the range and the complexity of the articulation and phonological disorders found in hearing-impaired school-aged children.

1. Age of onset of hearing loss (prelingual, postlingual).
2. Age at detection of hearing loss.
3. Type of hearing loss (permanent sensorineural, acquired permanent sensorineural, intermittent conductive loss).
4. Degree of loss of hearing sensitivity (mild, moderate [conductive or sensorineural] severe, profound, total sensorineural).
5. Age at fitting and full-time use of amplification.
6. Individual response to the use of residual hearing.
7. Other concomitant organic factors (visual impairment and illness, eg, meningitis, rubella, cerebral palsy).
8. Individual ability to exploit sensory input: use of residual hearing (where available), vision, and touch.
9. Method and quality of early intervention program.
10. Age at initiation of intervention.
11. Parental ability to cope, involvement in early education, and style of interaction.
12. Consistency and appropriateness of individual educational planning and treatment.
13. Knowledge and skill of the professionals in the integration of knowledge of audition, amplification, communication, speech, and language development.
14. Child's cognitive and sociologic abilities and learning style.

There may be vast differences in oral expressive performance among hearing-impaired children of school age. Oral expression performance will influence placement as well as learning and treatment decisions in the early school years. Some children by upper elementary school age will have sufficient mastery of an adult-like phonological system to be understood by familiar speakers and even strangers. Many other hearing-impaired children reach upper elementary school with persistent articulation and phonological disorders and poor speech intelligibility.[14] Given the amount of attention speech teaching receives in the education of hearing-impaired children, these results cannot be explained just by differences in population characteristics (eg, age of onset of hearing loss, type and degree of hearing loss, age at initiation of intervention, type of early intervention). Because the professional's task is to reduce and remediate the impact of sensory loss on speech and spoken language development to the greatest degree possible,[2,3,9,16,17] it is important to know and understand more about the type, quality, and appropriateness of treatment available to address individual student's learning needs during the school-aged years.

This chapter will present an overview of the history, pathophysiology, differentiating characteristics, assessment, treatment, and specific treatment related to articulation and phonological disorders of school-aged hearing-impaired students with sensorineural hearing losses in the severe and profound range. The information will be framed in the context of current perspectives, issues, and challenges facing clinicians and teachers.

History

Historically, the speech of the hearing impaired has been a subject of interest to linguists, phoneticians, acousticians, speech physiologists, speech–language pathologists, audiologists, educators of the deaf, parents, and the hearing impaired themselves. There are a number of excellent sources that provide a historic perspective on the teaching of speech to the deaf.[3,5,6,15,18,19] The goal of achieving intelligible speech production for the majority of hearing-impaired children remains a viable one in most programs for the hearing impaired regardless of degree of hearing loss and differences in educational/philosophic approaches and methods. Several advances in the past 20 years have contributed to the attainment of that goal.

By the mid 1970s, the availability of highly adjustable, powerful, personal hearing aids and portable classroom FM units enabled most hearing-impaired students to have consistent access to amplification.[11,12] Prior to this time, with some programmatic exceptions, vision and touch were the primary sensory input and feedback modalities used in teaching speech to the hearing impaired.[8] The auditory modality however is the primary input channel for spoken language learning.[4,11,12,16,18] Today, most hearing-impaired school-aged students wear amplification, yet there are still many unanswered questions related to the appropriateness of settings of individual amplification, maintenance of amplification, monitoring of residual hearing, and the use of residual hearing in the learning process.[11,17,20–23]

Ling's[5] seminal text on the theory and practice of teaching speech to the hearing impaired emphasized the use of residual audition as a viable sensory input modality in teaching speech, even for the profoundly deaf. The major contribution of his work was the synthesis of available information on speech for the deaf, on speech acoustics, and the suggestion of numerous strategies for teaching speech with an emphasis on exploiting hearing first, then vision and touch. A task analysis for determining best sensory input and feedback modalities is presented in Ling's monograph. Ling[5] and Ling and Ling[12] emphasized the need for professionals to have an adequate knowledge of acoustic phonetics and hearing aid function so they could exploit to the maximum each student's residual auditory function.

In the past 10 years the cochlear implant has begun to provide a new sensory input source for some hearing-impaired students.[24,25] Reports available to date with school-aged children are difficult to compare due to problems in matching children based on type of sensory device, type and amount of speech perception ability, and speech production practice. However, the cochlear implant appears to help some profoundly hearing-impaired children increase aspects of speech production performance over the first several years' postimplant experience. Further investigation concerning the outcomes of postimplant rehabilitation will address issues such as use of electrically stimulated hearing in speech perception and production and who should receive an implant and when.

Intelligibility Ratings

Much has been written about the possibility and desirability of helping hearing-impaired students achieve speech with a level of intelligibility sufficient for them to be understood in a face-to-face conversation with a stranger.[2,4,5,11,20,26] Enormous effort is expended during school years toward this goal. Yet the results of two large-scale studies by Jensema, Karchmer, and Trybus[27] and Wolk and Schildroth[28] indicate that despite considerable effort, intelligibility ratings of half of the school-aged hearing-impaired students have not varied over time. One of the most significant findings of the Wolk and Schildroth study[28] was the relationship between degree of hearing loss and intelligibility. The greater the degree of hearing loss, the less the intelligibility. Overall, students with less than severe losses were rated as 86.1% intelligible, while only 24.7% of those students with losses greater than 91 dB (profound) were intelligible. Other large population school-based studies have indicated this same general pattern, which is, all things being equal, the more hearing you have the easier it is to acquire intelligible speech (Table 9–1).[5-7,19-29]

However, all things are not equal when considering the speech of the hearing impaired. Wolk and Schildroth[28] concluded that the relationship between intelligibility and hearing loss did not hold when the student's mode of communication was considered. An examination of profoundly deaf students whose communication was only by speaking revealed that 73.0% were rated as intelligible. This finding is consistent with reports by other investigators and clinical reports that found that profound hearing loss does not preclude intelligible speech.[10,21] Among students with profound losses who used sign language only, 4.8% were reported intelligible, and among those who spoke and signed 24.7% were intelligible. These findings are encouraging because they support the view that profound deafness need not be a barrier to the acquisition of spoken language and intelligible speech. The poorer speech intelligibility scores reflected in the sign language-only communication groups could reflect a reluctance to speak due to

Table 9–1. Degree of Hearing Loss Compared with Speech Intelligibility

Results by Degree of Loss: Total Sample	Intelligibility	JKT (1978)	W&S (1988)
Less than 70 dB (mild–moderate)	Very intelligible or intelligible	86.2%	86.1%
71–90 dB (severe)	Very intelligible or intelligible	54.8%	59.0%
Greater than 90 dB (profound)	Very intelligible or intelligible	22.5%	24.7%
Results of Total Sample	Not intelligible	55.2%	55.0%

intelligibility problems or other reasons. However, it is likely that different communication expectations and amount of time spent speaking in a speaking-only environment versus a sign language-only or sign and speaking environment would account for some of the differences in intelligibility.

Taken as a whole the above findings do not represent an optimistic picture. Many professionals have written about their concern with the discouraging findings reported in these studies.[5,6,12,20,29–32] While it is difficult but not impossible for a child with severe-to-profound hearing loss to learn to speak intelligibly, this observation is not what is discouraging. What is most disconcerting is that the existing information on spoken language learning and intelligibility improvement in the hearing-impaired population has not been adequately accessed and applied in service delivery programs.

The principal professionals involved in the education of the deaf, teachers of the hearing impaired, speech-language pathologists, and audiologists, have expressed uncomfortableness and dissatisfaction about their preparation to serve the hearing-impaired population.[2,9,16,17,21,22,33,34] These professionals report the need for more information on the use of amplification, auditory learning techniques, speech development, speech remediation, spoken language development, and intervention with the hearing-impaired population. Clearly, there needs to be an improvement in personnel preparation programs and more and better in-service programs for practicing professionals.

Despite the findings cited above, there is reason for optimism. The same professionals who expressed concern over the discouraging findings reflect a strong resolve that the results of such studies must not discourage professionals from continuing to include work on articulation, voice, and spoken language intelligibility in the hearing-impaired population as part of their education and intervention.[5,6,12,20,29,31,32]

The next sections will review information on the differentiating characteristics of speech of the hearing impaired.

Pathophysiology

Among the various populations who demonstrate disordered phonological systems, the hearing impaired may be one of the most interesting and most challenging to work with. The auditory channel is the usual and most efficient sensory modality used in learning to speak.[4,5,16,35,36] Oller[37] indicated that the study of hearing-impaired children who have suffered an organic auditory sensory deficit constitutes a "natural" experiment in the role of audition in speech and spoken language development. However, all aspects of the human speech chain should be considered when attempting to understand the nature and treatment of phonological disorders of the hearing impaired.[1,38,39] These aspects include: the auditory system; the speech production system (respiratory system, phonatory system, and articulatory system); and the cognitive-linguistic system.

The cause of sensory hearing loss lies in the peripheral auditory mechanism in the cochlea.[15,38] Such sensory hearing loss can distort or preclude the transmission of signals along the auditory pathway. The amount of interference is related to the degree of loss-of-hearing sensitivity and frequency configuration of the loss.[1,5,11,15,38,40] Damage in the cochlea may vary with etiology, but most children, even those with profound losses, have some cochlear reserve or potential that responds to high sound levels provided by amplification. The frequency discrimination function of the cochlea cannot be repaired and hearing-impaired students must learn to make sense of the distorted signal that is transmitted to the brain.[5,15]

Boothroyd[15] made a point of differentiating sensory and neural impairment. Neural impairment influences how the nerve signal from the cochlea travels to and is integrated in the cortex. When damage is at the site of the cochlea (sensory), there may also be measurable loss of hearing sensitivity and discrimination ability.[15] The different effects of neural and sensory impairments are difficult to separate and may become clearer to the clinician through diagnostic aural rehabilitation. Possibly those students who seem to be "good" hearing-aid users may have only cochlear involvement, and those who are identified as "poor" hearing-aid users may have greater neural involvement.

By school-aged most hearing-impaired children have benefitted from aural habilitation. Ongoing diagnostic evaluation of an individual student's hearing continues to be important. School-aged hearing-impaired children can suffer from additional cochlear degeneration, cochlear damage from disease or trauma, as well as ear infections and intermittent conductive losses.[11,15,18] Studies of the effects of long-term wearing of amplification on auditory physiology are inconclusive; however, school-aged hearing-impaired children have the same potential to suffer from exposure to loud sounds as hearing children.[11,12,15]

Several additional perspectives on auditory pathophysiology and aural rehabilitation that are pertinent for the school-aged population are as follows:

1. A hearing-impaired child's potential use of residual hearing cannot be predicted from the pure-tone audiogram. While degree of loss of hearing sensitivity has been shown to have a positive correlation with speech intelligibility in school-aged children, there are individuals whose impressive auditory–oral performance "defies" their pure-tone audiogram. There are other individuals who, for lack of appropriate amplification or auditory–oral learning opportunities, do not seem to have maximized the use of their residual hearing potential and perform as more deafened than they really are.

2. It is accepted that most hearing-impaired students can benefit from amplification, even those with profound losses. Ongoing diagnostic auditory–oral (re)habilitation will inform both the professional and the student about the benefits or nonbenefits of using amplification.

3. The simple act of wearing hearing aids *will not be* sufficient for severe-to-profound hearing-impaired students to maximize the potential use of residual hearing for speech perception.[11,12,13,20,22]

4. Hearing-impaired students must learn how to listen to acoustic differences among speech sounds in manner, place, and voicing cues and among prosodic features. The linguistic aspects of prosodic features carry a heavy meaning load in English.[22] As an acoustic phenomenon, prosodic features are not readily available to hearing-impaired students through vision or tactile cues.

5. Once hearing loss has been detected, the aided audiogram should be of primary interest in planning aural (re)habilitation. Ling and Ling[12] provided useful information relative to optimum hearing-aid fitting and clinical monitoring of hearing-aid function and student responses to speech.

6. Most of the research on intelligibility of the school-aged hearing-impaired population does not report information on the aided audiograms or on the use of audition in the comprehension of speech and spoken language.

7. It can be hypothesized that the range of articulatory and phonological disorders among hearing-impaired school-aged students reflects to some extent poor exploitation of residual hearing.[5,6,10,11]

The hearing-impaired listener's ability to attend to the incoming acoustic message and to monitor the acoustic feedback of his own voice influences development of his phonological system.[4–6,10,11,17,41] It is generally accepted that most severe-to-profound hearing-impaired children would not learn to talk without hearing aids and assistance in learning how to listen and speak.[2,5,7,12,16,17,25,26,28]

Speech Physiology

Most children with prelingual and postlingual sensorineural hearing loss have normal respiratory, phonatory, and articulatory physiological function that can support articulatory and phonological development.[5,11,15] Hearing-impaired children therefore have the potential to develop motor control of phoneme production, voicing, timing, and coordination of the physiological correlates of speech. One of the goals of early auditory–oral habilitation is to promote phonological development by capitalizing on the hearing-impaired infant's early vocalization in the presence of amplification.[10,16,17,42,43] The hearing infant develops increasing control over his vocal production system, including phrase length vocalization, duration, timing, intensity, and intonational patterns during the first year of life. By contrast, poor control over these aspects of vocal production are archetypal problems in speech of the hearing impaired at school-aged and in adulthood. Many young hearing-impaired children do not experience a period of vocal play during which control of vocal productions patterns can be practiced without the stress of language deficits. It has been suggested that encouraging vocal play during early intervention may help offset and prevent the appearance of the often extreme vocal production problems found in many hearing-impaired speakers.[5,10,12,14,17,42,43]

Extensive literature exists describing voice abnormalities in hearing-impaired students. Some physiological studies have demonstrated vocal pathology in middle-school children and young adults. These pathologies include partial vocal fold atrophy,[44] abnormal oscillatory patterns,[45] velopharyngeal insufficiency,[46] and respiratory dysfunction to support speech.[47] Physiological change in the speech production system can develop with years of improper vocal production related to auditory sensory pathology.[2,5,17,46] A number of investigators have indicated that these physiological pathologies may be avoided and reduced by early speech development or through remediation in the early school years.[4,5,10,12,16,17,20]

Linguistic investigations over the past 25 years have increasingly assumed that there are `universal' abilities in the cognitive, linguistic, and communication domains that are innate to human beings.[4,10,12,16,46,48,49] Studies of language development of hearing-impaired children over the past 20 years lead to the conclusion that the majority of hearing-impaired children are also born cognitively intact, and they are prepared to learn spoken language.[4,10,12,16,17,42,43,48]

Differentiating Characteristics

Investigators describing speech characteristics of school-aged severe-to-profound hearing-impaired speakers have focused more on the segmental aspects (speech sound production errors at the word and syllable levels) and suprasegmental aspects (prosodic features) than on identification of phonological processes, patterns, and rule systems. This section of the chapter will focus on characteristics that differentiate articulation patterns of severe-to-profound hearing-impaired children from those of hearing children, followed by remarks about phonological characteristics.

A variety of perceptual and instrumental procedures have been used to analyze the segmental aspects of speech (vowels and consonants), suprasegmentals (prosodic features), and vocal characteristics of the hearing impaired.[8,50] The majority of perceptual studies have utilized live judgment or audio/videotaped speech, phonetic transcription, and rater judgments. Acoustic studies have been particularly useful for measuring duration, frequency, and amplitude information for both phonetic syllabic production and for the suprasegmental (prosodic) aspects of speech. Other studies have used physiological instrumentation to assess aerodynamic and biomechanical mechanisms and function within and across the respiratory, phonatory, and articulatory systems.

Vowels

The production of vowels in running speech requires tongue flexibility and accuracy in moving from one height and position to another. Tongue movement, shape of the oral cavity, and constrictions of the air flow create the acoustic formants that listeners use to discriminate vowels.[40,50] In their seminal study, Hudgins and Numbers[51] found that deaf students had problems in producing a range of differentiated vowels and diphthongs. Numerous investigators have reported perceptual, acoustic, and instrumental studies conducted during habitual hearing-aid wearing that have described vowel error patterns, substitutions, nasalization, neutralizations, dipthongizations, and prolongations.[27,32,51–53]

Levitt and Stromberg[9] analyzed existing data in an attempt to develop a quantitative description of typical vowel errors to better understand the underlying patterns. Ten error types were identified according to vowel (front, central, back, and schwa-like vowel) and error type:

1. Tense-lax substitutions [i for I]
2. Substitution of the intended vowel by neighboring vowel in the vowel quadrilateral (near-neighbor)
3. Substitution by a schwa-like vowel
4. Substitution by a vowel (other than a near-neighbor) that is closer to the center of the vowel quadrilateral

5. Substitution by a vowel that is further away from the center of the vowel quadrilateral (far-neighbor substitution)

6. Substitution by a vowel that is on the opposite side of the vowel quadrilateral (far-neighbor substitution)

7. Substitution of a diphthong by a vowel (usually by a major component of the diphthong or a near-neighbor of the major component [diphthongization])

8. Substitution of a vowel diphthong or excessive diphthongization of the vowel

9. Omission of the intended vowel or diphthong

10. Unidentifiable distortion

This schema describes the surface or phonetic level difficulties many hearing-impaired speakers have in attempting to produce vowels. Acoustic- and physiological-based studies are consistent with the findings from the perceptual studies. These studies provide information related specifically to auditory, visual, and tactile sensory input used by the hearing-impaired speakers.

Monson[7,54] found that hearing-impaired speakers inappropriately produced the second formant (anterior constriction of the tongue), and concluded that the magnitude of the second formant range was a good indicator of an individual student's vowel articulation ability. Tye-Murray,[55] using cineflurography and x-ray microbeam, reported that some deaf speakers used excessive jaw movement to establish different vowel shapes instead of appropriate tongue movement. The less flexible tongue movement reduces the formation of the acoustic vowel formants necessary to discriminate vowels. As the second formant (F2) carries the most acoustic information for vowel differentiation, both Tye-Murray and Monson concluded that lack of differentiation among tongue movements across vowels gives the listener the acoustic perception of vowel neutralization or schwa likeness. Stevens, Nickerson, and Boothroyd[46] used a nasal accelerometer and found that hearing-impaired students evidenced inadequate velopharyngeal control and produced vowels with inappropriate nasality.

Consonants

School-based studies have reported data on consonant errors in the hearing impaired. There is general agreement that consonant errors reflect problems with the voiced-voiceless distinction, substitutions of one consonant for another (voiced-voiceless, nasal-oral, fricative-stop), omission of initial and final consonants (eg, /s/ deletions), distortions (nasal emission, too great or too little plosive effort), inappropriate nasalization of consonants, and final consonant deletions.[7,9,56]

Coarticulation gestures have been studied in hearing-impaired individuals. Waldstein and Baum[57] concluded that in the case of anticipatory coarticulation [ʃi, ʃu, ti,tu,ki,ku], profoundly hearing-impaired students seemed to move their articulators in preparation for the upcoming vowel later than normal hearing children. In the case of perseveratory coarticulation [iʃ, uʃ, it,ut,ik,uk], the hearing-impaired students demonstrated less articulatory precision, probably due to the effects of the mechanical-articulation properties of the task.[58] In general, high correlations between segmental production and speech intelligibility have been reported.[26,53,59]

Suprasegments

It is also important to understand the impact of hearing loss on the student's suprasegmental or prosodic speech characteristics, which also contribute to intelligibility. Prosodic aspects of speech are commonly defined as including pitch (fundamental frequency and variation/intonation), intensity (loudness and stress), duration (rate and rhythm), and vocal quality.[40] These temporal and tonal features of speech extend over the phoneme segments, thus providing information that augments and supports the semantic and syntactic message.[22,40,46,49]

Numerous investigators since Hudgins and Numbers have described the prosodic characteristics (suprasegmentals) of the hearing-impaired school-aged child and young adults using acoustic and physiological measures.[7,46,47,60-62] This literature includes the study of lung volumes during speech, aerodynamic function during consonant production, vocal fold movement patterns, vocal harshness, nasality and velopharyngeal function, tongue movement, and jaw movement.

There is general agreement that hearing-impaired speakers demonstrate one or more of the following vocal production characteristics that reflect the interrelationships of prosodic features and physiological correlates of speech: aerodynamic function, biomechanical function, and articulation.[7,46,50,62]

1. Inadequate breath control
2. Excessive and inappropriate pausing
3. Inappropriate pitch register
4. Hypernasality
5. Pharyngeal resonance
6. Excessive tenseness/harshness
7. Inappropriate duration of stressed and unstressed syllables
8. Inappropriate rate of syllable articulation

A review of studies on physiological and acoustic aspects of phoneme production by hearing-impaired persons is available in McGarr and Whitehead.[50]

Phonological patterns of severe-to-profound hearing-impaired school-aged children have not been studied in the same way as the segmental productions of these speakers. No large-scale, longitudinal developmental studies have been performed on the emerging phonological systems of these children, in part due to problems of heterogeneity. Cole[10] and Ling and Ling[12] suggested that young severe-to-profound hearing-impaired children who are learning through the use of residual hearing would be expected to mark the same developmental phonological processes as hearing children. The ages, stages, and manifestations of these processes have not been studied in depth in the hearing-impaired population.

Similarly, there are no longitudinal studies and little information on the phonological process errors of school-aged hearing-impaired children. Smit[63] indicated that hearing children with phonological problems that persist into school age exhibit a range of errors that include unusual, bizarre, and idiosyncratic error types.[63] School-aged hearing-impaired students' range of phonological disorders includes developmental errors as well as idiosyncratic, unusual, and bizarre errors.[5,14,15,26,29,32,41,45,64] For hearing-impaired students, persistent phonological pattern problems in running speech would be related to perceptual input and feedback issues, level of neuromotor control of articulation, habituation of error patterns, and linguistic and phonological rules knowledge.

Characterizing phonological processes is difficult with the hearing impaired because of the overall complexity of factors involved in trying to produce an intelligible spoken message. For example, a 10-year-old hearing-impaired student may know that plurals in English are marked by the addition of final /s/, /əz/ and /z/, and is able to articulate /s/ and /z/ in syllabic contexts. However, this student cannot perceive /s/ at all through residual hearing and consistently omits /s/ in final position for plurals in conversation. In this case, the student has a consistent pattern of final consonant deletion for /s/. Should such a problem be characterized as an articulation problem, a phonological process problem, or a language-based problem? In either event, treatment should focus on the facilitation of the student's production of /s/ in final position contexts and practice in the context of pluralization.

Sufficient research information already exists to guide the treatment of phonological disorders of the hearing impaired. While there are still questions about specific articulatory and phonological production factors, the following findings are agreed on by most investigators:

1. There is remarkable similarity in articulatory errors and vocal production patterns among severe-to-profound hearing-impaired persons.
2. Despite similarities in speech difficulties across speakers, there is a remarkable degree of variability in the intelligibility level and in articulatory and prosodic problems of hearing-impaired persons.

Assessment

Assessment of phonological disorders of school-aged hearing-impaired students can represent quite a challenge. The clinician should consider interrelated factors that contribute to the overall intelligibility.[2] The clinician has to describe and attempt to understand the interrelationships between each student's increasing linguistic and communicative competency and each student's own speech sound system: that is, the use of his articulation system (motor speech sounds); the use of suprasegmentals (intonation, stress, and pausing); and the use of phonological processes and idiosyncratic phonological patterns.[14,17,64,65] It is important to analyze both the segmental and the suprasegmental characteristics. As noted above in the section on differentiating characteristics, hearing-impaired speakers often have vocal production problems that underlie the ability to produce phonemes and mark prosodic patterns.[2,5,7,39,45–47,50–52] Clinicians should assess the student's potential to use acoustic perceptual information to monitor input and output of the spoken message.

This section of the chapter will not critique assessment instruments but will rather present a framework and some perspectives on assessment. The following outline suggests parameters to be considered in an assessment.[2,5,20,22,26]

1. Information on audition:
   - Current audiograms: pure tone and aided responses in each ear
   - Knowledge of the amplification system worn by the student—both personal aids and FM devices
   - Information on other sensory aids: cochlear implants and vibrotactile aids
   - Assessment of the student's ability to detect and discriminate features of manner, place, and voicing
   - Assessment of the student's ability to identify and comprehend words and phrases auditorily
   - Assessment of the student's ability to discriminate suprasegmental information: voice/voiceless, intensity, duration, and pitch differences
   - Assessment of the student's ability to discriminate and use linguistic aspects of prosody for language comprehension (see item 4 below)
   - Assessment of student's ability to use semantic and syntactic knowledge to predict sentence meaning and to make informed guesses

2. Information on the use and integration of sense modalities:
   - Audition (as above)
   - Visual awareness and speech-reading ability
   - Understanding and use of tactile and orosensory cues

3. Oral-peripheral exam noting any extraneous and interfering facial movements and excess effort (jaw dropping, tongue contortions, overexaggerated lip-rounding).

4. Motor speech evaluation of the phonetic repertoire
   - Vowels and diphthongs (tongue flexibility)
   - Consonants by manner, voicing, and place
   - Noting of deletions, substitutions, and distortions

5. Aspects of prosody (suprasegmental features) and voice:
   - Vocal quality and ability to sustain phonation
   - Ability to initiate, control, and release the breath stream to sustain phrases
   - Ability to make intensity changes in overall voice and make stress differentiation within words and phrases
   - Ability to maintain an age- and sex-appropriate pitch register and the ability to vary intonation contours to mark discourse functions and to indicate effect

6. Phonological evaluation, preferably with a spontaneous conversational sample. The linguistic aspects of prosody should be assessed in at least sentence length context. Vowel and consonant co-articulatory information will supplement the phonetic evaluation. Phonological patterns should be noted.

7. Impression of intelligibility: rating scale, descriptive scale, or percentage rating

8. Pragmatic skills as listener and speaker. Speech occurs in spoken communication; therefore, the influence of linguistic and communicative competencies are part of the overall assessment process:
   - Student confidence level, self-esteem

- Knowledge of conversational frame, conversational mechanisms, and paralinguistic features
- Extended script knowledge
- Use of different sense modalities to monitor the speaker

9. Language assessment: Analysis of semantics and syntax will highlight areas where articulation or prosodic problems are affecting the comprehension of the student's message and vice versa. Speech remediation and practice should occur in linguistic context as much as possible. Familiarity with the student's language should provide numerous contexts for practice.

10. Student self-evaluation
    - Motivation for change in speech patterns
    - Self-awareness of problems in speech and spoken language production
    - Analysis of comfortable and uncomfortable conversational situations
    - Elements of speech that the student would like to target

Although the list of the above parameters to be considered in an evaluation can be overwhelming, informed analysis of evaluation results should facilitate the establishment of appropriate and reasonable teaching targets. While a variety of assessment procedures exist to assist in such an assessment, no completely satisfactory assessment package has been created for hearing-impaired students that incorporates a complete perspective on articulation and voice physiology in the population.[3,5,19]

Articulation (phonetic inventory) is one of the easiest aspects of speech to describe. A variety of instruments standardized on hearing children have been used to assess articulation of school-aged hearing-impaired children.[26] These instruments have been criticized as not providing information essential for evaluating the hearing-impaired child.[66] Such instruments typically do not include elicited vowel and diphthong productions[5,6] or assess the nonsegmental aspects of speech.[5] Instruments that do not include the assessment of vowels and/or suprasegmentals may not lead to appropriate treatment for most hearing-impaired students.[2,5,17,26]

The difficulty with a number of these procedures is that the target phoneme is elicited only once in initial, medial, and final positions. Speech is a dynamic process and sound productions may fluctuate across context. Contexts are a major influence on speech sound production in normally developing children but have an even more noticeable influence in the hearing impaired.[1] For example, it is common for students to produce a correct production in citation form, but inconsistently produce the target phoneme in conversational speech.[5]

Fortunately assessment instruments designed to elicit a phonetic inventory with hearing-impaired individuals are available.[5,6,29,53,67,68] Some of these instruments have been created for research purposes and may not be widely used clinically. Ling's Phonetic Level Evaluation (PLE) has probably become the most widely used articulation test created for the hearing impaired. The PLE is arranged to follow Ling's sequential model: nonsegmental aspects of speech, vowels, diphthongs, consonants, and consonant clusters are evaluated as motor speech targets in multiple syllable repetition at the rate of three syllables per second. Features of manner, place, and voicing are also noted. Several targets are

selected for teaching, usually consisting of suprasegmentals, vowels, and consonants. A review of Ling's speech program can be found in Ling[5,17] and a summary in Perigoe.[69]

Shaw and Coggins[66] conducted a study to determine the reliability of the PLE.[5]
Three areas were found to be problematic: (1) Interobserver agreement was low;
(2) the coding system is complex and may confound the accuracy of the raters; (3)
the instrument may not be sensitive to the skills of children who are still in the
acquisition process.

The Shaw and Coggins study highlights the problems with speech measurement tools designed to aid in treatment decisions. The more validity and reliability are controlled, the less the test seems to respond to the dynamic aspects of
speech. The author's experience corroborates the findings of the Shaw and
Coggins study; the bias of familiar listeners is reflected in the scoring responses
of clinicians using the PLE. This "familiar listener" phenomenon generally
results in an overgenerous evaluation. The hearing evaluator's own speech production is the yardstick with which a hearing-impaired speaker's phonological
productions are compared.

Assessment of phonemes and prosodic features in context and of vocal production patterns should be part of a thorough diagnostic evaluation. Subtelny,
Whitehead, and Orlando[70] created an instructional package to train listeners to
identify vocal production and prosodic difficulties in college-age hearing-
impaired speakers. Students with a wide range of oral expressive ability are presented to the listener reading the same paragraph. The instrument provides a
numeric index that indicates degree of problem and provides limited suggestions
for targeting and treatment of voice and suprasegmental problems.

A number of in-house instruments have been developed for prosodic feature
evaluation including short sentences that vary in discourse function and stress
marking.[29] These instruments have limited linguistic content and produce limited
clinical information. The preferred method would be an analysis of speech patterns in a spontaneous conversational sample. Such samples provide information
on an individual's use of prosodic features (vocal quality, rhythm, stress, and
intonation contours) as well as phonetic repertoire based on conversation and
information. Additionally, the same sample can be used for a language analysis
and for generating specific linguistic contexts for practice. Ling[5] detailed a
phonological analysis procedure based on a language sample of 50 utterances
from a variety of conversational contexts. Unfortunately, the instrument is quite
time consuming and provides only minimal guidance in the selection of treatment for targets. A short form of Ling's analysis together with some ideas for target setting are included in Ling's text.[17]

Parker and Rose,[41] among others, proposed that some hearing-impaired speakers do not simply produce "errors," but produce such sounds in a "regularized
deviant idiosyncratic phonological system." They argue that there is a systematic
relationship between the individual hearing-impaired student's "errors" and the
adult hearing model that they are attempting to realize. The phonological assessment instrument used by Parker and Rose can define contrasts in individual students' speech repertoires that enhance intelligibility for a familiar listener (eg,
{potato} realized with [b], {box} realized with [£], me realized with [v^b]. They sug-

gested that for some speakers "correction" of systematic phonological realizations may actually reduce intelligibility. They provide strong support for the analysis of speech at the phonological level whether the goal be maintenance of a phonological system or remediation.

Several additional perspectives on current issues relative to assessment are presented below:

1. Although the current thinking in developmental phonology and language indicates that a combination of cognitive-linguistic and motor speech tasks might be the best assessment strategy, many tools for the hearing impaired retain an articulation error/segmental approach to assessment.

2. Professionals often assess the nonsegmental aspects of speech (vocalization, duration, intensity, and pitch) divorced from linguistic context. This has created problems in translating the information into intervention targets.[24, 64]

3. Due to an overattention to assessment at the articulatory level there is frequently a lack of attention to speech in context and the dynamic interaction of speech physiology.

4. No assessment procedure currently exists that offers the clinician a useful and timely way to assess aspects of prosody in linguistic context and their physiological correlates.

Treatment

The treatment of the articulation and phonological skills of the school-aged hearing-impaired student must occur in the overall context of that individual's hearing, speech, language, and communication abilities. Clinicians face the challenge of establishing and implementing individual treatment plans that optimize sensory input and optimize instruction.[13,17,20,32] This section will not attempt to critique all treatment approaches utilized with hearing-impaired school-aged students but will rather present information on treatment from several different perspectives.

A number of sources provide approaches, sample lesson plans, suggested stages of practice, teaching strategies, and instructional materials for remediation of articulation and phonological disorders in school-aged hearing-impaired students.[3,5,15,17,18,20,22,30,32,71–76] Most of these materials suggest using residual audition to facilitate speech and language remediation with the hearing impaired. Specific instructional techniques on the use of audition, vision and touch are available.[3,5,11,12,17,20,22,35,63,73,77,78]

While information is available concerning treatment of articulation and phonological disorders in the hearing impaired, there is a lack of information on expectations for change and efficacy of various instructional methodologies.[15,17,19,26,32] Ling[17] (p 288) reiterated in his updated text that "there are now many more articles on the . . . characteristics than on prevention or remediation of abnormal patterns . . . of speech."

Available research reflects some of the methodological problems involved in clinical research in this area. McGarr[29] obtained detailed comparative intelligibility data on the same set of school-aged hearing-impaired students at two different points in time. All the students received speech remediation assistance, but the general approaches and specific instructional strategies varied across school sites and were not controlled. After 3 years of speech training, very few changes in segmental production were reported and the pattern of speech intelligibility (two thirds of subjects were rated unintelligible to barely intelligible) remained similar over 4 years. Similarly, Subtelny and Snell[32] reported no changes in the aural–oral communication abilities of some late adolescent and young adult college-aged students.

In contrast, other investigators have used a systematic auditory–oral Ling-type approach to speech remediation and have found changes in suprasegmental patterns, speech perception, and articulation for the majority of students studied.[36,74,79]

Treatment approaches and protocols used in schools vary greatly. Comparison of programmatic information is difficult due to the dirth of research concerning efficacy of treatment and heavy reliance on anecdotal writing concerning efficacy of treatment approaches.

Although there is much more to be understood about treatment issues, these are aspects of learning that should be considered when planning and implementing treatment:

1. Target selection and variety of targets
2. Student motivation level, self-evaluation, and self-responsibility
3. Prognostic impressions and time frames for remediation
4. Perception and production: consideration of sense modalities
5. Stages of practice: articulation and phonology
6. Linguistic and conversational practice and rehearsal contexts
7. Active, dynamic involvement of the student

Selection of targets should be based on the diagnostic parameters mentioned and supplemented by student involvement as appropriate.[62,64] Student motivation and setting of realistic expectations have long been of concern in the treatment of hearing-impaired college-aged adults.[62] The adult client is involved in discussion about the directions of the intervention and such a discussion provides information about the student's self-awareness and motivation level.

This author's experience has shown that school-aged children at first react with surprise when asked to give an opinion about their own speech and communication needs (eg, What things are difficult for you when you are speaking with people? What would you like to have some help with?). Once students understand that their active participation is being encouraged they tend to react positively to the opportunity to involve themselves in the assessment and planning process. Maintaining high motivation over many years of speech "work" is not easy for either the clinician or student. While the professional maintains responsibility for analysis, definition of what may or may not be achievable, and treatment approach, a discussion of oral communication problems and needs with the client may make treatment more meaningful and help maintain motivation for both professional and student.

Several targets[5,17,20,30,62] or a cluster[10] of targets (from amongst articulation, prosody, vocal production, and phonological rules problems) should be chosen for concurrent and interdependent work. It is useful to select targets that reflect several stages of practice such as elicitation of a new phoneme, correction of confusions or errors among several existing phonemes, and fine tuning of aspects that are closer to mastery.[5,20,26,30,62]

The treatment plan should include prognostic impressions about the student's phonological outcomes and determine probable time frames for change. It is often difficult to establish time lines or reasonable expectations for improvement in speech patterns of school-aged hearing-impaired children because so many students do not seem to improve over time.[27–29] The provision of speech remediation is usually a long-term matter (eg, lasting throughout school-aged years), but long-term speech remediation has not been shown to facilitate changes in segmental repertoire or in conversational intelligibility for many students.[5,6,27–29] Approaches that involve intensive learning with a focus on rapid remediation of speech have been proposed.[2,5,10,20,26,30,72,74,79] Professionals need to consider exploring intensive cycles of speech remediation that might occur several times during a school year in contrast to long-term continuous treatment. Expectations for short- and long-term change and the efficiency of particular remediation approaches could be better evaluated with controlled learning and treatment times.

To optimize the student's use of sensory input and information for self feedback, professionals should consider the appropriate sense modality (audition, vision, touch) or combinations relevant to perception and production of each phonetic or prosodic target. Clarifying auditory confusions (contrasts) or teaching auditory discrimination should occur prior to and as part of articulation and phonological work.[5,20,22,30,35,62,73,77–80]

Students should be actively involved in the learning process. They should judge the appropriateness of their speech productions during practice rather than depending only on clinician feedback. Clinician feedback should facilitate improved subsequent attempts. Many school-aged students are often reluctant to perform home practice because they do not feel confident to judge for themselves whether a production is appropriate or not. Many students can learn to improve their ability to self monitor using auditory, visual, orosensory tactile, and linguistic information. Several examples follow:

AUDITORY CUES

Students can develop confidence in listening to their speech by sorting out what they hear and discriminate well, what they hear and discriminate with difficulty, and what they cannot discriminate at all. For example, most students with aided residual hearing up to 1000 Hz should be able to learn to discriminate the nasal/oral contrast,[5,12,17,20,81] which is /ba/ versus /ma/. /m/ is a continuous sound with the acoustic nasal murmur occurring at about 300 Hz. This acoustic information contrasts significantly from the plosive burst created by the production of the /b/. Once a student has learned to perceive the differences, he can become more responsible for monitoring the production of those sounds through hearing.

VISUAL CUES

Many hearing-impaired students with poor speech intelligibility produce speech sounds and utterances with overexaggerated jaw movement, the "jaw-drop" phenomenon.[5,17,20,62] Some students are unaware of this and can tune in to their production by watching themselves in a mirror. However, it is not possible to take a mirror with you when you leave the treatment area, so remediation of this problem works best with an orosensory tactile cue (see below).

OROSENSORY TACTILE CUE

Students with the jaw-drop problem can learn to monitor the excursion of their jaw during speech practice by gently touching the underside of the chin with the back of their hand. If necessary, the student can immobilize the arm by resting the elbow on a table as well.

LINGUISTIC CUES

A student who is improving phonological use of the /s/ to mark plurals or possessives should be able to predict the occurrence of the phoneme in an utterance based on linguistic knowledge and should be able to use auditory and orosensory tactile information to monitor his productions in practice at home.

The range of treatment skills of professionals, their comfort level with addressing complex phonological disorders, and the level of service provided varies greatly across programs. There are several general treatment issues that merit comment.

1. A conceptual separation of work on articulation and voice production aspects from phonological rules seems to have occurred.[64]

2. Remediation of vocal production patterns and control of prosodic features in context still seems to remain the most challenging area of treatment.

3. Even when prosodic aspects of speech are targeted for remediation, practice occurs apart from meaningful context.

A Specific Treatment for Voiceless Fricatives

It was suggested in this chapter that the analysis of speech problems has focused too much on the articulatory aspects and on the movement and positioning of the articulators. Professionals frequently do not analyze the speech problem with the physiological and phonological systems in mind.[64] A treatment approach described below emphasizes an analysis of the problem considering articulatory, acoustic, and physiological correlates of fricative production.[1]

Contrastive Features

What are the contrastive features in voiceless fricatives that can be used to facilitate production? Voiceless fricatives are created by air friction as the air flows from the lungs, passes through open vocal folds, /h/, and is mediated by the articulators in the oral cavity that create points of constriction at different places (/f/ labiodental; /ʃ/ palatal; /s/ alveolar). The friction is caused by air being forced through the constrictions. The friction that is created at the differing points of constriction create the acoustic formants that distinguish the consonants from each other.

Typical Problems for the Hearing Impaired

Typical articulatory production errors of hearing-impaired students would be the reduction of a fricative to a stop (eg, /fa/ reduced to /pa/; /sa/ reduced to /da/); substitution of an affricate (eg, /tʃ/ or /da/ for /ʃ/); glottal friction reduced to a glottal stop (eg, /ʔ/ for /h/); "slushy" and overly broad production of /ʃ/ or /s/ (eg, sometimes similar to a lisp); and/or overexaggeration of movement in the production of /f/ (eg, jaw dropping for every /fa/ syllable). It is evident from such patterns that many school-aged children know quite a bit about place and manner of the fricative group even though they have not acquired control over monitoring input, production, or use. While there may be a range of individual articulation and phonological issues involved in the representation of fricatives, analysis that considers the interrelated aspects of the speech chain gives rise to a common problem. The underlying physiological problem for all of these errors relates to the amount of air pressure achieved at the point of constriction or the stopping of the airflow at some point in the vocal tract.[44,45,62] Frequently, this problem can be traced to the student's initiation of breath at the respiratory level and/or inability to direct the breath stream through the open vocal folds, across the pharynx, and into the oral cavity.

Phonological analysis of students' use of fricatives in language indicates fairly predictable pattern problems. Two broad categories of students can be mentioned: (1) those who have age-appropriate linguistic knowledge and knowledge of the phonological rules of English but have interfering articulatory problems; and (2) those with relatively poor linguistic knowledge and knowledge of phonological rules, which interacts negatively with articulation problems. Typical phonological patterns of school-aged hearing-impaired students would include deletions or reduction to a stop in final /s/, /əz/, and /z/ for marking plurals; and omission, distortion, reduction of /h/, /s/, /f/, /ʃ/ in word and sentence contexts in all positions.

Treatment Targets

Which fricative sounds should be taught first? When a student has not mastered fricative manner of production by elementary school age (or older school age or young adulthood) the easiest approach to teaching fricatives is to target voiceless fricatives first, starting with /h/ and then consonants in final position.[5,17] Instruction should be initiated on voiceless fricatives prior to voiced fricatives to reduce the articulatory load associated with voicing. The result is whispered speech[5,20,40] that highlights the acoustic aspects of speech production. When /h/ is produced without an accompanying vowel one hears the undifferentiated breath flow, that is, a whisper. Among the voiceless fricatives the glottal fricative /h/ would be targeted first because it provides a facilitative context for oral fricative production.

Among the oral fricatives, /f/, /ʃ/, and /s/ would be targeted early and in final position. The /s/ carries a very heavy grammatical load in English and thus the reason for targeting it as one of the early fricative remediation targets.

Intensive Treatment

How rapidly can remediation occur? It is possible to elicit appropriate place and manner of production in whispered speech of all four voiceless fricatives in one intensive session[64] with students of various ages (8, 15, and 22 years of age). Such students would already have an understanding of place of articulation differences for the fricative group even if they were not producing appropriate friction. Other students who show less understanding of the point of constriction differences for the various voiceless fricatives might require more attention to place of production. In this latter case, the elicitation of the voiceless fricatives in whispered speech might occur over several sessions. The goals and stages to be detailed below are useful for either situation.

Perceptual Input and Feedback Issues

Auditory feedback is of course the principal problem of the hearing-impaired student. The clinician should verify from the aided audiogram, detection, and discrimination tasks whether the student could benefit from using audition during fricative remediation. For students who have very limited hearing in the high frequencies and habituated errors in production of fricatives, visual and orosensory feedback information will need to be used during remediation.

AUDITION

1. Students with aided hearing to only 1000 Hz will not be able to detect or discriminate fricatives.
2. Students with aided hearing up to 2000 Hz should be able to detect and discriminate /ʃ/ from other fricatives (by elimination) and from other consonants by manner contrast.
3. Students with aided hearing up to 4000 Hz should be able to detect and discriminate /s/ and /f/ from other fricatives and other consonants by manner, but will not necessarily be able to discriminate /s/ and /f/ from each other.

VISION

Students with no usable audition or limited high frequency audition are able to contrast /f/ from /s/ and /ʃ/ by the different shape and placement of the articulators. However, this information alone is not usually sufficient to facilitate the production of fricatives and the control of an adequate breath stream. In fact, reliance on visual teaching strategies may confound the student's learning.

TOUCH

Tactile information can be used to facilitate the remediation of the fricatives. This includes hot/cold breathstream contrast, width of the breathstream, and directionality of the breathstream for each fricative. It is suggested that students feel their breathstream on the back of their hands. To highlight the sensation, the students can wet the backs of their hands.

*   /h/ = warm on exhalation with slightly open mouth; cold on inhalation; broad breath stream unmediated from the lungs, directionality pointing forward and slightly downward from the mouth
*   /f/ = cool on exhalation especially in contrast to /h/; narrow breath stream in contrast to /h/ and /ʃ/; quite sharp directionality pointing downward from the mouth

- /ʃ/ = warm on exhalation, similar to /h/; broad, strong breath stream; relatively forward directionality especially contrasted with /h/
- /s/ = cool on exhalation especially in contrast to /h/ and /ʃ/; narrowest breathstream; downward pointing directionality

TREATMENT

The following notes will only address treatment of voiceless fricatives in the whispered condition, the first stage of remediation, with suggestions for practice. The principal goals for the first level of remediation of voiceless fricatives are noted below:

1. Achieve relaxed and controlled repetition of /h/ alone and with a whispered vowel /u/, /a/, /i/.
2. Elicit appropriate place of production of /f/, /ʃ/, and /s/ in final position using /h/ as a "crutch."
3. Student produces voiceless fricatives in whispered syllables in initial position.
4. Student to monitor production of whispered syllables, repeated on one breath (eg, /fafafafa/).

STAGE 1

Build success by having the student learn to direct breath flow uninterrupted from the lungs through the vocal tract (eg, producing /h/ with no following vowel). A surprising number of students with "breath and fricative" problems may choke or feel distressed when asked to exhale and inhale for /h/. This dilemma highlights the paradox of students whose respiratory breathing is normal but who have never coordinated breath flow to support speech nor developed a useful orosensory and proprioreceptive feedback system. Cole and Paterson[20] suggested panting as a strategy for helping the student conceptualize and then control respiration for speech.

STAGE 2

Production of /h/ in a controlled manner usually can be achieved in a few minutes when tactile strategies are used by the student to monitor his own and the clinician/teacher's breathstream. Beware of lightheadedness when first asking a student to repeat /hʌ-hʌ-hʌ/. The goal of the first level of repeated practice is for the student to self initiate on command, to monitor the breath, and to reinitiate the breath flow without seizing up.

STAGE 3

The next step is to add the production of a *whispered* vowel to each of the exhalations (eg, hahaha:). The same quality of breath flow should be maintained for each successive initiation. Start with one syllable, /ha/, then ask the student to produce several with control of initiation, cessation, and reinitiation of the breath stream. Rhythmic counting or tapping can be useful in helping the student maintain control. The student continues to monitor the warmth, breadth, and directionality of the breathstream with his hand. Once this has been mastered (by most students in several minutes), repeat the same exercise but with /hi/ and /hu/ so that the extremes of the vowel triangle will be practiced.

STAGE 4

The next step involves a choice. If the student has proceeded this far and has shown understanding of the place of production of the other three targeted fricatives, continue to elicit appropriate place and use of breath flow in a relaxed and easy context. If the student has succeeded quite well but has been taxed enough for one session, stop, repeat the first steps in the next session, and then go on to the other fricatives. These steps should be accomplished in one or three sessions with most school-aged students.

When the choice is to target oral fricatives, elicit /f/ first in final position. The difference between producing /ha/ and /f/ in final position simply involves the lifting of the lower jaw and contacting the lower lip to the upper teeth. This can be accomplished easily and gently if a facilitating context is used. It is easier to produce a subsequent sound if you are producing a like sound. The student repeats the "crutch" /ha ha ha/ and then while holding the final /ha/ closes the jaw. If the student does not stop the breath flow, an /f/ will be produced (eg, /hahahaf:/). Repeat this strategy until the student can find the /f/ easily. Then have the student produce an /f/ syllable at the end of the "starter phrase" (eg, hahahafa). This sequence will be whispered. The next task is to repeat the above sound sequence until the student initiates /fa/ without the "crutch." It is recommended that the facilitating /ha/ syllables be reduced one at a time until the student can keep the breath flow going and appropriately time labiodental closure for /fa/.

Space prohibits the specification of all the repeated steps for other fricatives in the first level of whispered production. However, once the place and appropriate breathstream have been obtained in the whispered condition teacher and student need to go back to the beginning with /h/ and produce the same syllables with voiced vowels and more appropriate rapid articulation.

Practice in familiar linguistic contexts should also be included when this strategy is implemented. For example, the student and teacher could have a pretend dialogue based on answering who, how, how many, how much, and how far questions. The student would be expected to ask the questions and initiate the production of each with an appropriately produced /h/ plus whatever the following vowel would be. The goal is to provide immediate success in production. Each student's ability will be different, but it would be acceptable for the student to do one of many things (eg, whisper the question word, whisper the entire phrase, elongate the breath flow for /h/ or use the /hahahafa/ crutch as a starter).

Conclusion

This chapter provided an overview and a perspective of current issues related to articulation and phonological disorders in the school-aged hearing-impaired population with a focus on the severe-to-profound hearing-impaired population. The assumption was that a perspective on history, characteristics, assessment, and treatment needs, including real-life rehabilitation and educational issues, would help provide an understanding of the challenges faced by this population.

Many hearing-impaired students have not been able to significantly alter their speech and spoken language. Many professionals believe that we could do better by these students if the gap between the existing research and the application of that information by clinicians and teachers could be closed.

While speech and spoken language may not be the communication choice for some hearing-impaired and deaf students, it would be the preferred choice for others, especially with positive outcomes from teaching and remediation. The provision of articulation and phonological treatment services to this population can be improved if knowledge is shared across the relevant professions. It is encouraging that many experienced professionals are willing to question familiar practice and seem willing to take the risk of considering alternative ideas.

Suggested Readings

Boothroyd A: *Hearing Impairments in Young Children*. Washington, DC: AG Bell Association, 1988.
Calvert DR: Speech in perspective. In Luterman DM (ed): *Deafness in Perspective*. San Diego: College-Hill Press, 1986, pp 166–191.
Calvert DR, Silverman SR: *Speech and Deafness*. Washington, DC: AG Bell Association, 1983.
Cole EB, Gregory H (eds): Auditory learning. *Volta Rev Monograph* 1986; 88:1–22.
Hochberg I, Levitt H, Osberger MJ (eds): *Speech of the Hearing-Impaired*. Baltimore: University Park Press, 1983.
Kretschmer RR, Kretschmer LW: *Language Development and Intervention with the Hearing-Impaired*. Baltimore: University Park Press, 1978.
Kretschmer RR, Kretschmer LW: Language in perspective. In Luterman DM (ed): *Deafness in Perspective*. San Diego: College-Hill Press, 1986, pp 131–166.
Ling D: *Speech and the Hearing-Impaired Child: Theory and Practice*. Washington, DC: AG Bell Association, 1976.
Ling D: *Foundations of Spoken Language for Hearing-Impaired Children*. Washington, DC: AG Bell Association, 1989.
Markides A: *The Speech of Hearing Impaired Children*. Manchester, UK: Manchester University Press, 1983.
Schow RL, Nerbonne MA: *Introduction to Aural Rehabilitation*, 2nd ed. Austin, TX: Pro-Ed, 1988.
Stoker R, Ling D (eds): Speech production in hearing-impaired children and youth: Theory and practice. *Volta Rev* 1992; 94:xx–xx.

References

1. Bernthal JE, Bankson N: *Articulation and Phonological Disorders*, 2nd ed. Englewood Cliffs, NJ: Prentice Hall, 1988.
2. Boothroyd A: Evaluation of speech. In Hochberg I, Levitt H, Osberger MJ (eds): *Speech of the Hearing-Impaired*. Baltimore: University Park Press, 1983, pp 181–193.
3. Calvert DR, Silverman SR: *Speech and Deafness*, 2nd ed. Washington, DC: AG Bell Association for the Deaf, 1983.
4. Fry DB: The role and primacy of the auditory channel in speech and language development. In Ross M, Giolas TG (eds): *Speech Disorders in Children*. Baltimore: University Park Press, 1978, pp 15–43.
5. Ling D: *Speech and the Hearing-Impaired Child: Theory and Practice*. Washington, DC: AG Bell Association, 1976.
6. Markides A: *The Speech of Hearing-Impaired Children*. Manchester, UK: Manchester University Press, 1983.
7. Monson RB: General effects of deafness on phonation and articulation. In Hochberg I, Levitt H, Osberger MJ (eds): *Speech of the Hearing-Impaired*. Baltimore: University Park Press, 1983, pp 23–34.
8. Hochberg I, Levitt H, Osberger MJ (eds): *Speech of the Hearing-Impaired*. Baltimore: University Park Press, 1983.

9. Levitt H, Stromberg H: Segmental characteristics of the speech of hearing-impaired children: factors affecting intelligibility. In Hochberg I, Levitt H, Osberger MJ (eds): *Speech of the Hearing-Impaired*. Baltimore: University Park Press, 1983, pp 53–73.

10. Cole EB: Promoting emerging speech in birth to 3-year-old hearing-impaired children. *Volta Rev* 1992; 94:63–77.

11. Ross M, Giolas R (eds): *Auditory Management of Hearing-Impaired Children*. Baltimore: University Park Press, 1978.

12. Ling D, Ling, AH: *The Foundations of Verbal Learning for Hearing-Impaired Children*. Washington, DC: AG Bell Association, 1978.

13. Perusse M, Bernstein A, Ling Phillips A: Incorporating speech development into an education program. *Volta Rev* 1992; 94:79–94.

14. Calvert DR: Speech in perspective. In Luterman DM (ed): *Deafness in Perspective*. San Diego: College-Hill Press, 1986, pp 166–191.

15. Boothroyd A: *Hearing Impairments in Young Children*. Washington, DC: AG Bell Association, 1988.

16. Kretschmer RR, Kretschmer LW: *Language Development and Intervention with the Hearing-Impaired*. Baltimore: University Park Press, 1978.

17. Ling D: *Foundations of Spoken Language for Hearing-Impaired Children*. Washington, DC: AG Bell Association, 1989.

18. Schow RL, Nerbonne MA: *Introduction to Aural Rehabilitation*, 2nd ed. Austin, TX: Pro-Ed, 1988.

19. Moores DF: *Educating the Deaf*, 3rd ed. Boston: Houghton-Mifflin, 1987.

20. Cole EB, Paterson MM: Assessment and treatment of phonologic disorders in the hearing-impaired. In Costello J (ed): *Recent Advances in Speech Disorders*. San Diego: College-Hill Press, 1984, pp 93–127.

21. Markides A: The use of residual hearing in the education of hearing-impaired children–a historical perspective. *Volta Rev* 1986; 88:57–66.

22. Paterson MM: Maximizing the use of residual hearing with school-aged hearing-impaired children. *Volta Rev* 1986; 88:93–106.

23. Bess FH, McConnell FE: *Audiology, Education and the Hearing-Impaired Child*. St. Louis: C.V. Mosby, 1981.

24. Dawson PW, Blamey PJ, Rowland L, Dettman SJ, Clark GM, Busby PA, Brown AM, Dowell RC, Rickards FW: Cochlear implants in children, adolescents, and prelinguistically deafened adults: Speech reception. *JSHR* 1992; 35:401–417.

25. Geers AE, Tobey E: Effects of cochlear implants and tactile aids on the development of speech production skills in children with profound hearing impairment. *Volta Rev* 1992; 94:135–163.

26. Subtelny JD: Integrated speech and language instruction for the hearing-impaired adolescent, vol. 9. In Lass N (ed): *Speech and Language Advances in Basic Research and Practice*. New York: Academic Press, 1983, pp 43–102.

27. Jensema CJ, Karchmer MA, Trybus RJ: *The Rated Speech Intelligibility of Hearing-Impaired Children*. Gallaudet, Office of Demographic Studies, 1978.

28. Wolk S, Schildroth AN: Deaf children and speech intelligibility: A national study. In Schildroth AN, Karchmer MA (eds): *Deaf Children in America*. San Diego: College-Hill, 1986, pp 139–159.

29. McGarr NS: Communication skills of hearing-impaired children in schools for the deaf. In Levitt H, McGarr NS, Geffner D (eds): *Development of Language and Communication Skills in Hearing-Impaired Children*. Rockville, MD: ASHA Monographs, 1987; 26:91–107.

30. Ling D, Milne M: The development of speech in hearing-impaired children. In Bess F, Freeman BA, Sinclair JS (eds): *Amplification in Education*. Washington, DC: AG Bell Association, 1981, pp 98–108.

31. Gatty JC: Teaching speech to hearing-impaired children. *Volta Rev* 1992; 94:49–61.

32. Subtelny JD, Snell KB: Efficacy of a distinctive feature model of therapy for hearing-impaired adolescents. *JSHD* 1988; 53:194–201.

33. Hochberg I, Schmidt JL, Solomon LM, Schiavetti N, Godsave N, Burgess E: Improving speech services for hearing-impaired children in the schools: A consortium model for meeting continuing education and preservice training needs. *LSHSS* 1983; 14:181–194.

34. Woodford CM: Speech-language pathologists' knowledge and skills regarding hearing aids. *LSHSS* 1987; 18:312–322.

35. Cole EB, Gregory H (eds): *Auditory Learning*. Washington, DC: AG Bell Association, 1986.

36. Boothroyd A: Speech perception and sensorineural hearing loss. In Ross M, Giolas TG (eds): *Auditory Management of Hearing-Impaired Children*. Baltimore: University Park Press, 1978, pp 117–144.

37. Oller D: Metaphonology and infant vocalizations. In Lindblom B, Zetterstrom R (eds): *Precursors of Early Speech*. New York: Stockton Press, 1986, pp 21–35.

38. Borden GJ, Harris KS: *Speech Science Primer*, 2nd ed. Baltimore: Williams and Wilkins, 1984.

39. Perkins WH, Kent RD: *Functional Anatomy of Speech, Language, and Hearing*. Boston: College-Hill, 1986.

40. Pickett JM: *The Sounds of Speech Communication.* Baltimore: University Park Press, 1980.
41. Parker A, Rose H: Deaf children's phonological development. In Grunwell P (ed): *Developmental Speech Disorders.* London: Churchill Livingston, 1990, pp 83–107.
42. Cole EB: Listening and Talking: *A Guide to Promoting Spoken Language in Young Hearing-Impaired Children.* Washington, DC: AG Bell Association, 1992.
43. Paterson MM: *The First Fifteen Days of Hearing Aid Wearing: Microanalysis of Interactions Between a 15 Month Old Hearing-Impaired Child and Her French-Canadian Father.* Unpublished doctoral dissertation, University of Cincinnati, Cincinnati, OH, 1990.
44. Mahshie JJ, Contour E: Deaf speakers laryngeal behavior. *JSHR* 1983; 26:550–559.
45. Metz DE, Whitehead RL, Whitehead BH: Mechanics of vocal fold vibration and laryngeal articulatory gestures produced by hearing-impaired speakers. *JSHR* 1984; 27:56–62.
46. Stevens KN, Nickerson RS, Boothroyd A, Rollins AM: Assessment of nasalization in the speech of deaf children. *JSHR* 1976; 19:371–392.
47. Forner L, Hixon TJ: Respiratory kinematics in profoundly hearing-impaired speakers. *JSHR* 1977; 20:373–407.
48. Kretschmer RR, Kretschmer LW: Language in perspective. In Luterman DM (ed): *Deafness in Perspective.* San Diego: College-Hill Press, 1986, pp 131–166.
49. Clark E, Clark E; *The Psychology of Language.* New York: Harcourt Brace Jovanovich, 1977, pp 515–558.
50. McGarr NS, Whitehead RL; Contemporary issues in phoneme production by hearing-impaired persons: Physiological and acoustic aspects. *Volta Rev* 1992; 94:33–45.
51. Hudgins CV, Numbers FC: An investigation of the intelligibility of the speech of the deaf. *GenPsychMon* 1942; 25:289–392.
52. Angelocci AA, Kopp GA, Holbrook A: The vowel formants of deaf and normal-hearing eleven to fourteen-year-old boys. *JSHD* 1964; 29:156–170.
53. Smith C: Residual hearing and speech production in deaf children. *JSHR* 1975; 19:795–811.
54. Monson RB: Acoustic qualities of phonation in young hearing-impaired children. *JSHR* 1979; 22:270–288.
55. Tye-Murray N: The establishment of open articulatory postures by deaf and hearing talkers. *JSHR* 1991; 34:453–459.
56. Calvert DR: Articulation and hearing impairment. In Lass NJ, McReynolds LV, Northern JL, Yoder DE (eds): *Speech, Language and Hearing.* Philadelphia: Saunders, 1982, pp 638–651.
57. Waldstein RS, Baum SR: Anticipatory coarticulation in the speech of profoundly hearing-impaired and normally hearing children. *JSHR* 1991; 34:1276–1285.
58. Baum SR, Waldstein RS: Perseveratory coarticulation in the speech of profoundly hearing-impaired and normally hearing children. *JSHR* 1991; 34:1286–1292.
59. Markides A: The speech of deaf and partially hearing children with special reference to factors affecting intelligibility. *Br J Commun Dis* 1970; 5:126–140.
60. Dagenais PA, Critz-Crosby P: Comparing tongue positioning by normal-hearing and hearing-impaired children during vowel production. *JSHR* 1992; 34:35–44.
61. Thomas-Kersting C, Casteel RL: Harsh voice: Vocal effort perceptual ratings and spectral noise level of hearing-impaired children. *J Commun Dis* 1989; 22:125–135.
62. Whitehead RL, Barefoot S: Airflow characteristics of fricative consonants produced by normally hearing and hearing-impaired speakers. *JSHR* 1983; 26:185–194.
63. Smit AB: Phonologic error distributions in the Iowa-Nebraska articulation norms project: Consonant singletons. *JSHR* 1993; 36:533–547.
64. Paterson MM: *Teaching Speech to the Deaf: More than an Articulation Problem.* Short course, San Diego, AG Bell Association for the Deaf International Convention, 1992.
65. Ling D: Speech evaluation and phonological processes in hearing-impaired children. *Taralye Bull* 1990; 10:16–22.
66. Shaw S, Coggins TE: Interobserver reliability using the Phonetic Level Evaluation with severely and profoundly hearing-impaired children. *JSHR* 1991; 34:989–999.
67. Monson R, Moog JS, Geers AE (eds): *CID Picture Speech Intelligibility Evaluation (SPINE).* St. Louis: Central Institute for the Deaf, 1988.
68. Moog JS: *The CID Phonetic Inventory.* St. Louis: Central Institute for the Deaf, 1989.
69. Perigoe CB: Strategies of the remediation of speech of hearing-impaired children. *Volta Rev* 1992; 94:95–118.
70. Subtelny JS, Whitehead RL, Orlando NO: Description and evaluation of an instructional program to improve speech and voice diagnosis of the hearing-impaired. *Volta Rev* 1980; 82:85–95.
71. Geers A, Tobey E: Effects of cochlear implants and tactile aids on the development of speech production skill in children with profound hearing impairment. *Volta Rev* 1992; 94:135–163.
72. Haycock GS: *The Teaching of Speech.* Washington, DC: AG Bell Association, 1933.

73. Subtelny JS, Lieberth A: *Speech and Auditory Training: A Program for Adolescents with Hearing Impairments and Language Disorders.* Tucson, AZ: Communication Skill Builders, 1985.
74. Osberger MJ, Johnstone A, Swarts E, Levitt H: The evaluation of a model speech training program for deaf children. *J Commun Dis* 1978; 11:292–312.
75. Secord W: *Eliciting Sounds: Techniques for Clinicians.* Columbus, OH: Charles E. Merrill, 1981.
76. Waling S, Harrison W, Brewster B: *A Speech Guide for Clinicians and Teachers of Hearing-Impaired Children.* Tucson, AZ: Communication Skill Builders, 1987.
77. Erber N: *Auditory Training.* Washington, DC: AG Bell Association, 1982.
78. Stoker R, Ling D (eds): Speech production in hearing-impaired children and youth: Theory and practice. *Volta Rev* 1992; 94.
79. Novelli-Olmstead T, Ling D: Speech production and speech discrimination by hearing-impaired children. *Volta Rev* 1992; 86:72–80.
80. Whitehead BH, Barefoot SM: Improving speech production with adolescents and adults. *Volta Rev* 1992; 94:119–134.
81. Paterson MM: Integration of auditory training with speech and language for severely hearing-impaired children. In Sims D, Walter G, Whitehead RL (eds): *Deafness and Communication: Assessment and Training.* Baltimore: Williams & Wilkins, 1982, pp 93–106.

Part IV
Cultural Factors

10

The Phonology of a Sociocultural Variety: The Case of African American Vernacular English

WALT WOLFRAM, PH.D.

Introduction

There are several reasons for including a discussion of vernacular dialect phonology in a book on the phonological characteristics of special populations, although the basis for distinguishing the population in this case is markedly different from the pathophysiological one used to define the special populations discussed in other chapters. In this instance, the distinguishing criterion is sociocultural, as the use of African American Vernacular English (AAVE) is primarily associated with a sociolinguistically defined subset of African Americans.

It is only fitting that AAVE phonology be discussed as the paradigm case of vernacular dialect phonology because focus on AAVE launched the modern era of social dialectology. Although the description of various American English dialects has preoccupied American dialectologists for over a century now, the intensified debate about the status of AAVE in the late 1960s opened a number of critical issues about language diversity for the field of speech and language pathology.[1-4] Historically, AAVE is the vernacular variety that caused the speech and language profession to confront the deficit-difference controversy over language variation, and many current instances of sociolinguistic application in assessment and treatment have taken their cue from the discussion of AAVE.[5-7]

AAVE is also the native English vernacular variety that is arguably the most distant from Standard English in its phonological structure, so that descriptive and applied details discussed for this variety can be generalized readily to other socioculturally defined varieties of English. AAVE shares phonological characteristics with a wide range of vernacular varieties of English at the same time that its constellation of features uniquely sets it apart from them.

Finally, AAVE has undergone some unique sociohistoric development—development that figures into the phonological depth and breadth of differences encountered in this variety. The distinctive sociolinguistic situation of AAVE is not simply a matter of descriptive curiosity; it also impacts on evaluation and treatment issues as they relate to language variation. AAVE thus provides an ideal case for examining descriptive and applied issues related to socially situated "special" populations of speakers.

History

Hypotheses about the historic origin of AAVE have been reduced to two major alternatives, although the identification of ancestral sources for the particular phonological traits of AAVE phonology is often blurred by a complex set of sociolinguistic conditions that have affected its development over the years.

According to the *Creolist Hypothesis*, AAVE developed from an ancestral *creole language*, a special language developed in communicative situations in which the vocabulary from one language is imposed on a specially adapted, restricted grammatical structure. Creolists posit that the creole predecessor of AAVE, so-called Plantation Creole, was fairly widespread during slavery and persisted to some extent in the antebellum South as well. Furthermore, it is noted that Plantation Creole was not a unique development that arose in the mainland South; instead, this Creole shows continuity with well-known creoles of the African diaspora such as Krio, spoken today along the coast of West Africa in Sierra Leone, and English-based creoles of the Caribbean, such as Jamaican Creole. In the United States, Gullah (more popularly called "Geechee"), the Creole still spoken by a small number of African Americans in the Sea Islands off the coast of South Carolina and Georgia, is considered a direct descendent of an earlier, much more widespread creole. Those who endorse the Creolist Hypothesis maintain that this creole was fairly widespread among African Americans on Southern plantations, but that it was not spoken to any extent by European Americans.

Phonologically, Creole languages typically manifest syllable structure and sound inventory processes that make them phonologically more "natural" or "unmarked" (ie, phonetically more plausible or physiologically "easier" to produce) than their respective donor languages, although their phonology may, at the same time, remain influenced by the phonological traits of their ancestral languages. Thus, syllable structure processes in Creoles result in more "simplified" canonical sequences, making processes such as consonant cluster reduction, final consonant deletion, and unstressed syllable deletion relatively common.[8] Analogously, natural substitution processes such as stopping, vocalization of liquids, and final devoicing are commonly applied to the phonological inventory of the source languages in the creolization process.

It is important to note that Creolists do not typically maintain that present-day AAVE still qualifies as a Creole-like phonology. Instead, AAVE underwent a *de-Creolization process*, in which it lost many of its Creole characteristics through contact with mainstream, standard varieties. However, this process was neither instantaneous nor complete, leaving traces of a Creole predecessor that are still evident in present-day AAVE phonology.

The major alternative to the Creole Hypothesis is referred to as the *Anglicist*

Hypothesis, so-called because the origin of AAVE is proposed to be rooted histori-cally in varieties of English spoken in the British Isles, much like European American varieties of American English. The Anglicist position maintains that communication patterns of African Americans in the United States were roughly comparable to those of other immigrant groups. It is maintained that slaves brought with them to North America a number of different African languages or even pidgins and Creoles spoken at the time in West Africa. Over the course of a couple of generations, African Americans simply learned the regional and social varieties of the surrounding European American speakers, becoming phonologi-cally absorbed. Given the historic concentration of African Americans in the South, Southern-based vernacular varieties would thus be the formative influ-ence on the phonological development of AAVE. Any differences that cannot be explained on the basis of regional and social factors are postulated to result from the differential preservation patterns of British dialect features brought to North America by the colonists. For example, the pronunciation of *ask* as [æks] in AAVE is often mentioned as a retention of a verb form found in older English *acsian*. Although the Anglicist Hypothesis appeals to Southern American English, and, by extension, to the primary British dialects influential in the development of Southern American English as the historic basis for the development of AAVE phonology, this position does not completely rule out the possibility of some ves-tigial effects from ancestral African languages on AAVE phonology. However, these effects would at this point be quite subtle and negligible in their influence on the overall AAVE system.

The synchronic empiric evidence indicates that AAVE phonology certainly shows a strong affinity with Southern-based vernacular varieties. Of course, we cannot simply assume that the transmission of traits was unilateral; in fact, there is evidence that some features of present-day Southern European English (for example, the absence of contracted forms of the copula, such as *they nice* for *they're nice*) came originally from their African American counterparts.

At the same time that AAVE shares the vast majority of its structures with Southern-based vernacular varieties, it has several phonological traits that seem unique in AAVE. For example, the extent to which final consonant cluster reduc-tion and final consonant devoicing are applied in AAVE, as discussed in the next section, suggests that a simple Anglicist explanation for the AAVE phonological system is not completely adequate. However, most segmental remnants of Creole-postulated source features tend to be quantitative rather than qualitative at this stage in the development of AAVE, making them quite subtle in their effect.

In examining the similarities found between AAVE and Creole phonologies, we must be careful not to assume that these similarities necessarily indicate direct descendance. There are several different sociolinguistic situations and an underlying set of principles governing phonological variation and change that may converge in their effect on a phonological system, thus complicating the pic-ture of historic attribution.

For example, processes such as interdental fricative stopping (eg, [θ] → [t]; [d] → [d̪]), unstressed syllable deletion, and other natural phonological processes characterize a range of independent vernacular varieties of English—varieties that clearly have no Creole predecessor. As it turns out, certain natural changes may accelerate in the lower social classes while they are resisted by the upper classes, in spite of their phonological reasonableness. High-status groups have the most investment in maintaining a language variety the way it is. Low-status groups have less investment in maintaining the current state of linguistic structures; thus, they are more susceptible to the application of natural phonological processes. In fact, an important principle of sociolinguistic stratification involves the inhibition of natural changes by high-status groups. The effects of Creolization and the sociolinguistic *inhibition principle,* both of which move toward more phonological naturalness, certainly may converge. As we can see, sorting out the specific source for a particular AAVE phonological characteristic involves considerable understanding of sociolinguistic change and variation along with an appreciation for sociohistoric circumstance.

The historic development of AAVE raises a number of important issues about phonological change and historic attribution that do not necessarily lead to definitive answers. Nonetheless, we conclude that the most reasonable historic explanation for AAVE phonology appeals to a predominant Southern vernacular contact source, enhanced by some Creole vestiges and some possible independent phonological developments.

Distinguishing Characteristics of AAVE Phonology

Before presenting some of the specific phonological characteristics of AAVE phonology, it is necessary to understand how sociocultural varieties of English distinguish themselves from each other. This discussion is critical to our understanding of normal phonological behavior for vernacular dialect speakers; furthermore, it impacts on assessment and treatment considerations for such speakers.

The popular belief is that the varieties of English are distinguished by categoric phonological distinctions–that ALL members of one social group *always* use a certain variant while ALL the members of a different group *never* do. This caricature holds, for example, that speakers of vernacular dialects always manifest the [ð] → [d] stopping process in items such as *this* and *that,* or the nasal fronting process [ŋ] → [n] in unstressed syllables, such as the *-ing* in *swimming* or *taking* while speakers of standard varieties NEVER do. In reality, individual speakers, as well as groups of speakers, indicate variable usage of alternate phonological forms. Thus, one speaker may apply the stopping process in 90% of all those cases where it might have applied (that is, items that have an initial [ð] correspondence in the standard variety), another speaker apply it 50% of the time, and still another speaker apply it to 20% of all cases phonologically eligible for the application of the process. Furthermore, if we consider the scores of central tendency for socially grouped sets of speakers, we find they are typically differentiated by the relative frequency with which certain phonological processes or rules are applied rather than invariant use of one form or another. For example, in one of the early studies of the fluctuation of [Iŋ] and [In] (*swimming* versus *swimmin'*) fluctuation, Shuy, Wolfram, and Riley[9] found that upper-middle-class speakers used the [In] variant in approximately 20% of all cases where it might have been used, lower-middle-class speakers in 40%, upper-working-class in 50%, and lower-class in 80% of all cases.

Inherent fluctuation of phonological variables is characteristic of vernacular varieties of English even when the differences involve *group-exclusive distribution,* which is, patterns of sociocultural distribution in which certain traits are limited to particular groups. Thus, voiced fricative stopping before nasal segments (eg, [sEbm] *seb'm* for [sEvIn] *seven* or [Idʌt] for [Izʌt] *isn't*) is a group-exclusive phonological process in that it is only found among some social and regional varieties of English (Southern-based varieties of European American English and AAVE). However, the typical usage pattern among AAVE and Southern European American Vernacular English speakers is variable in that the same speaker may produce both [sEb m] and [sEvIn] as an inherent part of his phonological system. Vernacular varieties are rarely typified by the categoric application of a phonological process or rule. The recognition of so-called *inherent variability* is an important part of understanding the authentic nature of AAVE phonology because very few of the traits of AAVE phonology involve the categoric application of processes.

Although the fluctuation of phonological forms is inherent within the system, the relative frequency of particular variants may be constrained systematically by two types of factors. First, linguistic factors such as phonological environment and the internal composition of sounds may increase or decrease the frequency rates for variants in a patterned way. These types of constraints are referred to as *internal constraints* on variability. Second, social factors such as status, gender, and so forth may systematically affect the relative frequency of a form. These are referred to as *external constraints* on variability.

A classic example of a phonological process revealing systematic internal and external effects on variability is syllable-final consonant cluster reduction, where final stop clusters are matched for voicing (that is, both members of the cluster are either voiced or voiceless such as *mist, messed, find,* or *cold,* compared with *colt, jump,* or *runt,* where members of the cluster do not match in voicing). In Table 10–1, we show the mean scores of cluster reduction for groups of speakers from several representative varieties of English found in the United States. The relevant social factors here are status, region, and ethnicity; the relevant linguistic factors are a following consonant versus nonconsonant phonological environment and morphemic boundary (that is, clusters that are part of a single morpheme as in *mist* [mIst] versus clusters that are spread over two morphemes such as *miss+ed* [mIst]).

Table 10–1 shows that consonant cluster reduction is an inherently variable process and that varieties of English are differentiated on the basis of the relative frequency of its application. At the same time, it demonstrates that there are internal constraints on its variability. Thus, for all social and ethnic groups, the highest incidence of cluster reduction occurs when the cluster is part of a single morpheme and occurs before a consonant; the lowest incidence of cluster reduction always occurs when a cluster spreads over two morphemes and occurs before a vowel. This type of systematic variation must be kept in mind in considering the distinguishing characteristics of AAVE phonology; otherwise, the profile of AAVE that emerges will be distorted and exaggerated.

Table 10–1.   Comparison of Consonant Cluster Reduction in
Several Representative English Dialects

| | Language Variety | | | |
| | Followed by Consonant | | Followed by Vowel | |
	Not -ed Mean % Red.	-ed Mean % Red.	Not -ed Mean % Red.	-ed Mean % Red.
Northern white middle class	66	36	12	3
Northern white working class	67	23	19	3
Southern white working class	56	16	25	10
Northern black middle class	79	49	23	7
Northern black working class	97	76	72	34
Southern black working class	88	50	72	36

(Adapted from Wolfram[10] p 199)

The sociocultural and regional differences revealed in Table 10–1 indicate that AAVE is sensitive to the kinds of social factors that typically affect other English varieties—stratificational factors such as status, region, age, and gender and interactional factors such as conversational participants, roles, contextual settings, and so forth. For example, we have found that Eastern Seaboard varieties of AAVE phonology tend to have both the voiceless [θ] → [f] and the voiced [ð] → [v] cognates of interdental labialization in medial and final position (eg, [bæf] *bath* [smuv] *smooth*); whereas Midwest varieties of AAVE are more likely to have only the voiceless cognate. Furthermore, in varieties of AAVE phonology found close to the South Carolina and Georgia coastal areas, the influence of Gullah Creole phonology has resulted in some incidence of [t] for final [θ] in items like *bath* (ie, [bæt]).

Similarly, we note that Southern-based varieties of AAVE that are surrounded by regional *r*-less varieties of English tend to be more extensively *r*-less than their Northern counterparts, although Northern-based varieties certainly participate in the postvocalic *r*-less pattern. And, of course, there are status-based differences in the extent to which *r*-lessness is manifested based on social factors such as status, gender, age, and participation in various social networks. We certainly have to recognize regional and social varieties in any discussion of the structures of AAVE phonology.

While evidence exists supporting regional dialect differences within AAVE phonology, there is probably less regional variation involved in AAVE than in the regional versions of comparable European American varieties. There are several sociohistoric reasons that explain the contraction of regional differences. In the first place, the heavy historic concentration of African Americans in the South prior to the two world wars and the segregated interactional and communication network patterns that accompanied the Northern and urban migration following the wars mitigated many of the basic North–South distinctions found in comparable European American varieties. Furthermore, for reasons that range from historic segregation to ethnic solidarity, African Americans are not participating in a number of the dialect changes taking place in surrounding regional European American varieties, such as the shifting vowel system found in Northern cities[10] (p 85). The effect of this sociolinguistic situation results in the maintenance of a common core of phonological characteristics and a degree of insularity from surrounding regional European American varieties.

In the following section, some of the common structures of AAVE phonology are summarized. It is essential to keep in mind the inherently variable nature of these processes, as discussed above, and to recognize some of the major social and linguistic variables that constrain the relative frequency of the processes. Furthermore, it is necessary to understand that the vast majority of these features are NOT unique to the phonology of AAVE. Many of the structures are shared with more general versions of vernacular English varieties and the majority are shared by Southern European American vernacular varieties. To a large extent, AAVE phonology is not defined by its unique structures but by the particular constellation of structures and the extent to which various variable processes are applied.

Although different models of phonological description might be used to profile the phonological characteristics of AAVE, a natural phonological process model is used here because familiarity with this model is now fairly widespread among speech and language pathologists. This model may at first glance seem to imply an idealized standard English variety as the sole basis of comparison. However, the motivation for underlying units posited as the input for particular processes, in most cases, can be justified quite independent of their correspondence with comparable units in standard varieties of English. Hence, they are considered a regular part of unimpaired AAVE phonology.

Phonological Structures of AAVE

In the following outline, a selection of the major phonological structures of AAVE phonology is presented. These are broken down into three major categories: (1) syllable structure processes; (2) substitution and assimilation processes; and (3) prosodic features. This inventory should not be considered exhaustive because it is selective and limited in phonological detail. Where appropriate, primary internal constraints on variability are included in the outline.

Syllable Structure Processes

FINAL CONSONANT CLUSTER REDUCTION

Word-final consonant clusters ending in a stop may delete the final member when both members of the cluster are either voiced (eg, *find, cold*) or voiceless (*act, desk*). The process affects clusters within a single morpheme (eg, [mIst] *mist*) and clusters spread across two morphemes (eg, [mIst] *missed*), as indicated in the following list.

Single Morpheme	Across Morphemes
[st] *test, post, list*	*missed, messed, dressed*
[sp] *wasp, clasp, mask*	
[sk] *desk, mask, risk*	
[ʃt]	*finished, latched, cashed*
[zd]	*raised, composed, amazed*
[ʒd]	*judged, charged, forged*
[ft] *left, craft, cleft*	*laughed, stuffed, roughed*
[vd]	*loved, lived, moved*
[nd] *mind, find, mound*	*rained, fanned, canned*
[md]	*named, foamed, rammed*
[ld] *cold, wild, old*	*called, smelled, killed*
[pt] *apt, adept, inept*	*mapped, stopped, clapped*
[kt] *act, contact, expect*	*looked, cooked, cracked*

Variable Constraints on Cluster Reduction.
   Following consonant > nonconsonant (eg, *best pear > best apple*)
   single morpheme clusters > double morpheme clusters (eg, *mist > missed*)
   unstressed syllables > stressed syllables (eg, *breakfast > fast*)
Plural Formations.   Words ending in *sC* may pluralize with the regular syllable plural [Iz], as in [tEsIz] *tests* or [dEsIz] *desks.*
Other Suffixes.   Most varieties of AAVE retain a cluster when a suffix beginning with a vowel is added (eg, [tEstIn] *testing*); however, some varieties of AAVE, particularly Southern-based rural ones, may apply reduction in such cases as well (eg, [tEsIn] *testing* [prIdIkəbl] *predictable*).

FINAL CONSONANT DELETION

Final consonant singletons may be deleted to a limited extent. Some instances of final consonant deletion may be lexically determined.
   (eg, [fayv] → [fa] *five*
       [mæn] → [mæ̃] *man*
Variable Constraints on Final Singleton Deletion.
   Final nasals > nonnasals (eg, *man > cat*)
   following consonant > nonconsonant (eg, *cat near > cat away*)
   coronal > noncoronal consonant (eg, *cat > cup*)
   voiced > voiceless consonant (eg, *bad > bat*)

UNSTRESSED SYLLABLE DELETION

Unstressed initial and medial syllables may be deleted.
   (eg, [rImEmbə] → [mEmbə] *remember*
       [sEkrətEri] → [sEktEri] *secretary*)

SYLLABLE REDUCTION

[ay], [aw], and [oy] diphthong sequences followed by a syllabic liquid may be

unglided and collapsed into one syllable.

    (eg, [tayə] → [tar] *tire*

       [flawə] → [flar] *flower*

       [oyɬ] → [ol] *oil*)

CR REDUCTION

Initial θr sequences followed by a round vowel such as [u] or [o] may delete the *r*.

    (eg, [θru] → [θu] *through*

       [θro] → [θo] *throw*)

Unstressed *Cr* clusters may delete the *r*.

    (eg, [sÉkrətEri] → [sÉkətEri] *secretary*

       [prəfEsɚ] → [pəfÉsə] *professor*)

HAPLOLOGY

Reduplicated syllables may delete part of or the complete syllable.

    (eg, [mIsIsIpi] → [mIzsIpi] *Mississippi*

       [sIŋIŋ] → [sIŋ] *singing*)

DEPALATALIZATION

Palatal glide [j] may be deleted in a *CjV* sequence.

    (eg, [kəmpjuɚt] → [kəmputə] *computer*

       [fIgjɚ] → [fIgə] *figure*)

Variable Constraint on Depalatalization:

Unstressed > Stressed (eg, *figure > music*)

METATHESIS

The sequence of selected final *s* + **Stop** sequences may be transposed. For the most part, the items affected by this process are lexically defined.

    (eg, [æsk] → [æks] *ask*

      [græsp] → [græps] *grasp*)

Neutralization and Assimilation Processes

FRICATIVE STOPPING

1. Syllable-initial interdental fricatives may be stopped, particularly if the fricative is voiced.

    (eg, [ðoz] → [doz] *those*

      [ðo] → [do] *though*)

Variable Constraint on Stopping:

Voiced > Voiceless (eg, *though > thought*)

2. Voiced fricatives preceding nasals may be stopped.

    (eg, [sEvIn] → [sEbm̩] *seven*

      [Izn̩tɚ] → [Idn̩t] *isn't*)

3. Voiceless interdental fricative contiguous to a nasal may be stopped.

    (eg, [tEnθ] → [tEnt] *tenth*

      [nəθIŋ] → [nətn̩] *nothing*)

UNSTRESSED NASAL FRONTING

In unstressed syllables, velar nasals such as [Iŋ] may be fronted to [In].
  (eg, [swImIŋ] → [swImIn] *swimming*
      [gEtIŋ] → [gEtn] *getting*)

NASALIZATION

Nasalized vowels may be used for final **V + Nasal** sequences.
  (eg, [mæn] → [mæ̃] *man*
      [rImen] → [rImẽ] *remain*)
  Variable Constraints on Nasalization:
  Coronal > Non-Coronal (eg, *man > stem*)
  Pause/Consonant > Vowel (eg, *man by > man at*)

LABIALIZATION

In syllable-final position, interdental fricatives may become labiodental fricatives.
  (eg, [bæθ] → [bæf] *bath*
      [smuð] → [smuv] *smooth*)
  Variable Constraints on Labialization:
  Voiceless Interdental > Voiced Interdental (eg, *bath > smooth*)

LIQUID VOCALIZATION

There are several environments in which postvocalic *r* and *l* may be vocalized; the liquid may be vocalized or be deleted completely.
R Vocalization.   The complete set of *r* vocalization patterns is most typically found in Southern-based AAVE varieties; Northern varieties are sometimes limited to the first two types.
1. Syllabic *R* in Unstressed Syllables
    (eg. [fev] → [fev] *favor*
        [bIg] → [bIg] *bigger*)
2. Vowel + Consonantal *R*
    (eg, [fIr] → [fIə] *fear*
        [kar] → [kaə] *car*)
3. Stressed Syllabic *R*
    (eg, [wʒˆk] → [wək] *work*
        [fʒˆ] → [fə] *fur*)
4. *VrV* ambisyllabic sequences
    (eg, [dUrIŋ] → [dUIn] *during*
        [kærəI] → [kæU] *Carol*)
L Vocalization.
1. Postvocalic *l* may vocalize to [u] or [U]
    (eg, [bEl] → [bEU] *bell*
        [nIkł] → [nIkU] *nickel*)
2. Preceding a labial consonant [l] may be deleted
    (eg, [hElp] → [hEp] *help*
        [wUlf] → [wUf] *wolf*)
Variable Constraints on Liquid Vocalization:

Following Pause/Consonant > Vowel (eg, *car near > car at*)
Unstressed Syllable > Stressed Syllable (eg, *compare > fanfare*)

FINAL STOP DEVOICING

In syllable-final position, voiced obstruents may be devoiced. The length of the preceding vowel, however, remains unaffected, so that items such as *bud* and *butt* typically do not become homophonous. Phonetically, a glottal stop may be used for /d/.

(eg, [bæːd] → [bæːt] or [bæːʔ] *bad*
    [pIːg] → [pIːk] *pig*)

str Backing. Initial *str* clusters may back [t] to [k], particularly in rural Southern varieties of AAVE. In some deep South rural varieties, this process may even be applied to initial *tr* clusters as well.

(eg, [strit] → [skrit] *street*
    [strim] → [skrim] *stream*
    [tri] → [kri] *tree*)

Variable Constraint on *str* Backing:
High Front Vowels > Non-High Front Vowels (eg, *stream > strap*)

VOWELS

AAVE vowel production shares many traits with more generalized Southern varieties of English, including the following:

Glide Reduction.   [ay] and [oy] glides may reduce the glide of the diphthong.

(eg, [taym] → [tam] *time*
    [sayd] → [sad] *side*)

Variable Constraint on Glide Reduction:
Following Voiced Segment > Voiceless Segment (eg, *ride > right*)

Vowel Merger.   Preceding restricted phonological environments, the distinction between certain vowel contrasts may be reduced or eliminated.

1. [I] and [E] may be neutralized preceding nasals
    (eg, [pIn] *pin* or *pen*
        [kIn] *kin* or *Ken*
    Variable Constraint on Neutralization:
    Coronal > Noncoronal (*pin/pen > him/hem*)

2. tense-lax vowel merger preceding liquids *l* and *r*
    (eg, [pUl] *pool* or *pull*
        [pIl] *pill* or *peel*
        [mæri] *Mary, marry,* or *merry*)

Centralizing.   Between sibilants, back and front vowels may be centralized.

(eg, [sIstə] → [sɨstə] *sister*
    [sIzəz] → [sɨzəz] *scissors*)

Prosodic Features

STRESS

Most characteristic stress differences in AAVE involve primary stress placement, often moving forward primary stress placement to the initial syllable.

(eg, [po'lis] rather than [pəli's] "police"
[ǰu'lay] rather than [ǰəlay'] "July").

INTONATION

AAVE intonation tends to include a higher pitch range and more rising and level final contours than other varieties of English. A creaky voice "falsetto" register is also used, particularly by men.

Issues in Evaluation

Several important issues need to be raised with respect to the phonological assessment of AAVE speakers. An initial concern is the determination of standards of phonological normalcy. Historically, of course, Standard English phonology was used as the exclusive metric for determining normal phonological development and this norm was conventionally instantiated in most standardized assessment instruments. It is clear that an AAVE speaker judged on the basis of Standard English phonological norms would be penalized simply for being different, although the severity of the penalty is disputable. In scoring a group of AAVE speakers with clinically unremarkable histories according to Standard English test norms on three widely used articulation tests, Cole and Taylor[11] found that over half of the subjects were identified as phonologically impaired. When the scores were adjusted to give credit for appropriate AAVE phonological responses, none of the subjects was identified as phonologically impaired. Washington and Craig,[12] however, comparing preselected groups of communicatively unimpaired (as assessed by classroom teachers) and communicatively impaired low socioeconomic African American children found that the overall classification of impairment did not change when articulation scores were adjusted to give credit for phonological responses in AAVE.

The degree of penalty for not recognizing AAVE phonological responses may be in question, but it is clear that the only equitable approach to assessing vernacular dialect speakers is one that takes into account the local norms of these speakers.[13,14] The scoring procedures of a number of current standardized articulation tests (for example, Goldman-Fristoe, Fisher-Logemann) now have been amended to recognize vernacular dialect phonologies so that these speakers are not penalized simply for being dialectally different.

The fact that a number of AAVE phonological characteristics converge with processes that are found during the developmental stages of Standard English has certainly added fuel to the unwarranted interpretation that AAVE speakers simply speak underdeveloped versions of Standard English phonology. For example, cluster reduction, stopping, labialization of interdental fricatives, and many other of the processes presented in the AAVE phonological profile certainly converge with the output of processes observed during the developmental stages of Standard English phonological acquisition. The explanation for this similarity, however, is not to be found in developmental retardation, but in the universal set of phonological naturalness and marking principles that guide phonological variation and change toward a more natural state in different types of language situations. These situations include internal language change over time and space, normal first and second language acquisition, and even phonological disorders. So the observation of convergence in the processes of vernacular dialect phonology and developmental phonology is a valid one, but the traditional interpretation is unjustified. To say that the process of cluster reduction in AAVE phonology results from a fossilized phonological delay in acquiring English would be akin to a claim that the present-day English reduction of the earlier English [xt] clusters (ie, [xt] → [t]) in words such as *right* and *bright* results from the habituation of inadequate learning of English phonology by modern generations of speakers. Phonological systems are dynamic systems that are always in the process of change and AAVE has simply followed a universal and natural course of change in arriving at its current state.

The evaluation of phonology in AAVE is further compounded by the fact that so many of the distinguishing features of the dialect involve systematically constrained variable processes rather than categoric ones. For example, as shown in Table 10–1, the "normal" AAVE range of consonant cluster reduction is quite different depending on the phonological context and composition of the cluster. For example, cluster reduction involving a cluster spread over two morphemes in the phonological context of following a vowel (eg, *missed out*) may only affect about a third of all eligible cases (see Table 10–1); whereas cluster reduction for a single morpheme cluster in the context of a following consonant affects nine of 10 cases. Thus, a speaker of AAVE applying cluster reduction to bimorphemic clusters at a level significantly higher than the mean (eg, two standard deviations above the mean) may have an impairment involving clusters, even though the application of final cluster reduction is a regular process applied within AAVE phonology.

Unfortunately, most information about AAVE phonology in children derives from the elicitation of single-word responses to picture stimuli, often using standardized articulation tests that tap single or limited tokens of particular phonological forms. Such data simply cannot provide access to the inherently variable nature of most AAVE phonological structures—data needed to determine the normal developmental stages of AAVE phonology and the authentic difference between phonologically unimpaired and impaired AAVE speakers.

Present research[15, 16] reveals that a number of differences between unimpaired and impaired AAVE speakers involve the relative incidence of process application rather than the categoric presence or absence of a particular process. For example, Seymour, Green, and Hundley[15] showed that both unimpaired and impaired speakers of AAVE reveal final consonant deletion, but that the impaired group simply applies the process at a significantly higher rate than unimpaired speakers. The picture of impairment is complicated further by the fact that inherent variability is constrained by internal and external factors. As Stockman[16] has shown, final consonant deletion is sensitive to its phonetic composition and surrounding phonological context (eg, deletion is favored when the consonant is a coronal one).

Finally, it cannot simply be assumed that all stages and rates of development in the acquisition of AAVE phonology will necessarily follow a route that is isomorphic with the developmental progression of other English varieties. For example, Wolfram[17] showed that the development of vowel nasalization (eg, [mæ̃] for [mæn] *man*) in AAVE follows the general pattern found in nasal vowel language such as French rather than that found in oral vowel systems.[18] In this development, an initial stage of general final consonant absence (eg, [mæ]) gives way to an intermediary stage of primary segment presence (eg, [mæn]) that, in turn, develops into a stage of variable vowel nasalization (eg, [mæn] and [mæ̃]) that is systematically constrained by linguistic environment and external social factors.

It is quite clear that the evaluation of AAVE speakers' phonological status is much more involved than it appears at first glance. Theoretically and descriptively, it is necessary to consider the variable nature of processes and systematic constraints on variability in the determination of normalcy. However, this perspective cannot be accommodated methodologically without gathering a sufficient amount of data for the analysis of variable patterns. On a practical evaluation level, this vantage point underscores the necessity of obtaining adequate language samples of natural language use to complement the imposing limitations of the traditional single-item elicitation task in phonological assessment.

Treatment Issues

An understanding of the structure of AAVE phonology is just as essential in remediation as it is in the evaluation process. Clinicians need to consider several different factors related to dialect in the context of therapy, including the selection of items for treatment, the shaping of phonological behavior in therapy, and the determination of normative target forms. It should go without saying that this discussion of treatment issues assumes that the targeted remediation population discussed in this section is limited to clients who are diagnosed as being impaired in terms of the norms of their indigenous community of speakers.

There are three fundamental ways in which dialect variation and phonological impairment may interact. For convenience, these are referred to as *types I, II, and III* impairments. In a *type I* impairment, normative phonological structures are qualitatively and quantitatively held in common across dialects so that the normative forms in both a standard and vernacular variety are the same. For example, in syllable-initial position, the norms for stops, nasals, and sibilants in AAVE phonology appear to be no different from the norms of other native-based American English varieties. Thus, velar or palatal fronting (eg, [tæt] for *cat* [sɪp] for *ship*) are considered nonnormative productions regardless of the native American English dialect of a speaker.

Type II impairments involve a cross-dialectal qualitative difference in a normative form or process. For example, the correspondence of syllable-final labiodental fricatives for the interdental fricatives of other varieties (eg, [tuf]/[tuθ]) and the [skr]/[str] (eg, [skrit]/[strit]) sequential correspondence involve normative processes not shared by most socially favored American English varieties. Given the universal principles that govern phonological change and variation, some of the nonnormative productions may, of course, be identical across dialects even though the normative productions are not. Thus, an AAVE speaker and a Standard English speaker may converge in producing nonnormative [tus] for "tooth" or [swit] for "street") even though the normative models for the respective phonological varieties differ (eg, [tus] for [tuθ] in Standard English and [tus] for [tuf] in AAVE).

Type III impairments involve forms qualitatively shared, but quantitatively differentiated cross-dialectally. For example, a standard and vernacular variety may share a form or a process, but simply differ in the relative occurrence. As shown earlier, syllable-final cluster reduction characterizes a wide range of English varieties, but the degree of process application distinguishes AAVE phonology from other English dialects. In this instance, the significant "overextension" of a variable process in terms of different quantitative norms would constitute an impairment.

Although it is logically possible for vernacular dialect speakers to manifest only one of the above types of nonnormative behavior, moderate-to-severe cases of phonological impairment would typically involve all three types. Furthermore, given the hierarchy of natural principles underlying all phonological variation and change, an implicational relationship would be expected to hold among these three types of impairment in which a type I impairment implies a type II, and a type II implies a type III impairment (ie, type I ⊃ type II ⊃ type III). That is, if a client indicates a type I impairment he or she also will be expected to indicate a type II, but not necessarily the converse.

Treatment for type I impairments does not involve differential norms in the remediation process and, other things being equal, probably should be given priority in treatment. In treating type II and type III disorders, special considerations have to be given to differential norms—norms that may involve both qualitative and quantitative dimensions.

One of the difficult problems that arises in dealing with type II and type III impairments is the selection of appropriate target norms for remediation. For example, suppose an AAVE speaker reveals final consonant deletion at a rate significantly above the AAVE norm.[16] Eventually, the [θ]/[f] will have to be targeted along with other final consonants in the remediation process. In deciding an appropriate target sound for the speaker, two factors must be considered, one relating to the clinician and the other relating to the client.

Although it might be suggested that the clinician use a target norm that is appropriate for the dialect, there are important sociolinguistic considerations that militate against this choice. To begin with, most clinicians are speakers of Standard English varieties, and using vernacular dialect norms would involve forms with which they are not comfortable. More importantly, vernacular-speaking clients often are perceptually aware of Standard English norms even if they do not use these socially favored forms themselves.[15] Clients may therefore view any attempt by a clinician to use a model other than Standard English as pretentious and inappropriate. This is particularly true given sociolinguistic expectations for a therapeutic setting and the differential status of the interaction involving the clinician and client in this setting.

The form considered appropriate for the client in a productive response is, however, another matter. Because phonological disorders are defined according to the norms of the community, these norms must be kept in mind when correcting a disorder. Even if a clinician uses a Standard English model, a client may select a sociolinguistically appropriate model on the basis of community norms, thus modifying the target provided by the clinician. It is thus quite possible for a client suppressing final consonant deletion to produce a final [f] for [θ] even though the norm provided by the clinician is limited to [θ]. This sociolinguistically sensitive vernacular accommodation must be taken into account in determining the suitable remediation of a form.

The remediation of type III disorders clearly calls for a practical understanding of the role of systematic variation in phonology. For example, if a normative level of final consonant cluster reduction in a given linguistic environment is approximately 33%, the mean and normal variance must be taken into account when establishing a criterion for correct production. Attention to quantitative levels of production in remediation obviously calls for more attention in a clinical setting to speech styles in which variation is inherent, such as spontaneous conversation. It also calls for more extended quantitative tabulations in treatment and assessment profiles because normalcy is so often defined on the basis of relative frequency levels for natural process application rather than categoric absence or presence. Although such a quantitative orientation certainly complicates the task of the clinician, it seems unavoidable if dialectally divergent populations are to be treated in a realistic and equitable way.

Conclusion

The focus is almost exclusively on AAVE phonology in this discussion, but issues and principles discussed here may be applied to any number of vernacular varieties. It is evident that the consideration of a population defined on the basis of a dialect involves acquiring a particularized descriptive base with respect to the phonological characteristics of the variety. This descriptive foundation, in turn, has an important impact on evaluation and treatment issues. The variable nature of many vernacular phonological forms calls for clinicians to understand the systematic nature of phonological fluctuation and to integrate this understanding into the practical diagnostic and remediation paradigm.

Throughout the discussion it was assumed that the speech and language pathologist is focusing on the diagnosis and remediation of phonological disorders for speakers who manifest authentic impairments in terms of vernacular dialect norms. The issue of teaching Standard English phonology as a second dialect involves a quite different set of considerations—considerations that range from underlying philosophic orientation to practical methodological sociolinguistic issues. While some of the practical methods used in teaching second dialect phonology may coincide with strategies used in a remediation paradigm, the goals and motivation for such a program are quite distinct from treating a genuine impairment. Furthermore, a program focused on learning Standard English as a second dialect must be injected with a fundamental understanding of basic sociolinguistic issues such as the legitimate nature of dialect diversity and language prejudice, along with a pragmatic rationale for acquiring a second dialect. These are issues most appropriately addressed outside of a clinical setting. In a clinical setting, speech and language pathologists would do well to restrict themselves to the appropriate treatment of authentic cases of phonological impairment. This is a significant challenge in its own right.

Suggested Readings

Bailey G: Phonological characteristics of African American vernacular English. In Mufwene SS, Rickford JR, Bailey G, Baugh J (eds): *Structure of African American Vernacular English*. Routledge (forthcoming).

Cole L, Deal VR (eds): *Communication Disorders in Multicultural Populations*. Rockville, MD: ASHA (forthcoming).

Seymour HN: Assessment of phonological disorders among Black English speakers. In Cole L, Deal VR (eds): *Communication Disorders in Multicultural Populations*. Rockville, MD: ASHA (in press).

Seymour HN, Ralabate: The acquisition of a phonological feature of black English. *J Commun Disord* 1985; 18:139–148.

Seymour HN, Seymour CM: A therapeutic model for communicative disorders among black English speaking children. *JSHD* 1977; 42:247–256.

Seymour HN, Seymour CM: Black English and Standard American English contrasts in consonantal development of four- and five-year-old children. *JSHD* 1981; 46:274–280.

Stockman IJ: *Constraints on Black Children's Final Consonant Deletion* (forthcoming).

Williams R, Wolfram W: A linguistic description of social dialects. In Jeter IK (ed): *Social Dialects: Differences Versus Disorders*. Rockville, MD: ASHA, 1977, pp 11–31.

Wolfram W: Language variation in the United States. In Taylor OL (ed): *Nature of Communication Disorders in Culturally and Linguistically Diverse Populations*. San Diego: College-Hill Press, 1986, pp 301–332.

References

1. Raph JB: Language and speech deficits in culturally disadvantaged children: Implications for the speech clinician. *JSHD* 1967; 32:203–214.
2. Baratz JC: A bi-dialectal task for determining language proficiency in economically disadvantaged Negro dialects. *Child Dev* 1969; 40:889–901.
3. Taylor OL: Social and politic involvement of the American Speech and Hearing Association. *ASHA* 1969; 11:216–218.
4. Wolfram W: Sociolinguistic premises and the nature of nonstandard dialect. *Speech Teach* 1970; 176–186.
5. Cole L, Deal VR (eds): *Communication Disorders in Multicultural Populations*. Rockville, MD: ASHA (forthcoming).
6. Taylor OL (ed): *Nature of Communication Disorders in Culturally and Linguistically Diverse Populations*. San Diego: College-Hill Press, 1986.
7. Taylor OL (ed): *Treatment of Communication Disorders in Culturally and Linguistically Diverse Populations*. San Diego: College-Hill Press, 1986.
8. Holm J: *Pidgins and Creoles*. Cambridge, MA: Cambridge University Press, 1988, p 2.
9. Shuy RW, Wolfram W, Riley WK: *Linguistic Correlates of Social Stratification in Detroit Speech*. USOE Final Report No. 6-1342, 1967.
10. Wolfram W: *Dialects and American English*. Englewood Cliffs, NJ: Prentice Hall, 1991.
11. Cole PA, Taylor OL: Performance of working class African American children on three tests of articulation. *LSHSS* 1990; 21:171–176.
12. Washington JA, Craig HK: Articulation test performances of low-income African American preschoolers with communication impairments. *LSHSS* 1992; 23:201–207.
13. Seymour HN, Seymour CM: Black English and Standard American English contrasts in consonantal development of four- and five-year-old children. *JSHD* 1981; 46:274–280.
14. Haynes WO, Moran MJ: A cross-sectional developmental study of final consonant production in southern black children from preschool through third grade. *LSHSS* 1989; 20:400–406.
15. Seymour HN, Green L, Hundley R: *Phonological Patterns in the Conversational Speech of African American Children*. Paper presented at ASHA Convention, Atlanta, 1991.
16. Stockman IJ: *Constraints on Black Children's Final Consonant Deletion* (forthcoming).
17. Wolfram W: Language variation in the United States. In Taylor OL (ed): *Nature of Communication Disorders in Culturally and Linguistically Diverse Populations*. San Diego: College-Hill Press, 1986, pp 301–332.
18. Ruhlen M: Nasal vowels. In Greenberg JH (ed): *Universals of Language*. Stanford, CA: Stanford University Press, 1978; 2:203–242.
19. Williams R, Wolfram W: A linguistic description of social dialects. In Jeter, IK (ed): *Social Dialects: Differences Versus Disorders*. Rockville, MD: ASHA, 1977, pp 11–31.
20. Bailey G: Phonological characteristics of African American Vernacular English. In Mufwene SS,

Rickford JR, Bailey G, Baugh J (eds): *Structure of African American Vernacular English. Routledge* (forthcoming).
21. Seymour HN, Seymour CM: A therapeutic model for communicative disorders among black English speaking children. *JSHD* 1977; 42:247–256.
22. Seymour HN: Assessment of phonological disorders among Black English speakers. In Cole L, Deal VR (eds): *Communication Disorders in Multicultural Populations*. Rockville, MD: ASHA (in press).

11

Phonological Differences Among Speakers of Spanish-Influenced English

EMILIO PEREZ, PH.D.

Introduction

With the growing number of Hispanics in the United States, speech–language pathologists will likely encounter many children who speak Spanish only, have limited English proficiency, or are bilingual and will require or elect speech–language services. It will frequently be the case that speech–language pathologists who are not bilingual, who do not have the academic or clinical training, and who are not familiar with linguistic differences among Spanish-influenced English speakers will be providing services to these children. An understanding of the varieties of Spanish-influenced spoken English and a description of phonological differences among speakers of Spanish-influenced English may thus be helpful to speech–language pathologists. In addition to information of this nature, assessment procedures and intervention approaches and strategies appropriate to Hispanic clients are also outlined in this chapter.

Speakers of Spanish-Influenced English

Spanish is the second most commonly spoken language in the United States. Currently, there are 23.4 million individuals of Hispanic origin in the United States.[1] This group is expected to become the largest minority population in the United States by the year 2020.[2] It is anticipated that this phenomenon may occur earlier than anticipated, however, because the predictions for 1990 have already been surpassed.[1]

The composition of the Hispanic population in the United States is quite diverse, with the largest segment coming from Mexico. Other countries contributing to the American Hispanic population include: Puerto Rico, Cuba, Dominican Republic, and Spain; as well as Guatemala, El Salvador, Nicaragua, Costa Rica, Honduras, and Panama in Central America; and Columbia, Venezuela, Ecuador, Peru, Chile, Bolivia, Paraguay, Uruguay, and Argentina in

South America.[1,3] For further information on the origins of the Hispanic population in the United States, see Langdon and Cheng.[4]

The majority of Hispanic children in the United States come from homes where Spanish is spoken by parents, extended family members, and siblings. How much of the second language children learn depends on how accepting of the second language the parents and extended family members are, how much siblings and other relatives interact in the second language, and how long a child has been in school. The use of two languages may vary significantly from one family to another and within a family from one child to another.

Hispanics in the United States may be monolingual and speak only Spanish (generally immigrants); likewise, be monolingual and speak only English (first-generation Americans and their children); have limited English proficiency (immigrants and first-generation Americans); or be bilingual. The level of bilingual skill varies tremendously among Hispanics, including both high and low levels of proficiency in both English and Spanish or dominance of one language over the other. The language dominance may also vary with respect to speaking and writing.[5] Those who are bilingual may or may not speak with a noticeable Spanish accent. Many public schools, especially in areas with large Hispanic populations, have programs for the monolingual Spanish speaker as well as for the Limited English Proficient (LEP) speaker.[6-10] Often, the LEP Hispanic student is provided with speech–language services in the public schools. Hispanics with noticeable Spanish accents who do not have communication disorders may elect to have speech–language intervention for accent reduction.[11] However, there are differences of opinion as to whether such intervention should be elective or mandatory.[12,13]

The dialect found in speakers of Spanish-influenced English stems from a variety of sources. One influencing factor is the articulatory basis of their first language, which is the physiological articulatory patterns habituated during the process of learning the phonology of the first language. For example, the dentalization of the /t/ and /d/ in Spanish will invariably lead to dentalization of the English /t/ and /d/ that are apical. A second major influence is the variety of Spanish spoken by parents and other relatives. For example, Castilian Spanish is quite different from Mexican Spanish and even more different from the variety of Spanish spoken in the Philippines. Further, some of these varieties of Spanish have been influenced by native aboriginal languages spoken in Central and South America and in the Philippines. The geographic area in which the family settled in the United States is another influence in the dialect spoken. The variety of Spanish-influenced English spoken in Harlem, for example, has been influenced by Black English Vernacular and in the southern states by Southern English. How well the Spanish-influenced English speaker has learned to master the English language is also dependent on the length of residency in the United States, attendance or disruption of schooling, type of classrooms attended, uses of language, and health and developmental factors.[14] Age of the child, age when training in the second language began, level of acquisition of the first language, and the socioeconomic status of the language learner also affect second language learning.

Phonological Differences

In the tables that follow are phonological characteristics of Spanish-influenced English as compared with phonological characteristics of General American English (GAE). Whenever possible, differences among speakers from different countries or linguistic communities in the United States are noted. To date, Anderson and Smith[15] and Iglesias and Anderson[16] have presented phonological process usage among Spanish-speaking Puerto Rican children, and Hidalgo[17] has described phonological differences between Mexican and Chicano varieties of Spanish. Information on dialects other than Chicano and Puerto Rican Spanish is scarce.[18] Zentella[18] cites the urgent need for more research on dialectal variations within the growing and diverse Hispanic population in the United States.

It is important to understand that the phonological differences listed below are not all inclusive in terms of the dialects observed across Spanish-influenced English speakers. Individual differences *alone* would account for some variation, not to mention the major influences discussed above.

Vowel Differences

The most notable phonological differences are with respect to the vowel system. In Spanish, there are five vowels /a/, /e/, /i/, /o/, and /u/ that are used in their pure forms. In GAE there are at least 15 different vowels. Consequently, with the Spanish-influenced English speaker, the small vowel inventory causes confusion and often adjacent American-English vowels are substituted for each other. Apparently, the confusion of adjacent vowels is also common in the Mexican-Spanish and Chicano-Spanish dialects[17] and not uncommon in dialects of American English[19].

Table 11–1 illustrates the vowel substitutions that are frequently made by speakers of Spanish-influenced English with examples.

As illustrated in Table 11–1, most substitutions are adjacent vowel substitutions, for example, I/i, æ/ɛ, U/u, and vice versa. Monophthongization, the reduction of a diphthong to a single vowel, also occurs where diphthongs are most often used in American English simply because these vowels are produced in their pure form in Spanish, for example, /eI/ and /oU/. The central diphthongs /Ir/, /ɛr/, /ar/, / r/, and /Ur/ are often made with a one-tap or multiple trill of the apical or uvular type. Diphthongs like /aI/ and /ju/, on the other hand, present no problem because in Spanish the two vowels in a diphthong are more widely spaced and have rising and falling stress patterns as in American English.[20]

Consonant Differences

Consonant differences may be described in terms of phonological processes and may result from a number of factors. There are some consonants that occur in English that do not occur in Spanish and vice versa. For example, the English consonants /v/, /θ/, /ð/, /z/, and /ʒ/ do not occur in Spanish, although they may occur as allophonic variations of other phonemes, for example, when the intervocalic /d/ becomes /ð/. As seen from this example, some allophones of stops cross manner-of-articulation boundaries and become fricative, such as

Table 11–1.   Vowel Substitutions in Spanish-Influenced English
as Compared to GAE

Substitutions	Examples	GAE	Spanish-Influenced English
Front vowels			
I/i	Eat, feet, bee	/it/, /fit/, /bi/	/It/, /fIt/, /bI/
i/I	Is, sit	/Iz/, /sIt/	/iz/,/sit/
e/eI	Ace, bake, pay	/eIs/, /beIk/, /peI/	/es/, /bek/, /pe/
æ/ɛ	Excuse, head	/ɛkskjuz/, /hɛd/	/ækskjuz/, /hæd/
eI/ɛ	Present	/prɛzənt/	/preIzənt/
ɛ/æ	At, ham	/æt/, /hæm/	/ɛt/, /hɛm/
Back vowels			
U/u	Ooze, food, to	/uz/, /fud/, /tu/	/Uz/, /fUd/, /tU/
u/U	Should, foot	/SUd/, /fUt/	/Sud/, /fut/
o/oU	Oat, coat, so	/oUt/, /koUt/, /soU/	/ot/, /kot/, /so/
o/ŋ	All, ball	/ŋl/, /bŋl/	/ol/, /bol/
Central vowels			
a/ʌ	Up, color	/ʌp/, /kʌlɚ/	/ap/, /kalɚ/
ɛr/ɝ	Early, bird, sir	/ɝˈlI/, /bɝˆd/, /sɝˆ/	/ɛrlI/, /bɛrd/, /sɛr/

when /b/ becomes [β] or [v] and /g/ becomes [γ] as they occur in the intervocalic position. The following Spanish consonants do not occur in English: /n/, /λ/, /γ/, /χ/, /ř/, and /β/. These sounds will often be substituted for similar English consonants. Additionally, some sounds that occur in both languages are produced with different distinctive features, for example, the /t/ and /d/ are dentalized and unaspirated in Spanish but are apical and aspirated in English.

Another factor responsible for consonant differences is that some phonological rules in Spanish and English differ. Most notably is the fact that only /s/, /n/, /r/, /l/, and /d/ occur in the final consonant position in Spanish. The /d/ is the only stop that occurs in the final position in Spanish and it is frequently deleted. The fact that relatively few Spanish consonants are used in the final consonant position is a reflection of syllable structure differences. In Spanish, the majority of nouns, for example, are polysyllabic and of the CVC(C)V(C) and VC(C)V types.[21] These nouns will most often end in open syllables. Consequently, while final consonant deletion is not a great problem in Spanish with its few final consonants, it may be a problem when learning English with its many final consonants.

As in most languages, consonant clusters are difficult to articulate in the stream of an utterance. For the Spanish-influenced speaker, the word-initial /st/ cluster, which does not occur in Spanish, poses a problem and will result in the addition of the vowel /ɛ/ before the /st/. As such, the consonants become abutting consonants rather than a cluster, which is, the /s/ arrests the first syllable while the /t/ releases the second syllable. Clusters are generally simplified and reduced to one or two consonants, such as /tar/ instead of /star/ and /skim/ instead of /skrim/. Cluster reduction is as common in Spanish-speaking children as it is with English-speaking children.[15]

Table 11–2 illustrates some of the processes operating in Spanish-influenced English.

As can be seen in Table 11–2, many syllable structure, substitution, assimilation, and other phonological processes may occur in the speech of a Spanish-influenced speaker. While many processes are listed, the list is not all inclusive because many dialects of Spanish-influenced English are yet to be described. Nonetheless, the list is inclusive of most phonological processes found in the speech of Spanish-influenced speakers.

Assessment of Phonological Differences

The question of whether assessment of speech–language disorders should be made in the native language, the second language, or both has been debated in the past. Because there is evidence that a language disorder in the first language will be reflected in the second language,[22-24] the consensus is to assess in both languages. Assessment of LEP individuals should be conducted by an examiner who is a fluent speaker of Spanish.[25] When this is not possible, an interpreter, preferably an interpreter with the same linguistic background as the client, should assist in the assessment. The role of the interpreter has to be made quite explicit at the onset of the assessment. If the interpreter is reading a test stimulus in Spanish, they may not embellish the stimulus in any manner to make it more understandable to the child or it will invalidate the test administration. Likewise, they must record, as accurately as possible, any response made by the child and may not elaborate on the child's response to make the response correct or acceptable.

Phonological tests have been developed for Spanish speakers, such as *Assessment of Phonological Processes—Spanish*[26] and *The Assessment of Phonological Disabilities.*[27] These tests include single-word stimuli to assess commonly used syllabic and substitution processes. A connected speech sample will also be necessary to observe the many variations of Spanish-influenced English. Variations are influenced by the speaker's background, language, and culture. These measures will yield target processes for intervention.

While articulation tests may be useful, they are only useful if each word is transcribed narrowly. Otherwise, the patterns of misarticulations may not be obvious to the observer. There are many articulation tests written in English. One such test that may be useful for the Spanish-influenced English speaker is the *Fisher-Logemann Test of Articulation Competence.*[28] This test assesses consonants in the traditional initial and final positions; however, all medial consonants are tested in the intervocalic position. Because Spanish has many consonants used in the intervocalic position, this test will assess articulation differences in a position greatly influenced by the first language. Another test that may be used for assessing articulation is the *Medida Española de Articulación* (MEDA),[29] which assesses the acquisition of phonemes in Spanish.

Because phonology is only one aspect of language, a thorough language assessment in both languages should also be carried out with Spanish-influenced children suspected of having phonological disorders. Langdon,[14,2] Langdon and Cheng,[4] and Adler[30] have published procedures for language assessment with bilingual/multicultural clients.

Table 11–2. Phonological Differences in Spanish-Influenced English as Compared to GAE

Phonological Processes	Examples	GAE	Spanish-Influenced English
Syllable structure processes			
Unstressed syllable deletion	Explain	/ɛkspleɪn/	/spleɪn/
Final consonant deletion	Girls, house	/gɝ^z/, /haʊs/	/gɝ^l/, /haʊ/
Cluster reduction	Stairs, best	/stɛrz/, /bɛst/	/tɛrz/, /bɛs/
Epenthesis	Spain, stamp	/speɪn/, /stæmp/	/ɛspeɪn/, /ɛstæmp/
Glottal omission	Hat, hand	/hæt/, /hænd/	/æt/, /ænd/
Substitution processes			
Stopping of fricatives	Thumb, they	/θʌm/, /ðeɪ/	/tʌm/, /deɪ/*
Deaffrication	Chop, match	/tʃap/, /mætʃ/	/ʃap/, /maʃ/
Affrication	Shop, ship	/ʃap/, /ʃɪp/	/tʃap/, /tʃɪp/†
Affrication of glide	You, yard	/ju/, /jard/	/dʒu/, /dʒard/‡, or /ʒard/§
Assimilation processes			
Dentalization	Two, do	/tu/, /du/	/t̪u/, /d̪u/‖
Labial assimilation	Very, voice	/vɛrI/, /vɔIs/	/bɛrI/, /bɔIs/
Prevocalic voicing	Sip, sink	/sIp/, /sIŋk/	/zIp/, /zIŋk/
Postvocalic devoicing	Chairs, cars	/tʃɛrz/, /karz/	/tʃɛrs/, /kars/¶
Other Processes			
Trilling	Around	/əraʊnd/	/ərʊnd/, or /ə̌raʊnd/, or /əraʊnd/#
Intrusive /h/	And, it	/ænd/, /It/	/hænd/, /hit/

*The /θ/ and /ð/ are not found in Spanish, although the /θ/ is substituted for the /s/ in Castilian Spanish.

†Occurs in Mexican and Chicano Spanish due to contact with English.[17]

‡May be used in some countries in South America, such as Venezuela and Peru.

§May be used in some countries in South America, such as Argentina and Chile.

‖The /t/ and /d/ are both dentalized and unreleased in Spanish.

¶The /z/ does not occur in Spanish.

#May be used by some variety of Puerto Rican English.

Intervention

Speech–language intervention approaches and strategies for Hispanics in the United States have varied widely depending on whether the child is: (1) monolingual speaking Spanish that is average for his age or delayed; (2) LEP; (3) bilingual with dominance in one language or the other or equally language-dominant; and (4) proficient in English but desires accent reduction. Information on phonological process intervention with Hispanics is almost nonexistent. Research is needed to find the best approaches/strategies for individuals who speak Spanish-influenced English.

Language Intervention

For the monolingual and LEP child who has age-appropriate language in Spanish, the bilingual classroom is the setting of choice.[3] There are several programs published for the LEP Hispanic child.[6–10] These programs are concerned with overall language learning in a bilingual class and include work on phonology. Speech–language services would only be offered if articulatory, voice, or fluency disorders existed. For the monolingual child with delayed language, instruction should occur in the native language, with some instruction in learning a second language.[31] Speech–language services may be required in the native language. For the bilingual child, many options exist. Primarily, the bilingual child would be placed in the regular classroom unless the child was significantly delayed in either language, in which case the bilingual classroom would be the appropriate setting.[31] Further, the bilingual child would receive speech–language services from a bilingual speech–language pathologist who could code switch when necessary to best serve the child. The bilingual child without a language delay in the regular classroom may require speech–language services only if they have articulatory, voice, or fluency disorders.

Phonological Intervention

Because so many Spanish-GAE differences involve confusions of adjacent vowels, voicing confusions, stopping, etc, a minimal-pair contrast approach lends itself well to intervention, especially if the contrasts are made semantically or syntactically. For example, this author and many Hispanics have avoided saying the word "sheet" knowing full well that due to vowel variation, another word would invariably come out. In fact, in working with a nurse from South America, she indicated that in making up a patient's bed she would invariably ask for "linen" to avoid saying the word "sheet."

The cycles approach[32] may also be used to eliminate phonological processes. This approach requires the student to follow various steps that include auditory bombardment with amplification and production training to develop a new kinesthetic image of the targeted pattern.[33] For the unintelligible student, this approach quickly leads to intelligibility after three cycles that last approximately 12 weeks each.

One approach to phonological intervention with Hispanic children of Puerto Rican decent was reported by Goldstein and Iglesias.[34] They used the spontaneous-imitation–spontaneous (S-I-S) method of production with six children ranging in age from 3 years 6 months to 4 years 8 months. In this procedure, illustrated words with the target process were presented to the children for a spontaneous production of each word. If the production of the target process on the first word was correct, then the next word illustration was presented. If the target production was incorrect, the clinician modeled the word for the child to obtain a spontaneous (delayed imitation) production. This procedure was used successfully in remediating weak syllable deletion and initial consonant deletion.

Dialect Reduction

Dialect-reduction assessment procedures[35] and programs have been developed for students in the classroom[36] or for anyone with a foreign accent who wishes to speak a dialect closer to GAE.[37,38] These programs provide step-by-step instructions for dialect reduction and include audio cassette tapes for laboratory or home practice.

The paired-stimuli strategy developed by Weston and Irwin[39] may also be used. With this strategy, a word in which the targeted sound is produced correctly is paired with other words having the target sound. For example, if the word "meet" is produced correctly, it may be paired with other words like "eat, east, ease, feet, beet, seat" etc. If a word with the targeted sound is not produced correctly, then a single word with the target sound may be learned and later paired with other words.

Regardless of which approach/strategy is used, the habituated physiological articulatory patterns learned in the first language will change. This will affect both languages. Initially, a slower rate will help in altering the articulatory patterns of the first language. Later, the rate should be increased to automatize the new articulatory patterns. This is not unlike what Van Riper[40] stated years ago in his traditional approach to articulation intervention.

Summary

With the growing number of Hispanics in the United States, many speech–language pathologists who are not necessarily bilingual will need to service that population. This chapter describes phonological differences among speakers of Spanish-influenced English and outlines assessment and intervention procedures.

References

1. Current Population Reports. *The Hispanic Population in the United States.* Washington, DC: Bureau of Census, 1990.
2. Bouvier L, Davis C: *The Future Population Composition of the United States.* Washington, DC: Demographic Information Services Center of the Population Reference Bureau, 1982.
3. Dalbor JB: *Spanish Pronunciation: Theory and Practice.* New York: Holt, Rinehart, Winston, 1980.
4. Langdon HW, Cheng LL: *Hispanic Children and Adults with Communication Disorders.* Gaithersburg, MD: Aspen Publishers, 1992.
5. Obler LK: Bilingualism and the brain. *Thesis* 1992; 6:14–19.
6. Biber D, Krashen S: *On Course: Bilingual Education's Success in California.* Sacramento, CA: California Association for Bilingual Education, 1988.
7. Cummins J: *Bilingualism and Special Education: Issues in Assessment and Pedagogy.* San Diego: College-Hill Press, 1984.
8. Keyes JL, Schulman R: *William H Taft High School, Project Adelante, O.E.E. Evaluation Report,*

1982–1983 (Final Report). New York: New York Board of Education, Office of Educational Evaluation, 1984.

9. Ruiz NT: *The Optimal Learning Environment (OLE) Curriculum Guide: A Resource for Teachers of Spanish-Speaking Children in Learning Handicapped Programs* (Unpublished manuscript). Davis, CA: 1988. University of California at Davis.

10. Ruiz NT: An optimal learning environment for Rosemary. *Excep Child* 1989; 56:130–144.

11. American Speech-Language-Hearing Association: Social dialects position paper. *ASHA* 1983; 25:23–24.

12. Adler S: *Cultural Language Differences: Their Educational and Clinical-Professional Implications.* Springfield, IL: Charles C. Thomas, 1984.

13. Adler S: Bidialectism: Mandatory or elective? *ASHA* 1987; 29:41–44.

14. Langdon HW: Language disorder or difference? Assessing the language skills of Hispanic students. *Excep Child* 1989; 56:160–167.

15. Anderson R, Smith BL: Phonological development of two-year-old monolingual Puerto Rican Spanish-speaking children. *J Child Lang* 1987; 14:57–78.

16. Iglesias A, Anderson N: Dialectal variations. In Bernthal JE, Bankson NW (eds): *Articulation and Phonological Disorders,* 3rd ed. Englewood Cliffs, NJ: Prentice Hall, 1993, pp 147–161.

17. Hidalgo M: Español mexicano y español chicano: Problemas y propuestas fundamentales (Mexican Spanish and Chicano Spanish: Fundamental problems and proposals). *Lang Problems Lang Plan* 1987; 11:166–193.

18. Zentella AC: Lexical leveling in four New York City Spanish dialects: Linguistic and social factors. *Hispania* 1990; 73:1094–1105.

19. Williams R, Wolfram W: A linguistic description of social dialects. In Jeter IK (ed): *Social Dialects: Differences vs. Disorders.* Rockville, MD: ASHA, 1977, pp 1–31.

20. Wise CM: *Applied Phonetics.* Englewood Cliffs, NJ: Prentice Hall, 1957.

21. Iglesias A, Cohen L, Butierrez-Clellen V, Marcano M: *The Phonological Complexity of Spoken Spanish.* Paper presented at the American Speech-Language-Hearing Association Convention, Washington, DC, November 1985.

22. Langdon HW: *Determining a Language Disorder in a Bilingual Spanish-Speaking Population* (Unpublished doctoral dissertation). Boston, MA: Boston University, 1977.

23. Linares-Orama N: Evaluation of syntax in three-year-old Spanish-speaking Puerto Rican children. *JSHR* 1977; 20:350–357.

24. Merino B: Language development in normal and handicapped Spanish-speaking children. *Hisp J Behav Sci* 1983; 5:379–400.

25. Langdon HW: Assessment and intervention strategies for the bilingual language-disordered student. *Excep Child* 1983; 50:37–46.

26. Hodson B: *Assessment of Phonological Processes—Spanish.* San Diego: Los Amigos Research Association, 1986.

27. Iglesias A: The assessment of phonological disabilities. In Goldstein B, Iglesias A (eds): *The Development and Treatment of Phonological Processes in Spanish-Speaking Children.* Paper presented at the American Speech-Language-Hearing Association Annual Convention, Atlanta, GA, November 1991.

28. Fisher H, Logemann J: *The Fisher-Logemann Test of Articulation Competence.* Boston: Houghton Mifflin, 1971.

29. Aldrich-Mason M, Figueroa-Smith B, Martines-Hinshaw M: *Medida Española de Articulacion.* San Ysidro, CA: San Ysidro School District, 1976.

30. Adler S: Assessment of language proficiency of limited English proficient speakers: Implications for the speech-language specialists. *LSHSS* 1991; 22:12–18.

31. Galvan M: Placement consideration. *Excep Child* 1983; 50:37–46.

32. Hodson BW, Paden EP: *Targeting Intelligible Speech,* 2nd ed. Austin, TX: Pro-Ed, 1991.

33. Hodson BW: *Phonological Assessment and Remediation: Expediting Intelligibility Gains.* Workshop presented at University of Arkansas at Central Arkansas, Little Rock, AR, 1993.

34. Goldstein B, Iglesias A: *The Development and Treatment of Phonological Processes in Spanish-Speaking Children.* Miniseminar presented at the American Speech-Language-Hearing Association Annual Convention, Atlanta, GA, November 1991.

35. Compton AJ: *Compton Phonological Assessment of Foreign Accent.* San Francisco: Carousel House, 1983.

36. Anderson JR: *Dialect Reduction and Accent Restructuring: Some Methods for the Bilingual Classroom.* Paper presented at the 73rd Annual Meeting of the Speech Communication Association, Boston, 1987.

37. Compton AJ: *Foreign Accent Improvement Series.* San Francisco: Carousel House, 1983.

38. Stern DA: *The Sound and Style of American English: A Course in Foreign Accent Reduction.* Los Angeles: Dialect Accent Specialists, Inc., 1987.

39. Weston A, Irwin J: The use of paired-stimuli in the modification of articulation. *J Percept Motor Skills* 1971; 32:947–957.
40. Van Riper C, Irwin JV: *Voice and Articulation.* Englewood Cliffs, NJ: Prentice Hall, 1958.

12

Asian/Pacific Students and the Learning of English

LI-RONG LILLY CHENG, PH.D.

Asian/Pacific Islanders (API) constitute a growing percentage of today's immigrants to the United States. Their arrival and subsequent residence here require that they learn English to attain whatever enticement attracted them, whether it be equitable opportunity, prosperity, or political/religious acceptance. They often find English and American culture difficult to master. API children not only must adjust to mainstream culture but to the American school system and its academic "survival of the fittest." Their most obvious obstacle is their non–English-proficient or limited–English-proficient (NEP/LEP) status.

This chapter provides: (1) basic background information about second-language learning; (2) specific information about Asian/Pacific Islander students and their languages, including phonological characteristics; (3) issues that need to be considered when evaluating speech of API children; (4) a case study of a child with an organic based disorder that initially was misdiagnosed is presented to exemplify some of the aspects that must be taken into consideration in the decision-making process. In addition, some recommendations for consideration by educators, specialists, and policymakers are presented. Those shaping education to meet the needs of all students—immigrant and United States born—should strive to fulfill the promise of equal opportunity.

API Languages Spoken in the United States

Demographics

In the last 2 decades, the United States has attracted a tremendous influx of immigrants from Pacific Rim countries including Mexico, Panama, El Salvador, Guatemala, Taiwan, People's Republic of China, Hong Kong, Vietnam, Laos, Kampuchea, and other Central and South American countries.[1] This group shift of immigrants represents a shift in backgrounds of this nation's immigration population—from European to Pacific Rim—and has changed the country's ethnic profile.

According to 1990 census figures, the United States grew 9.8% in total population between 1980 and 1990. The Anglo population grew by 6%, African American by 13.2%, Native American by 37.9%, Asian Pacific Islander by 107.8%, and Hispanic American by 53%. In 1990, it was reported that there were 199,686,070 European Americans, 29,986,070 African Americans, 22,345,059 Hispanics, and 7,273,662 Asian Pacific Islanders residing in the United States.[2]

School Projections

It is expected that by the year 2000 one third of all school-aged children will be from ethnic minority groups, and by 2020 39% of our school-aged population will be minorities.[2] In the state of California, sometime between the years 2000 and 2010, Hispanics will constitute over 30% of the general population, Asians 13%, African Americans 8%, and Anglos less than 49%.[3]

California, which educates one ninth of the nation's public school students, is a prime example of the increasing diversity taking place in the school population. Table 12–1 illustrates the state's projected ethnic/minority enrollment.

Background: Languages of the API Region

The languages of API originate from the following language families: Altaic, Paleosiberian, Dravidian, Sino-Tibetan, and Austro-Asiatic.[4] The Altaic family includes Turkish, Mongolian, Korean, and Japanese. Paleosiberian refers to language isolates spoken in eastern Siberia, representing a geographic grouping. Dravidian languages are spoken in the southern half of India, and Sino-Tibetan in China, Tibet, Burma, and other countries. Finally, Austro-Asiatic languages are spoken in much of Southeast Asia, including Vietnam, Cambodia, and Laos, as well as islands in Thailand, Burma, China, and India. Pacific Islander languages are Malayo-Polynesian and include Tagalog, Illocano, and Chamorro, and Papuan, the language of New Guinea. A summary of the languages is presented in Table 12–2.

Over 1200 indigenous languages are spoken among the 5 million inhabitants of the Pacific Islands. More than 500 languages are spoken on Papua New Guinea, for example. Although few people speak the native Hawaiian language today, many similar languages continue to thrive in the South Pacific. These include Fijian, French, Cook Islands, Maori, Samoan, Tongan, Bislamam Hindi, Pidgin,

Table 12–1.   Projected Population (%) of California's Ethnic School Enrollment

	1980	1990	2000	2010	2020
Anglo	59.8	51.5	44.9	39.2	35.0
Black	8.7	8.3	7.7	7.2	6.8
Hispanic	24.6	30.5	35.3	39.2	42.0
Asian	6.9	9.7	12.1	14.4	16.2
Total	100.0	100.0	100.0	100.0	100.0

Source: California Department of Education, Data Bical (1990).

Table 12–2. Common API Languages spoken in the United States

NEP/LEP (non–English-proficient and limited–English–proficient) Students Come from Various Language Backgrounds, Including the Following:

Language	Description
Arabic	Southwest Semitic language; a variety of dialects are spoken in Arabia, Jordan, Syria, Palestine, Egypt, Iraq, and parts of northern Africa
Bengali	Modern Indic language spoken in Bengal (East Bengal is Bangladesh; West Bengal is in Republic of India)
Chamorro	Language spoken in Guam, Saipan, and some Micronesian islands; belongs to the Austronesian language family
Chinese	One of a group of Sino-Tibetan languages and dialects spoken in China, including Mandarin, Cantonese, Amoy, Fukien, and Shanghai
Farsi	Language spoken in Southern Iran
French	Romance language spoken in France, Switzerland, southern Belgium, and other former French territories
German	West Germanic language spoken in Germany, Austria, and Switzerland and other former German territories
Hebrew	Semitic language of the ancient Hebrews
Hindi/Urdu	Hindustani language spoken in West Pakistan, where it is the principal language, and by Muslims in India
Hmong	Language spoken by the Hmong people from the mountain area of Laos
Ilokano (Ilocano)	Language spoken in the Philippines
Japanese	National language of Japan
Khmer	Mon-Khmer language of a people of Cambodia
Korean	Language of Korea, unclassified officially but containing many words of Chinese origin
Lao	Official language of Laos, a Tai language of a Buddhist people living in the area of the Mekong river in Laos and Thailand
Malay	Austronesian language of the Malays, a people inhabiting the Malay Peninsula, other parts of Malaysia, and Indonesia
Pilipino	National language of the Philippines
Portuguese	Romance language spoken in Portugal and Brazil and former territories
Punjabi	Indian language spoken in the Punjab, a region in northwest India
Samoan	National language of American Samoa, a region in the Pacific
Spanish	Romance language spoken in Spain, Central America, South America, and parts of the Caribbean
Tagalog	Austronesian language of a people native to the Philippines
Turkish	Turkic language of Turkey
Vietnamese	Language of Vietnam, belonging to the Mon-Khmer subfamily of Austro-Asiatic languages

Motu, Marshallese, Kiriati, Tavaluan, Chamorro, Papua New Guinean, Palauan, and a host of others. The lingua francas are English, Pidgin, French, Spanish, and Bahasa Indonesian.

Colonial Influences

Many nations of Asia/Pacific or Pacific/Asia share the experience of having been "discovered" by Portuguese, Spanish, British, German, and French conquistadors after the 16th century. The British empire, for instance, included India, Malaysia, and Hong Kong. The Spaniards occupied the Philippines, Guam, Saipan, and many other Pacific Islands, and the Portuguese occupied Taiwan and Macao.

Colonial influences introduced English as a second language in many API countries, including Malaysia, India, and the colonies of Hong Kong and Singapore. Spanish/American influences have left legacies of names and other language relics on Guam, the Philippines, and other Pacific Islands. Countries such as China, Japan, and Thailand, which were not colonized by Europeans, have not adopted English. Table 12–3 shows an East-West Center report of languages used in the Asia-Pacific Region by number of radio broadcasts. English and Mandarin Chinese are the two top languages used.

Second Language Learning

Research in second-language acquisition typically references the following concepts.

Transference

Transference is the carryover of phonological, syntactic, and morphologic patterns from an individual's first to second learned language. In *Mirror of Language,* Kenji Hakuta described the misuse of the word "mistake." "Oh no, I mistake," the subject declares, unable to relinquish the "verbness" of the word's application in her first language, Japanese.[5]

Table 12–3. Most Common Languages Used in the Asia/Pacific Region by Number of Broadcasts

Language	Number of Broadcasts
English	284
Chinese	179
Indonesian	61
Japanese	60
Vietnamese	41
Hindi	31
Urdu	29
Korean	28
Bengali	22
German	21
Total	756

Source: Pacific Dialogue, College of Professional Studies and Fine Arts, San Diego State University (1993).

During transference, knowledge of a familiar function (native language) crosses over to that which is unfamiliar (second language). This way, "the novel function is first executed through old, available forms."[6] Importantly, the transference process varies from one individual to the next. Although one Japanese learner of English misuses the word "mistake," another may use it correctly.

Interference

Because second-language learning depends on habits acquired during the process of first-language acquisition, it follows that "old habits must be unlearned or extinguished before new habits can be learned."[7] Interference results from unextinguished habits. More precisely, interference errors, which reflect acquisition of an earlier language, are absent from the normal development of those learning the language as a first language. Despite early perceptions of interference as a major influence on second-language learning, studies in the early 1970s showed that roughly a third of the errors made by second-language learners was traceable to first-language structures.[8-14] Most second-language errors are thought to reflect attempts to generalize and apply linguistic rules before they are mastered.[7] The frequency of interference errors in adults seems to taper off as their learning progresses.[15]

Recent definitions of interference refer to it as deficiencies present in early stages of second-language phoneme acquisition. Dulay, Burt, and Krashen[16] talk about two types of interference: psychologic and sociolinguistic. Psychologic interference refers to the use of old habits while learning new ones (transfer), whereas sociolinguistic interference takes place during linguistic borrowing and language switching (code-switching).

Code-switching

Code-switching is the use of more than one language during speech. Because it occurs naturally and intentionally in bilinguals, it is considered an important aspect of bilingualism.[17] Code-switching occurs at lexic, semantic syntactic, morphologic, and phonological levels of language and can be divided into two categories: conversational and situational.

Lexic-level and semantic-level code-switching are practiced when words or ideas are better expressed in one language than another. For example, the phrase "the whole enchilada" is commonly used to mean "the whole thing." Syntactic code-switching entails application of the syntactic rules of one language to another, as in this mix of Mandarin Chinese and English, the syntactic structure being correct in Mandarin but not English: I show you ta ["ta" means "it" (I show it to you)]. Morphology-switching alternates roots of one language with those of another. For example, in Mandarin "wo dzai chie*ing*," which means "I am cutting," is a switch from Mandarin morphology to English morphology because -ing is an English pattern. And, finally, phonological code-switching causes a young Taiwanese-speaking woman to call herself "Charlene" rather than "Shawlain" in adapting her pronunciation to the English phonology system.

Conversational code-switching is common among first- and second-generation immigrants, who use their dual-language knowledge to sharpen communication.

A native Shanghainese speaker will, for example, insert the Shanghainese exclamation "Aya!" into an English sentence for emphasis. Situational code-switching typically accompanies a change in setting. A second-language English speaker will code-switch differentially depending on the nature of the situation (casual or official, for example) or company.

Factors underlying code-switching behavior carry significant weight in the field of bilingualism. These include cultural experiences, bilingual linguistic competence, and social contexts of discourse. These factors not only reveal a great deal about acculturation but can be used to enhance the process of second-language acquisition.

Accent

Everyone speaks with an accent, whether Bostonian, Southern, or Cantonese. Accent may be defined as a regional/linguistic influence on an individual's pronunciation of words and phrases. One's pronunciation of English naturally falls under the influence of one's first language. For example, the phoneme /f/ does not appear in Taiwanese (Min) and, therefore, the word *food* may be pronounced as /*hood*/. There is German-influenced English, Mandarin-influenced English, Italian-influenced English, etc.

Interestingly, the French accent may be considered "charming," while a Cantonese accent might be deemed "undesirable." This hidden agenda is commonly, if unconsciously, shared among native speakers of English, socialized to believe that a British accent (Queen's English) is not only desirable but marketable and that a "French accent" is fashionable and classy. Because everyone speaks with an accent, attitudes regarding different accents and subtle social meanings behind them need to be examined. For more information on this subject, read Anisfeld, Bogo, and Lambert[18]; Gallois and Callan[19]; Giles[20]; Lyczak, Fu, and Ho[21]; and Ryan, Carranza, and Moffie.[22]

Some LEP students communicate adequately in English and use correct grammar, but withdraw from normal social discussions because of a fear of being perceived negatively by their peers because of their accent. While avoiding the stigma attached to speaking with an "accent," they are missing out on normal practice of English.

Accent Reduction

Despite the benefits of code-switching, instructional programs have been designed to train nonnative English speakers in phonology and effective communication—or accent reduction.[23,24] Attending students feel their English sounds un-American and frequently fail to acknowledge their hard-earned communication skills. Even after graduating from such programs, most individuals report feeling socially isolated and unable to communicate well, and thus frustrated.[25–27] They also report a "glass ceiling" in the workplace, where their vocational advancement is held back by an invisible, accent-based barrier and their ethnicity. The concept of accent reduction is not based in reality and implies a decrease in some area. The term enhancement better reflects the goal of such "accent reduction" programs in addition to being more positive and additive. The goal of such training programs is to improve intelligibility and to add features and fine tuning to their existing repertoire. Perhaps the term "accent reduction" should be changed.

Permeability

This concept provides a label for the sporadic and unstable nature of second-language acquisition. The emerging second language is subject to multiple contextual changes, including when, where, and how it is used.[28,29] Sociolinguistic factors are viewed as predominant stabilizers or agitators of phonological progress[30]; their variability may determine a learner's tendency to monitor speech or adjust it to an interlocutor or particular discourse domain.[31-33]

Variables in Second-Language Learning

Successful second-language learning depends on a number of variables, such as age, social context, and individual differences. "Cerebral dominance" theory purports that neurophysiological transformation (or lateralization) during puberty is accompanied by increasing rigidity in the "acquisition device" in the brain[34] that may be related to the fact that adult second-language learners rarely attain native-like pronunciation. Supporters of this theory believe that exposure to a foreign language before puberty enhances the learning of "proper" pronunciation.

Social context is another key variable in second-language acquisition. Sociolinguists purport that social factors also influence acquisition patterns, relying on ethnicity, nationality, and sexual identity to explain transference variability. For example, certain groups of English monolingual Chicanos in the Los Angeles area have retained Spanish phonology features as a means of establishing identity with other Chicanos. Hill[35] attributed the puberty cutoff for plasticity in language learning to an increased cultural awareness or the need for identification with a social group at this age. Individual factors thought to contribute to acquisition variability are personality and attitude, aptitude for phonetic mimicry, and language proficiency. Odlin[36] contended that students with relatively low anxiety levels experience greater facility with second-language acquisition. Students with high anxiety sometimes avoid potentially challenging phonemic structures and focus on the form rather than content of their messages, resulting in more errors at both phonemic and suprasegmental levels.

Another aspect of personality is seen in individuals who identify with native speakers of a foreign language. They are more apt to identify and retain distinct sounds and form associations between them. In addition, LEP students with more positive attitudes toward their new culture and language tend to acquire their second language more readily.[5]

Although the correlation between first-language aptitude and second-language acquisition has not been proven, research indicates that first-language aptitude can be used as a strong predictor for later success.[5,36] Another variable for acquisition success is the learner's proficiency or breadth of exposure to a second language. Research shows that transfer effects ebb progressively as the learner advances. Students rely less on phonological rules of the native language as they form generalizations about the new phonological system.[37]

According to a *California Perspectives* report,[3] the nine most spoken Asian/Pacific languages among LEP students in California were Vietnamese, Cantonese, Khmer, Hmong, Pilipino, Korean, Lao, Mandarin, and Japanese. The major API groups in California were Filipino, Chinese, Japanese, Vietnamese, Korean, Indian, Cambodian, Laotian, Hmong, and Thai. Their phonological systems can be described briefly as follows.[38] For more detailed descriptions, see Ruhlen.[4]

PILIPINO

27 phonemes: 16 consonant sounds, including the glottal stop ('), 5 vowel sounds, and 6 diphthongs; complex system of affixation: words consist of roots, either substantive, verbal, or adjectival and affixes that show respect, focus, and mode; root and affix determinants of word meaning; large-scale borrowing from Spanish and English.

CANTONESE

19 consonants, 52 vowels recognized by the Yale Romanization System (YRS); its seven to nine tones (exact number debated among linguists) change in category when used in particular sequences; no consonant blends.

MANDARIN

35 initial sounds and 32 final sounds; two sonorants (finals), namely /n/ and /ŋ/; four tones, a neutral tone, and varying pitch levels, durations, and directions; no consonant blends.

JAPANESE

Five vowels: /a/, /i/, /u/, /e/, /o/, varying in duration; silent /i/ and /u/ vowels when located between voiceless consonants such as /f/, /h/, /k/, etc.; 18 consonants, some doubled, as in /kk/ and /pp/; a single final consonant: /n/; numerous grammatical differences from English.

VIETNAMESE

Tonal, basically monosyllabic; pitch changes denoting different lexic meanings; no consonant blends; limited number of final consonants, including /p/, /t/, /k/, /m/, /n/, and /ŋ/.

KOREAN

19 consonants, eight vowels; varying combinations of consonants and vowels used in formation of syllables; no consonant clusters in initial or final positions of words; no contrast in vowel length; no labiodental, interdental, or palatal fricatives; three kinds of stops and fricatives: voiced, tense voiceless, and lax voiceless; /r/ and /l/ sounds belonging to same phonemic category in allophonic variation; no tonic word stress; significant syntactic differences from English.

CAMBODIAN/KHMER

85 initial consonant clusters, largely different from those of English; aspirated and nonaspirated stops; two fricatives; vowels divided into short and long; sen-

tential intonation patterns; steep fall in intonation on final syllables to denote simple, affirmative, negative, and interrogative statements; monosyllabic or disyllabic words, stress on second syllable; syllable types including variable combinations of consonants and vowels; large-scale technical lexic derivation from French; significant syntactic differences from English.

LAOTIAN/LAO

Unstressed; six tones (five denoting syllables), including high, rising, rising-falling, falling-rising, falling, and short; three syllable types (cvc, cvvc, cvv); vowel word-ends; numerous morphologic and syntactic differences from English.

HMONG

Consonants with aspirated and unaspirated forms; consonant clusters only in initial positions, including nasals + stops and nasals + stops + /e/; only one final consonant; six basic vowels; seven tones; /r/ as a stop rather than a liquid, thus sounding like /t/ or unaspirated like /d/.

Tables 12–4 to 12–8 outline the phonemic qualities of some Asian/Pacific languages spoken by LEP students.

API Students and English Acquisition

Difficulties in Acquisition

LEP students' first-language phonetic systems usually differ greatly from, or may even contrast to, the English system. After more than a decade of study, linguists have concluded that interference related to these phonological differences is due, in part, to the way sounds are perceived and produced in functional categories.[39–42] The following analysis of difficulties that Chinese speakers encounter while learning English will illustrate the challenge at large—namely, how educators and specialists can recognize natural interference and thereby adjust their techniques.

Mandarin speakers learning English may insert a schwa in consonant blends such as /beləkə/ for the word "black," or omit a consonant, pronouncing the word "strawberry" as /tr/ŋ/beri/. Japanese vowel word-ends and the syllable structure consonant-vowel (CV) may result in a vowel insertion after the final consonant or between consonants in clusters such as saying "spring" as /spiriŋ/; Mandarin speakers learning English may pronounce the word "milk" as /miluku/.

Mandarin and Cantonese Phonological Contrasts with English

Because there are no consonant clusters in Mandarin or Cantonese, English clusters of consonants are "difficult" for Chinese speakers learning English. English rules for syllabification and syllabic stress may also present a challenge because each Chinese character represents just one syllable. The switchover from Chinese to English phonology can produce truncated words and telegraphic speech. For example, "I want s-pa-ghe-tti."

Table 12–4. Tones in Mandarin

	Pitch-Level	Duration and Direction
First tone	High Half-high Mid Half-low Low	(high level →)
Second tone	High Half-high Mid Half-low Low	(rising ↗)
Third tone	High Half-high Mid Half-low Low	(falling-rising ✓)
Fourth tone	High Half-high Mid Half-low Low	(falling ↘)

English consonant clusters can occur in different positions:

1. double consonants
   - initial position: spy, bribe, clown
   - final position: ask, gasp
   - medial position: basket, mustard
2. triple consonants
   - initial position: splash, spring
   - final position: asks, lisps

In Mandarin, there are two finals (sonorants), namely, /n/ and /ŋ/; in Cantonese, there are seven finals: /m/, /n/, /ŋ/, and /p/, /t/, /k/, and /ŋ/. In English, however, all consonants except for the glides /w/, /j/, and /h/ appear in final position. Mandarin speakers learning English sometimes omit final consonants, finding it difficult to produce them. For example, office is produced as /ofi/.

Furthermore, Mandarin speakers frequently produce the English phoneme /tʃ/ in "chair" as /ʃ/, which is considered to be a minimal shift in place of articulation. Cantonese speakers frequently produce the English phoneme /ʃ/ in "social" as /s/ using what exists in Cantonese phonology in place of an English phoneme. These speakers may also substitute an English sound for one that does not exist in Chinese. For example, they may use "sin" for "thin," even though there is no /si/ in Mandarin. Other foreign speakers of English also experience difficulty in learning the /μ/ and /æ/ phonemes.

Table 12-5. Mandarin Initial Consonants

Manner of Articulation		Place of Articulation						
		Bilabial	Labiodental	Apicodental	Alveolar	Apicopalatal	Laminopalatal	Dorsovelar
		Upper Lip	*Upper Teeth*	*Lower Teeth*	*Alveolar Ridge*	*Hard Palate*	*Hard Palate*	*Velar*
		Lower lip	*Lower lip*	*Tongue tip*	*Tongue tip*	*Tongue tip*	*Tongue blade*	*Dorsum*
Stops	Voiceless Unasp.	p			t			k
	Asp.	p*			t*			k*
Affricates	Voiceless Unasp.			ts		tʂ	tɕ	
	Asp.			ts*		tʂ*	tɕ*	
Nasals	Voiced	m			n			(ŋ)
Lateral	Voiced			l				
Spirants	Voiceless		f	s		ʂ	ɕ	x
	Voiced					ʐ		

Unasp.; unaspiration; Asp.; aspiration.
*Occurs in the final position of a syllable only.

Table 12–6. Vietnamese Consonants

Sounds (IPA Symbols)	Spelling	Key Words (initial)	Key Words (final)	Initial	Final
p	p		dep (pretty)		x
b	b	ba (three)		x	
t	t	tai (ear)	hát (sing)	x	x (Northern)
tʻ	th	thu' (letter)		x	
d	d	den (black)		x	
ṭ	tr	tre (bamboo)		x	
c	ch	cha (father)	sách (book)	x	x (Southern and Central)
k	c, k	ca (sing) ký (sign)	bác (uncle)	x	x
kþ	c		hoc (study)		x
g	g, gh	gan (liver) ghét (hate)		x	
m	m	ma (ghost)	im (silent)	x	x
n	n	nó (he/she)	lan (orchid)	x	x (Northern)
ɲ	nh	nhà (house)	lính (soldier)	x	x (Southern and Central)
ŋ	ng, ngh	ngà (ivory) nghe (hear)	làng (village)	x	x
ŋ͡m	ng		lông (hair)		x
f	ph	phi (waste)		x	
v	v	v'ê (go back) (not in Southern)		x	
s	x	xa (far)		x	
z	d, gi, r	rong (seaweed) da (skin) già (old) (in Northern only)		x	
ʃ	s	sai (wrong) (not in Northern)		x	
ʒ	r	r'ông (dragon) (not in Northern)		x	
j	d, gi	da (skin) già (old) (not in Northern)		x	
x	kh	khen (praise)		x	
h	h	hè (summer)		x	
l	l	lê (pear)		x	
r	r	ru'ôi (fly) (in some dialects only)		x	
w	u, o	oà (burst out crying) hao (flower) guý (precious)		x	medial x
y	i	hai (two)		x	x

Table 12–7. Loan Words

Foreign Letter	Pilipino Equivalent Letter(s)	Foreign Loan Word	Pilipino Equivalent Word
c	k	calesa	kalesa (horse-driven cart)
ch	ts	chinelas	tsinelas (house slippers)
c	s	circo	sirko (circus)
ch	ts	cha	tsa (tea)
f	p	cafe	cape (coffee)
		fino	pino (fine, texture)
j	h	jota	hota (letter j)
		juez	huwes (judge)
j	s	jabon	sabon (soap)
ll	ly	cepillo	sepilyo (toothbrush)
ll	y	caballo	kabayo (horse)
ñ	ny	niña	ninya (girl)
q	k	tanque	tangke (tank
		maquina	makina (machine)
rr	r	carro	karo
v	b	virgen	birhen (virgin)
x	ks	taxi	taksi (taxi)
z	s	lapiz	lapis (pencil)
		zapatos	sapatos (shoes)

As with the Mandarin speaker, Cantonese-speaking individuals may confuse elements of the English vowel system and substitute the following words: snake/snack, raid/red, eat/it, boat/bought, sew/saw, roof/rough, and got/gut. In light of the fact that the following sounds are not part of Mandarin or Cantonese, errors can be found in the following examples: "s" (sun/*th*umb, Ka*ss*y/Ka*th*y, ba*s*/ba*th*), "f" (ba*f*/ba*th*), and "d" (*d*is/*th*is). Liquid sounds such as "r" and "l" are frequently confused (*r*ight/*l*ight, *cr*own/*cl*own, *l*ice/*r*ice). In addition, omissions of word endings and cluster reductions are common (gra/grace, ma/maze, wi/wife, fi/five, ca/cake, kee/keep, ba/bag, boo/boot, be/bed, fi/fish, spa/spray, custer/cluster, etc). Cantonese English-learners may also insert vowels into consonant clusters (be*l*ue/blue), perform a minimal place of articulation shift (t∫air/*ch*air), and shorten or lengthen vowels (s*ea*t/s*i*t). See Hodson[43] for further explanation on minimal place of articulation shift.

Some background knowledge in tonal language is helpful for clinicians who may need to work with speakers who use tones phonemically and make mark words with tonal patterns. The five tones of Mandarin determine the meanings of syllables. A difference in tone marks a difference in meaning:

Table 12–8.   English and Pilipino Vowels and Diphthongs

English		Pilipino	
/e/	bed	/e/	eto (here it is)
/i/	meet	/i/	ibn (bird
/I/	bit		
/ai/	bite	/ay/	kamay (hand)
/ei/	bait	/ey/	reyna (queen)
/æ/	bat		
/u/	but		
/ə/	lesson, bonus, normal		
/ʉ/	later, author, sugar, fur, fir, her		
/o/	hot		
/a/	car, father	/a/	araw (sun, day)
/ô/	or	/o/	oo (yes)
/o/	no		
/u/	pool	/u/	ulo (head)
/U/	pull		
/aw/	now	/aw/	ilaw (light)
/oy/	toy	/oy/	baboy (pig)
		/uy/	aruy (ouch!)
		/iw/	paksiw (a food cooked with vinegar)

- —/ba/ (first tone) means "eight"
- —/ba/ (second tone) means "to pull"
- —/ba/ (third tone) means "handle"
- —/ba/ (fourth tone) means "to give up"
- —/ba/ (neutral tone) means "okay"

Mandarin children normally acquire tone usage by 2 years of age. Table 12–9 shows the tones used by Cantonese speakers.

Mandarin speakers and others frequently misplace English word stress, for example, tele'vision or sepa'rately. Moreover, the intonational patterns of the English language differ from those of Mandarin and Cantonese, and variations convey different meanings (eg, statements from questions, demands from requests, excitement from sarcasm, enthusiasm from indifference). Because it may be difficult for Chinese speakers to learn these patterns as well as morphologic and syntactic skills of the English language, both the speaker and listener need to understand distinctions between languages to communicate optimally.

Clinical Considerations in Assessing API Students

Particular challenges arise when determining whether speech deviations are disorders, delays, or simply second-language difference. Speech-language pathologists

Table 12–9. Tones in Cantonese

Traditional Tone Class	Tone Values	Status	Examples
Upper even	55	Emic	/fan/"grade"
	54(53)	Etic	
Upper rising	25	Emic	/fan/"powder"
Upper going	33	Emic	/fan/"sleep"
Lower even	11	Emic	/fan/"burn"
Lower rising	13	Emic	/fan/"strive"
Lower going	22	Emic	/fan/"share"
High entering	5	Etic	/fan/"sudden"
Mid entering	3	Etic	/fat/"law"
Low entering	2	Etic	/fat/"punish"

must understand some basic structural rules of students' first languages to evaluate and effectively treat disorders.

Hmong is a low-incidence language whose phonology (very different from English) not only obstructs its speakers' learning of English but masks possible disorders. Language acquisition problems are difficult to assess and are often overlooked. And whereas most adult speakers understand two major dialects of Hmong, White (Hmoob Dawb) and Green (Hmoob Ntsuab), young children are less capable of comprehending both; their communication with bilingual paraprofessionals may therefore be obscured due to dialectal differences.

Knowledge of characteristics of students' native languages (Hmong, for example) allows clinicians to adequately assess and identify language disorders. Such knowledge is vital not only for assessment but for effective intervention as well. For information on the phonetic systems of the languages of the world, read Cheng[38] and Ruhlen.[4]

Case Study

Van, a 14-year-old Vietnamese refugee, entered school in the United States at age 13. He was placed in a sixth-grade English as a Second Language (ESL) program, where he remains. His younger brother Vy, age 9, attends ESL at the same school. Most of the students in the program are Spanish speaking, primarily from Mexico.

Van's ESL teacher reported that he had made limited progress after 6 months in the program. She found his speech somewhat "nasal" and difficult to understand. Being aware of a high occurrence of nasal consonants in Van's home language, Vietnamese, she concluded that he was LEP and that his ability to alter his "accent" was possibly impeded by his being a teenager.

After a year in the program, Van was still performing poorly. A newly hired speech–language pathologist reported after an initial screening that Van's speech (including pressure consonants—fricatives, plosives and affricatives—and high vowels) had a hypernasal quality. An oral-speech mechanism examination revealed normal palatal morphology and reduced oral air flow. Van was reported not stimulable when prompted to produce words and syllables with pressure consonants. The clinician recommended a medical examination.

A nasoendoscopic examination conducted by an otolaryngologist revealed a possible covert submucous cleft. After meeting great resistance from Van's parents, the doctor confirmed the diagnosis through dissecting Van's levators. Several sessions of postsurgical speech therapy helped Van to improve his speech and his academic performance also began to improve.

Clinicians need to consider a number of critical questions when they observe speech intelligibility problem in ESL/LEP students. In Van's case, they are:

1. How fluent was he in his home language, Vietnamese?
2. Could his parents, family members, and Vietnamese-speaking friends understand his native speech?
3. Was his speech (home language and school language) intelligible to most people?
4. Could he produce English consonants and nonnasal Vietnamese consonants and high vowels when stimulated to do so?
5. What English phonology differences exist between utterances of Van and Vy and between Van's speech and that of his parents?
6. What comments did former teachers make about his speech (according to his school record from Vietnam, if available)?
7. Does he have difficulty learning to read and write?

Van's case serves to highlight a number of aspects that need to be considered when making clinical decisions:

1. What are some of the primary characteristics that need to be considered when determining if a speech disorder exists?
2. How do we differentiate between interlanguage phonological transference and actual speech disorder?
3. When should a speech referral be made for an ESL/LEP student exhibiting difficulty with English phonology?
4. What is the role of the individual's language transference?
5. What is the length of time the student has been exposed to English?
6. How old was the student when he first learned English?
7. What are the phonological patterns in teenagers learning English as a second language?
8. What is the time span normally expected when English phonology should be mastered?
9. Were observations in multiple contexts used in making the diagnosis? In this instance the clinician picked up on the critical aspects of Van's speech when making the medical referral.

Challenges in Service Delivery

LEP populations are heterogeneous in terms of country of birth, native language, immigration experience, degree of acculturation, and socioeconomic status.[44] But they hold in common a lack of familiarity with the English language, culture, history, and contemporary experiences—and cultural stereotypes. Their characteristics range among the following[45]:

- Insufficient communication skills in English
- Varying experience with auditory comprehension
- Lack of metalinguistic awareness—Language communicates beyond its surface structure, subtly conveying messages "between the lines" and through speaker intonation. LEP students often have limited opportunities to develop the metalinguistic sophistication needed to differentiate literal from nonliteral English expressions.
- Presence of an "accent" in spoken English—Some students possess a noticeable accent that adversely affects their intelligibility.
- Lack of social knowledge—They lack experience communicating in American social contexts.
- Varying degrees of world knowledge—They come from all corners of the world and have different kinds of knowledge.
- Insufficient cultural literacy—Often, they have received little information on American customs and traditions but plenty on their own people. Their social and educational experiences differ greatly from that of their native-born peers.

EP API students are challenged by unfamiliar sociocultural rules. Some problem areas are:

- Turn-taking—Asian LEP children generally do not ask questions or interrupt lectures. Their cultures view education as a formal process best accomplished through observation, memorization, and pattern practice combined with reading factual information.[46] The American educational system, on the other hand, stresses critical thinking, discovery, and general openness. API students may appear passive and nonparticipatory.
- Paralinguistic rules—Although varying from culture to culture, non-Western behaviors are commonly misinterpreted. The Chinese withholding of expression, observation, and interaction results in limited eye contact and is often perceived unfavorably by Westerners. Another example is giggling, which signals embarrassment. When reprimanded, a Chinese student may giggle rather than respond verbally.
- Politeness—Humility is highly valued. When praised, Chinese often respond with embarrassment. When thanked, the culturally appropriate reply is, "No need to thank me."
- Social distance—They are taught to respect teachers and maintain a proper social distance from them. Questions such as "What is your honorable age?" and "Where is your esteemed office?" can be appropriate or rude depending on the age, public status, and marital status of the asker and the asked.

Possible Solutions

Clearly, a knowledge of cultural and pragmatic characteristics is essential for successful interaction and communication with LEP API students. For clinicians to identify phonological disorders, they must collaborate with native informants to ascertain students' native language competencies. Furthermore, clinicians must remember that linguistic interferences and differences are not deviancies.

Continued research on second language acquisition is needed. Furthermore, speech evaluation methods must be improved for LEP students of all backgrounds. Meanwhile, educators and clinicians can follow these recommendations for optimal practice:

- Increase knowledge of languages spoken by LEP students. Learning a few words and showing interest can provide an environment of mutual enthusiasm and motivation toward language learning. Increased knowledge of API languages allows identification of possible communication disorders.

- Work on bilingual acquisition. Areas that affect intelligibility are phoneme production, intonation patterns, words, and paragraphs.

- Provide opportunities for modeling American English. Training in cultural literacy goes beyond phonology, morphology, and syntax to include stress and intonation. Teachers should also discuss explicit similarities and differences between languages, taking into account what is appropriate and inappropriate, especially when using jargon or colloquialisms.

- Avoid and encourage students to avoid labeling "accents" because everyone speaks with some type of an accent.

- Identify and explain sociolinguistic rules. These include turn-taking and allocation, topic shift and maintenance, and ritualized behaviors such as complimenting, greeting, and leave-taking. Assumptions should not be made about what children know; for example, they may have never experienced birthday parties.

- Provide opportunities for language practice in multiple social contexts. Encourage students to join social activities, clubs, and student governments to be immersed in various forms of discourse. Also, reading children's literature, comic books, newspapers, magazines, crossword puzzles, poetry, and other materials will enhance their vocabularies while increasing familiarity with the social meanings of words. In the classroom, the buddy system allows LEP students to adjust to new environments and develop social circles. Newcomers profit best by being placed with socially outgoing children. Peer teaching or tutoring is also helpful because it is not intimidating and may appeal to students' previous styles of learning.

- Collaborate with ESL and resource teachers, language professionals, and other language/culture informants. This way therapy activities can be used to enhance classroom communication skills.

In addition, clinicians doing communication assessment of this population should consider the following factors:

- Consideration of students' native language phonological development: Research their home language phonological systems when problems are suspected; use families as a resource. Parental involvement not only will sharpen a teacher's understanding of the LEP home environment, but also will provide insight regarding appropriate assessment procedures.

- Base observations on a holistic perspective: Obtain medical, familial, educational, immigration, and psychological/adjustment details, which can provide critical missing links for assessment, diagnosis, and intervention.
- Observe multiple interactions. Peers, teachers, aides, siblings, parents, and even strangers provide useful information regarding LEP students' communication behaviors.
- Ensure a naturalistic, nonthreatening observation environment under culturally and pragmatically appropriate procedures: This may be a game, a project, conversation, or object sharing. Children may be asked to describe culturally familiar objects such as chopsticks, for example.
- Distinguish between disorders and common linguistic differences: Cultural-linguistic variations complicate this distinction. Clinicians need to pay close attention to nonverbal paralinguistic features, kinesics, and proxemics, as well as receptive and expressive language. They must also understand students' use of metalinguistic features, pragmatic use of language, and general use of content.

Cheng[44,47] provides a few helpful strategies for both faculty and students in their collaborative English teaching/learning process.

Concluding Comments

Immigrants to the United States enter the country's arena of opportunity with high hopes, but with certain disadvantages, the most critical being a lack of proficiency in English. Although immigrant parents often must compromise their goals by working below their skill level, their children can invest in education.

Increasing awareness by educators and clinicians of LEP students' languages and backgrounds and understanding of bicultural/bilingual acquisition sends to these childrens' homes the message of encouragement that education lends access to social and professional opportunities.

Education is the key to not only personal achievements but for national success as well. Quality education serves us all.

References

1. Trueba HT, Cheng LL, Ima K: *Myth or Reality: Adaptive Strategies of Asian Americans in California.* Washington, DC: The Falmer Press, 1993.
2. United States Bureau of the Census: *Census of the Population: Asian and Pacific Islander Population by State,* 1986.
3. Olsen L: Whose culture is this? Whose curriculum will it be? *Calif Perspect* 1991; 2.
4. Ruhlen M: *A Guide to the Languages of the World.* Stanford, CA: Stanford University, Language Universals Project, 1975.
5. Hakuta K: Mirror of Language: *The Debate on Bilingualism.* New York: Basic Books, 1986.
6. Werner H, Kaplan B: *Symbol Formation.* New York: John Wiley & Sons, 1963.
7. McLaughlin B: *Second Language Acquisition in Childhood. Preschool Children,* 2nd ed. Hillsdale, NJ: Lawrence Earlbaum Associates, 1984; 1.
8. Dulay H, Burt M: Goofing: An indicator of children's second language learning strategies. *Lang Learn* 1972; 22:235–251.
9. Brudhiprabha P: *Error Analysis: A Psycholinguistic Study of Thai English Compositions.* Masters thesis, McGill University, Montreal, Canada, 1972.
10. Ervin-Tripp S: Is second language learning like the first? *TESOL Q* 1970; 8:137–144.
11. George HV: *Common Errors in Language Learning.* Rowley, MA: Newbury House, 1972.

12. Lance D: *A Brief Study of Spanish-English Bilingualism: Final Report. Research Project Orr-Liberal Arts,* 15504, College Station, TX: Texas A&M, 1969.
13. Peddie R: Par Erruer: *Error Analysis and the Early States of Adolescent Foreign Language Learning.* Doctoral dissertation, University of Auckland, Auckland, New Zealand, 1982.
14. Richards J: Error analysis and second language strategies. *Lang Sci* 1971; 17.
15. Taylor B: Toward a theory of language acquisition. *Lang Learn* 1974; 124:23–37.
16. Dulay H, Burt M, Krashen S: *Language Two.* Oxford, UK: Oxford University Press, 1982.
17. Cheng LL, Butler K: Code-switching: A natural phenomenon vs. language "deficiency." *World Engl* 1989; 8(3):293–310.
18. Anisfeld M, Bogo N, Lambert W: Evaluational reactions to accented English speech. *J Abnorm Social Psychol* 1962; 65:223–231.
19. Gallois C, Callan G: Personality impressions elicited by accented English. *J Cross-Cult Psychol* 1981; 12:347–359.
20. Giles H: Communicative effectiveness as a function of accented speech. *Speech Monogr* 1973; 40:330–331.
21. Lyczak R, Fu G, Ho A: Attitudes of Hong Kong bilinguals toward English and Chinese speakers. *J Cross-Cult Psychol* 1976; 7.
22. Ryan EB, Carranza MA, Moffie RW: Reactions toward varying degrees of accentedness in the speech of Spanish–English bilinguals. *Lang Speech* 1977; 20:268–273.
23. Biederman PW: Dialectician puts accent on the stars. *Los Angeles Times* 1989; 23:J10.
24. Compton AJ: *Compton Phonological Assessment of Foreign Accents.* San Francisco, CA: Carousel House, 1983.
25. Heller SB: Teaching assistants get increased training: Problems arise in foreign student programs. *Chronicle High Ed* 1986; 29:9–11.
26. Molholt G: Computer-assisted instruction in pronunciation for Chinese speakers of American English. *TESOL Q* 1988; 22:91–111.
27. Weade R, Green JL: Talking to learn: Social and academic requirements for classroom participation. *Peabody J Ed* 1985; 62:6–19.
28. Larson-Freeman D: Second language acquisition research: Staking out the territory. *TESOL Q* 1991; 25:315–338.
29. Anderson PJ, Graham SM: *Issues and Myths in Second-Language Phonological Acquisition Among Children and Adults* (Unpublished manuscript). Wichita State University: Wichita, KS, 1993.
30. Beebe L: Sociolinguistic variation and style shifting in second-language acquisition. *Lang Learn* 1980; 30:433–447.
31. Krashen S: The monitor model for adult second language performance. In Burt M, Dulay H, Rinocchiaro M (eds): *Viewpoints on English as a Second Language.* New York: Regents, 1977.
32. Beebe L, Zuiengler J: Accommodation theory: An explanation for style shifting in second-language dialects. In Wolfson N, Judd E (eds): *Sociolinguistics and Second-Language Acquisition.* Rowley, MA: Newbury House, 1983, pp 195–213.
33. Selinker L, Douglas D: Wrestling with "context" in interlanguage theory. *Appl Linguist* 1985; 6:190–204.
34. Lenneberg E: *Biological Foundations of Language.* New York: John Wiley & Sons, 1967.
35. Hill J: Foreign accents, language acquisition and cerebral dominance revisited. *Lang Learn* 1970; 20.
36. Odlin T: *Language Transfer: Cross-Linguistic Influence in Language Learning.* New York: Cambridge University Press, 1989.
37. Major R: Foreign accent: Recent research and theory. *Int Rev Appl Linguist* 1988; 25:185–202.
38. Cheng LL: *Assessing Asian Language Performance.* Oceanside, CA: Academic Communication Associates, 1991.
39. Ojemann GA, Whitaker HA: The bilingual brain. *Arch Neurol* 1978; 35:410–412.
40. Sasanuma S: Impairment of written language in Japanese aphasics: Kana versus kanji processing. *J Chin Linguist* 1974; 2:141–158.
41. Tzeng OJL, Wang WSY: The first two R's. *Am Sci* 1983; 71:238–243.
42. Wang WSY: Phonological features of tone. *IJAL* 1967; 33:25–29.
43. Hodson BW, Paden EP: *Targeting Intelligible Speech.* Austin, TX: Pro-Ed, 1991.
44. Cheng LL: Faculty challenges in the education of foreign-born students. In Clark LW (ed): *Faculty and Student Challenges in Facing Cultural and Linguistic Diversity.* Springfield, IL: Charles C. Thomas, 1993, pp 173–183.
45. Cheng LL: Recognizing diversity: A need for a paradigm shift. *Am Behav Sci* 1990; 34:263–278.
46. Cummins J: The role of primary language development in promoting educational success for language minority students. In California State Department of Education, Office of Bilingual Bicultural Education (ed): *Schooling and Language Minority Students: A Theoretical Framework.* Los Angeles: Evaluation, Dissemination and Assessment Center, California State University, 1981, pp 3–49.
47. Cheng LL: Dick and Jane: A journey to cultural literacy. *Clin Connect* 1989; 3:4–5.

Index